THE NEUTROPHILS: NEW OUTLOOK FOR OLD CELLS

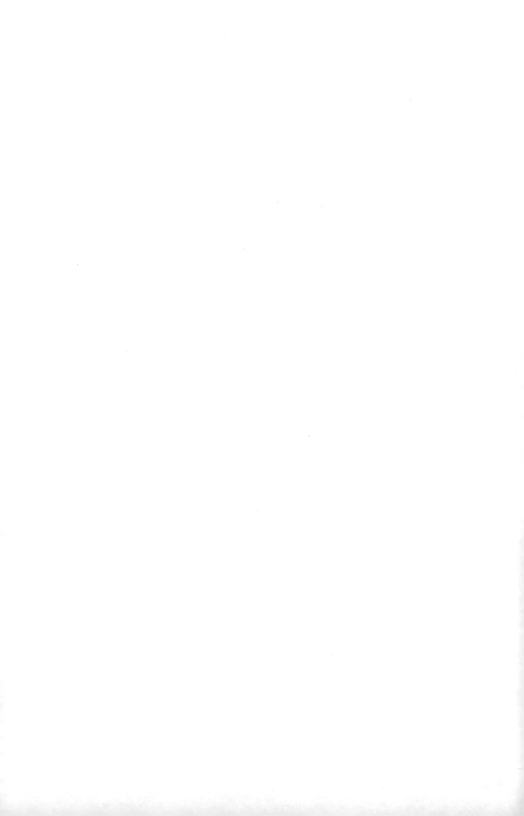

THE NEUTROPHILS: NEW OUTLOOK FOR OLD CELLS

Editor

Dmitry I Gabrilovich
Vanderbilt University School of Medicine

Imperial College Press

Published by

Imperial College Press
203 Electrical Engineering Building
Imperial College
London SW7 2BT

Distributed by

World Scientific Publishing Co. Pte. Ltd.
P O Box 128, Farrer Road, Singapore 912805
USA office: Suite 1B, 1060 Main Street, River Edge, NJ 07661
UK office: 57 Shelton Street, Covent Garden, London WC2H 9HE

British Library Cataloguing-in-Publication Data
A catalogue record for this book is available from the British Library.

THE NEUTROPHILS: NEW OUTLOOK FOR OLD CELLS

ISBN 1-86094-082-X

This book is printed on acid-free paper.

Printed in Singapore by Uto-Print

To my dad and first friend Isaak

PREFACE

This book is about one cell, the polymorphonuclear neutrophil. But at the same time this book is also about all human cells and the organism itself, since the neutrophil as no other cell is involved in maintaining homeostasis of an organism. It is not simply because of their abundance (more than 2×10^{10} cells in circulation), but mainly because these cells are able to perform numerous functions. They produce free radicals, phagocytize microorganisms, secrete a number of cytokines, kill tumor cells, neutralize viruses, etc. Over the past 100 years, this cell has witnessed times of intense interest and great expectations and periods when that interest waned. The major breakthrough in neutrophil research happened between the 1880s and 1920s (discovery of "polynuclear cells" by Paul Ehrlich and pioneering groundwork by Ilya Metchnikoff). The neutrophil was at the epicenter of intensive discussion about the nature of immunity and was considered by many as a most crucial player in immune response. Although studies of neutrophils continued in following years in brilliant works by Ado, Karnovsky, Becker and many others, this cell slowly but steadily was upstaged by lymphocytes and macrophages. With new information emerging about the roles of lymphocytes and macrophages in immune response, the appearance of new techniques to clone antigen-specific lymphocytes, identification of different lymphocyte subsets etc., the neutrophil was pushed out of the spotlight and on to the periphery of discussion. It was considered mostly as a vehicle for bacterial phagocytosis. Neutrophil had fallen out of fashion. *Sic transit gloria mundi.*

However, times change again. New major breakthroughs in neutrophil research started about 20 years ago and continue today. It took the appearance of new methods of molecular biology and biochemistry to revive interest in this cell. It turns out that the neutrophil has a fascinating biochemistry, able to secrete many factors and affect many physiological and pathological processes. This cell has become a very interesting model for investigation of general mechanisms of cell activation and metabolism, attracting the attention of many investigators. The number of publications in the scientific literature skyrocketed from 686 in 1966–1968 to 6837 in 1993–1995. For the same period of time the number of publications about lymphocytes increased 5 times and monocytes/macrophages 8 times (Source: Medline search based on keywords).

In preparing this monograph, authors tried to pursue two major aims. First, to provide readers with a detailed overview of the recent developments in neutrophil research, as well as to present some topics that have never been discussed in monographs before. Second, to draw the attention of a broad spectrum of researchers from other fields and clinical scientists to this incredible cell, to demonstrate how much neutrophil can give in return for exploration by inquisitive minds. This monograph consists of two blocks. The first, larger block, describes basic neutrophil biology and the second, smaller one, shows how our knowledge of neutrophil biology can be applied in practical medicine.

In the first chapter of this monograph, Dr. English discusses in detail the molecular basis of neutrophil activation, demonstrating why neutrophils may serve as a unique model for investigation of basic mechanisms of cell activation. Dr. Heinecke describes the current status of our knowledge of probably the most important functional feature of these cells — respiratory burst. Readers will find information about relatively new players in this field, as well as well known factors such as NADPH and myeloperoxidase. A very important characteristic of these cells is their ability to migrate to the site of infection or tissue injury. In the third chapter Dr. Zweier talks about mechanisms of neutrophil migration and the role of different receptors responsible for accumulation of these cells in tissues. Dr. Ferrante discusses the effect of fatty acids on neutrophil function, a new area of investigation that may potentially have a significant impact not only on our understanding of neutrophil biology, but also on clinical medicine. In the next chapter, Dr. Casatella presents an exhaustive overview of soluble factors released by neutrophils in response to different stimuli and their impact on functioning of other cells. Drs. Fanning,

Redmond and Bouchier-Hayes describe the mechanisms and significance of apoptosis, an important mechanism of neutrophil death. The first block concludes with an overview by Dr. Rot of chemokine receptors, an interesting element in neutrophil function.

Accurate use of laboratory techniques and correct interpretation of the results are critically important in clinical practice. In the opening chapter of the second block Dr. Virella discusses available methods for evaluation of neutrophil function. In the next chapter Dr. Roberts gives an overview of the role of neutrophils in the anti-viral response, discussing in detail neutrophil function in HIV and influenza virus infections. The last two chapters address how to improve defective neutrophil function in certain diseases. Drs. Dale and Nelson discuss the use of colony-stimulating factors in the treatment of neutropenia and infectious diseases. Benefits and possible pitfalls of neutrophil transfusion therapy are reviewed by Dr. Strauss.

This book is the result of the collective effort of a group of scientists. I am extremely grateful to the individual contributors to this book, who kindly found time in the midst of their active research and clinical duties to share with us their knowledge and thoughts.

Dmitry Gabrilovich
Vanderbilt University, Nashville, TN, USA

LIST OF CONTRIBUTORS

Dr. D. Bouchier-Hayes, Department of Surgery, Beaumont Hospital, Beaumont Road, Dublin 9, Ireland

Dr. Marco A. Cassatella, Institute of General Pathology, Medical School, University of Verona, Verona, Italy

Dr. David C. Dale, University of Washington Seattle, WA, USA

Dr. Denis English, Bone Marrow Research Laboratory Experimental Cell Research Program Methodist Research Institute Indianapolis, IN, USA

Dr. N.F. Fanning, Department of Surgery, Beaumont Hospital, Beaumont Road, Dublin 9, Ireland

Dr. Antonio Ferrante, Department of Immunopathology, The Women's and Children's Hospital and the University of Adelaide, 72, King William Road, North Adelaide, SA 5006, Australia

Dr. Dmitry Gabrilovich, Vanderbilt University, Nashville, TN, 37232-6838, USA

Dr. Jay W. Heinecke, Department of Medicine and Department of Molecular Biology and Pharmacology, Washington University School of Medicine, St. Louis, MO 63110, USA

Dr. Charles S.T. Hii, Department. of Immunopathology, The Women's and Children's Hospital and the University of Adelaide, 72, King William Road, North Adelaide, SA 5006, Australia

Dr. Zhi H. Huang, Department of Immunopathology, The Women's and Children's Hospital and the University of Adelaide, 72, King William Road, North Adelaide, SA 5006, Australia

Dr. Steve Nelson, Louisiana State University Medical Center, New Orleans, LA, USA

Dr. Deborah A, Rathjen, Department of Immunopathology, The Women's and Children's Hospital and the University of Adelaide, 72, King William Road, North Adelaide, SA 5006, Australia

Dr. H. Paul Redmond, Department of Surgery, Beaumont Hospital, Beaumont Road, Dublin 9, Ireland

Dr. Robert L. Roberts, Division of Immunology/Allergy, UCLA School of Medicine, Los Angeles, CA, USA

Dr. Antal Rot, Sandoz Research Institute, Vienna, Austria

Dr. Ronald G. Strauss, University of Iowa College of Medicine, Iowa City, IA, USA

Dr. Gabriel Virella, Department of Microbiology and Immunology, Medical University of South Carolina, Charleston, S.C., USA

Dr. Jay L. Zweier, Molecular and Cellular Biophysics Laboratories, Department of Medicine, Division of Cardiology and the Electron Paramagnetic Resonance Center, The Johns Hopkins University School of Medicine, Johns Hopkins Bayview Medical Center , Baltimore, MD, USA

CONTENTS

CHAPTER 1

MOLECULAR BASIS OF NEUTROPHIL ACTIVATION

Denis English[1]

1. A Cell of Discovery

Few cells have contributed as much to our understanding of the processes that mediate cellular activation — the so called *cellular signalling pathways* — as the neutrophilic leukocyte. On constant patrol for signals of foreign invaders, the neutrophil explodes into action at the first sign of an attack, firmly sealing the perimeter before marching deliberately into the contested territory, potently armed to neutralize most challengers. Comprised thousands of fortified cells working together to achieve a common goal, the **moving front** of neutrophils releases a avalanche of toxic agents upon these unwanted assailants, including **charged proteins, oxidants** and **hydrolytic enzymes**. Designed to purge the tissues of intolerable pathogens, these heavy armaments also damage neighboring tissue cells, perpetuating the inflammatory response. Every aspect of this sequence, from its inception in the capillaries to its cataclysmic end in the tissues, has been studied in minute detail. The cells are readily available from human or animal blood and readily employed in elaborate models constructed in the lab. As a result, we have gained an excellent understanding

[1]Correspondence to: Denis English, Ph.D. Bone Marrow Research, Laboratory Exptl. Cell Research Program Methodist Research Institute Indianapolis, IN, 46202; Phone: 317-929-2663, Fax: 317-929-2021

of the processes that result in microbial killing and tissue destruction effected by activated neutrophils. We have a good appreciation of the signals that prompt these cell into motion. And we have a fair understanding of the cellular processes involved in metabolic activation, the molecular events underlying neutrophil activation. In some cases, we have gained clues from studies with other cells, but many aspects of our understanding of the basic events that govern the initial stages of cellular activation have been gleaned directly from studies with neutrophils themselves.

Thus, the neutrophil has been a cell of discovery; a cell that responds dynamically and immediately to a diverse array of stimuli with activation of a multiplicity of pathways leading to an impressive cadence of responses. A cell that provides the first and most effective line of host defense against microbes penetrating the dermal barrier. A cell that presents a wealth of novel resources to the determined investigator. This essay will explore the pathways leading to those responses, and the mechanisms of their induction. In it, I will emphasize how unique contributions made from studies with neutrophils have resulted in increased clarity of known pathways and, in several notable instances, recognition of new avenues of cellular activation.

2. Signal Transduction: Communication Across the Plasma Membrane

2.1 *General considerations*

Neutrophils patrolling the capillaries are tipped off to signs of foreign invasion either by soluble agents that have permeated the underlying endothelial network or by changes on the surface of endothelial cells (Fig. 1.1). The initial response is **adherence** of the neutrophil to the vascular endothelium, followed by emigration, or **diapedesis**, through this vascular matrix. In response to an increasing gradient of attractive molecules known as *chemotaxins*, neutrophils migrate directionally toward the source of the tissue irritation, a process termed **chemotaxis**. During migration, cellular armaments are **primed** for later activation. Autocrine factors are synthesized, cytokines and other mediators are released, amplifying the inflammatory response.

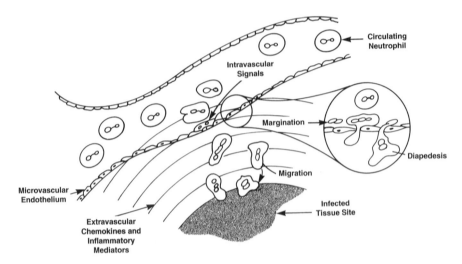

Figure 1.1. Margination, diapedesis and chemotactic migration of neutrophils from the circulation to sites of tissue infection. Triggered by soluble mediators released from the infected tissue as well as by "juxtacrine" factors deployed on the outside of the endothelial cell plasma membrane (1), circulating neutrophils adhere to the vessel wall and migrate through the endothelium into the infected area. Primed by cytokines and other inflammatory mediators, neutrophils arrive at the infected area in a highly reactive state, and respond vigorously upon ingestion of the invading organism.

Finally, the responding neutrophils encounter the offending pathogen. Promoted by signals on the surface of the microbial invader called *opsonins,* the neutrophil ingests its prey by the process of **phagocytosis**. Captured within a *phagocytic vacuole*, the predator triggers a barrage of cellular responses designed to bring a quick end to the threat of sustained infection (Fig. 1.2). **Exocytosis** results in the discharge of hydrolytic enzymes, charged proteins and other preformed cellular mediators into the phagocytic vacuole, making life uncomfortable for the detained prisoner. Simultaneously, components of a sophisticated antimicrobial system assemble at the periphery of the isolated prison. Operating within the retaining wall of the phagocytic vacuole, the newly functional system uses reducing agents available in the neutrophil cytosol to generate a flux of short lived, highly reactive oxidizing agents within the

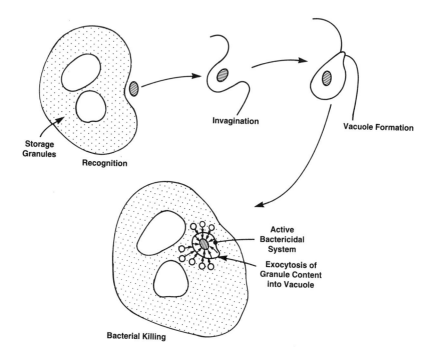

Figure 1.2.   Neutrophil phagocytosis. Upon recognition of opsonic factors coating the wall of the fated microorganism, the neutrophil cell wall invaginates, trapping the captured pathogen within a phagocytic vacuole. Contents of neutrophil storage granules are discharged into this biological prison, whose walls become electrified as a result of the assembly of a functional electron transport system which converts molecular oxygen into toxic free radicals. Few organisms escape this toxic barrage; those that do are capable of sustaining life-threatening infection, especially when other components of the immune system are compromised or depressed.

confines of the vacuole. This process, known as **oxidative activation** ensures that a viable detainee will not easily escape.

Each of the components of this sequence -adherence, chemotaxis, priming, mediator release, phagocytosis, exocytosis, and oxidative activation- is triggered by a **signal transduction pathway** which transmits information to the metabolic machinery of the cell. Initial events in individual signal transduction pathways, in turn, can be thought of as consisting of three distinct components, **sensation**,

transmission and **metabolic activation**, corresponding to the upstream, midstream and downstream biochemical processes involved (Fig. 1.3). The sensation phase of many signal transduction pathways commonly involves activation of cell surface receptors by soluble extracellular mediators. After the receptor encounters and binds the enticing stimuli, structural or biochemical changes on the receptor's intracellular domain communicate with downstream messengers of cellular activation. In addition to receptor ligation, surface perturbation resulting from juxtacrine interactions with adherent cells initiates

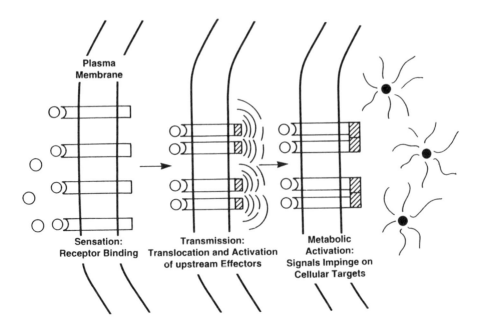

Figure 1.3.   Initial components of cellular signal transduction pathways. The initial event resulting in functional activation often involves binding of an agonist by a plasma membrane receptor, the sensation phase of cellular signalling. After receptor binding, translocation and activation of intracellular mediators results in the generation of second messengers or the activation of adaptor "proteins" which transmit the receptor driven response. The reactivity of these messengers results in metabolic activation as cellular targets spring into action. While some of the second messengers and adaptor proteins involved in cellular activation have been identified, many of the factors which mediate intracellular information transmission have yet to be discovered, and the investigation of cellular signalling is one of the most active and vibrant areas of modern research.

certain signal transduction pathways. In some cases, previous responses are sufficient triggers. For example, oxidative activation may be induced by certain inflammatory agents in the absence of phagocytosis, by adherence of neutrophils to activated endothelial cells or by phagocytosis alone.

While the search for new receptors and the extracellular signals which trigger them occupy the minds of many creative scientists, processes by which information is transmitted after receptor ligation is one of the most lively area of investigation in research today. These processes are governed by **G-proteins**, **protein kinases** and **phospholipases**. They lead to ion fluxes, morphologic alterations and metabolic activation. In some instances, the final response is dramatic; the light of a firefly, the contraction of a muscle, the movement of an individual cell. In others, it is subtle but none-the-less critical for homeostasis. In some cases, the manner by which initial sensing leads to information transmission is clear; in others it is not. Unfortunately, in most instances, **biochemical processes that link information transmission to the final downstream activation phase of signal transduction are not well defined.** As a result, descriptions of events such as *chemotaxin-induction of directed migration* or *agonist-induced superoxide release* often highlight these areas of uncertainty, precluding a cohesive appreciation of the mechanisms involved.

2.2 *Advantage: Neutrophil*

Precise definition of many cellular signal transduction pathways is hampered by the fact that biochemical changes induced by these pathways are readily reversible and not easily reconstructed in cell-free systems. While these obstacles are not insurmountable, they are formidable and often limit initial experimental approaches to studies with inhibitors and pharmacological probes. Unfortunately, what these agents are considered to influence in the cell is highly dependent on how much is known about them at the time of the study. Valuable information can be gained with inhibitors, especially when they fail to alter function but exert the anticipated effect on their cellular target. However, when functional inhibition is observed, it can be difficult to link this effect to inhibition of the targeted function, or even to be sure that the inhibitor is functioning as advertised. In any event, results gleaned from studies with inhibitors have played a major role in shaping our present understanding of cellular signalling pathways. Limitations of these studies explain why many gaps remain and many areas of uncertainty exist. New approaches using more specific biochemical and molecular probes will clarify many aspects of cellular signalling.

Certain characteristics of neutrophil physiology have facilitated study of the signal transduction pathways which activate the cell. First, the neutrophil responds quickly and dynamically to many different types of metabolic agonists. The cells migrate chemotactically and ingest their prey. Pioneers of the study of infectious disease followed these events microscopically. Modern researchers still do.

In addition, and perhaps more importantly, several key neutrophil responses result in stable biochemical changes that can be reproduced in cell-free activation systems. The best example of this is activation of the cells' plasma membrane NADPH oxidase, which produces the superoxide free radical at the expense of cytoplasmic NADPH. This enzyme is dormant in resting cells, but is activated during phagocytosis to generate oxidants within the phagocytic vacuole (Fig. 1.4). Pioneering studies by Bernard Babior, John Curnutte, Linda McPhail and others demonstrated that plasma membranes from resting neutrophils lacked appreciable oxidase activity, which was expressed in high levels in membranes from previously activated cells (2). As discussed below, development of a cell-free system to activate this enzyme in resting cell membranes led to an explosion of activity to dissect the mechanisms involved. These studies are still ongoing, and have yielded valuable information regarding the **final effectors** of cellular activation. How these mediators are induced by upstream effectors activated soon after receptor ligation remains to be determined, but promises to be the focus of fruitful investigation in the years ahead.

2.3 *Molecular probes*

In recent years, genetic approaches have been employed to facilitate definition of cellular signalling pathways. These studies typically involve biological

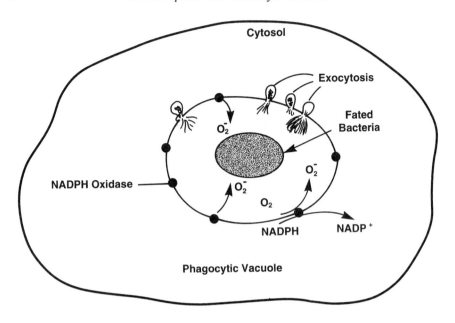

Figure 1.4.   Action in the phagocytic vacuole. Phagocytosis results in the assembly and activation of an NADPH oxidase in the walls of the phagocytic vacuole, an enzyme which exists in a dormant state in resting cell plasma membranes. The activated enzyme generates the superoxide free radical (O_2^-) from molecular oxygen at the expense of cytosolic NADPH, exposing microbes trapped within the vacuole to toxic reactive oxygen metabolites. While many aspects of the oxidase assembly and activation process have been clarified in recent years, many questions remain, and studies of oxidase activation continue to provide new insights into the identity and function of downstream effectors of cellular activation.

manipulation of the cellular environment to enhance, inhibit or limit the effects of specific proteins thought to play a role in information transmission. These proteins — including receptors, signalling enzymes, co-factors, regulators, and substrates — may be **over-expressed, knocked-out** or expressed in a **mutant form** to inhibit the effects of endogenous mediators. The effects of such genetic manipulation on agonist-induced responses are evaluated to clarify the role of the target protein in cellular signalling. Genetic approaches have yielded valuable information regarding specific signalling pathways, but their utility is limited by several factors. First, the target must be both known and cloned.

Nucleic acid probes to enhance or limit the effects of putative mediators cannot be generated in the absence of information pertaining to the identity and amino acid sequence of the mediator. Since the function and identity of the target is the focus of investigation, this information is often not available.

A second limitation of genetic manipulation pertains to the specificity of the approach. Since probes designed to mimic or neutralize specific molecules are employed, their influence is often assumed only to result from effects on the targeted molecule. However, it is clear that this is not always the case. Anti-sense DNA, used to prevent the transcription of certain genes, can influence multiple non-targeted functions in a manner that is often problematic and always unanticipated. Controlling for these effects with non-sense sequences addresses this problem, but does not resolve it completely since diverse sequences may retain individual non-specific properties. Similarly, vehicles used to transfect genetic materials, including virons and plasmid vectors, may influence the cellular environment in ways that have little to do with the gene being transferred. Again, controlling for non-specific effects with appropriately designed vehicles affords some measure of protection, but does not eliminate the problem entirely.

The most severe limitation of genetic engineering has a biological foundation; alterations effected by changing the genome are not apparent until the new genetic material is operational. Products of endogenous genes may be expected to contribute to or regulate cellular responsiveness as long as they exist, even if their expression in genetically engineered cells is inhibited. Thus, **transient transfection**, wherein new DNA is incorporated into a cell for only a few generations, can provide only limited new insight into protein functioning. **Stable transfection**, in which the genome is permanently altered as a result of viral DNA incorporation, can prevent this problem, but this approach is of little value for a cell, like the neutrophil, that does not divide. However, it may soon be possible to genetically manipulated neutrophils for experimental analyses by stable transfection of committed bone marrow progenitor cells. Mary Dinauer and colleagues have used this approach to produce neutrophils rescued from targeted disruption of genes involved in NADPH oxidase activation (3). Cells generated in a similar manner may be useful for studies of signalling pathways involved activation of other neutrophil functions.

2.4 *Metabolic agonists*

Several diverse stimuli are commonly used for investigation of neutrophil responses. These agents fall into several broad categories, including chemotaxins, phagocytic particles, membrane disruptive agents and physiological stimuli, such as immune complexes. In addition, reagents which activate diverse types of cells as a result of their ability to induce specific biochemical processes have been exploited in studies with neutrophils. For example, the protein kinase C activator, **phorbol myristate acetate (PMA)** is a potent stimulus of neutrophil oxidative activation and specific granule exocytosis. Unlike many other agents, it induces these effects in the absence of a discernable cytoplasmic Ca^{++} flux. **Diacylglycerol** similarly activates protein kinases and is known to induce both oxidative activation and directed migration of neutrophilic leukocytes. **Fluoride** ion, used at relatively high concentrations, activates G-proteins resulting in phospholipase activation and Ca^{++} mobilization. It has been used to investigate neutrophil oxidative activation and the potential role of G-proteins in the activation of neutrophil phospholipase D (4–6).

Chemotactic agents exert interesting and varied effects on neutrophil metabolism, and have provided valuable clues related to activation of pathways leading to exocytosis, adherence and oxidative metabolism, in addition to directed, or chemotactic, migration. Commonly used chemoattractants include: the complement fragment **C5a** which is generated in immune complex activated sera; chemotactic **interleukins** (IL-8) and other "**chemokines**", which are released from a variety of cells as a result of metabolic activation; certain **biologically active lipids**, such as arachidonic acid, platelet activating factor (PAF), leukotriene B4 (LTB4) and **phosphatidic acid**; and the synthetic tripeptide, **formyl-methionyl-leucyl-phenylalanine** (FMLP), which is thought to mimic the effects of chemotaxins released by invading bacteria. Many, if not all of these agents initiate their effects by ligating specific receptors on the exterior surface of the neutrophil plasma membrane. As discussed below, processes induced after receptor ligation which lead to directed migration are not well defined, and seem to vary considerably between the individual attractants. For example, responses to certain attractants (FMLP, C5a, PAF) are inhibited by preincubation of cells with the G_i-protein antagonist, **pertussis toxin**, while responses to other chemotaxins are inhibited by agents that prevent the functioning of intracellular **tyrosine kinases**. Recent studies by Gary Johnson, G.S. Worthen and colleagues implicate **phosphatidylinositol-3-kinase** (PI3K) as a mediator of neutrophil migration induced by IL-8 (7); the involvement of this enzyme in migration induced by other attractants, like its role in actin polymerization in other cell types, is not well defined. To further complicate matters, cellular responses to chemoattractants also depend on the concentration of the stimulus used and the manner of agonist presentation. Exposure of cells to relatively high levels of FMLP in the absence of a chemoattractant gradient results in vigorous initiation of the oxidative burst, exemplified by release of the superoxide free radical. Signalling pathways induced by FMLP which lead to oxidative activation are, in all probability, distinct from those that lead to directed migration.

Membrane disrupting agents have been useful agonists for studies of neutrophil activation. To this end, digitonin, saponin other detergents and exogenous phospholipases have been employed to induce functions in intact cells. These agents may exert their effects, at least in part, by promoting an influx of ionized Ca^{++} from the extracellular milieu. In this respect, the specific Ca^{++} **ionophore A 23187**, has proven useful for a wide range of studies with neutrophilic leukocytes.

Immune reactants and phagocytic particles activate neutrophils in ways that are not completely understood. The ability of immune complexes to induce oxidative activation, adherence and other functions results from Fc receptor ligation and resultant activation and translocation of intracellular receptor-associated tyrosine kinases and tyrosine phosphatases (8). Microbes coated with phagocytosis-promoting proteins or opsonins likely induce similar responses. In addition, the act of phagocytosis appears to induce membrane changes that potentiate the activation process, leading to enhanced oxidative responses, hyperadherence and exocytosis of granular material into the phagocytic vacuole. The manner in which these pathways intersect in order to emanate in an orchestrated response which efficiently subjects the ingested organism to antimicrobial assault is completely undefined.

3. Molecular Pathways of Cellular Activation

3.1 *G protein-coupled receptors*

Several neutrophil agonists, including FMLP, C5a, IL-8 and PAF, exert their effects by binding membrane receptors that activate heterotrimeric G-proteins. These signalling molecules are composed of α, β and γ subunits (9). G-protein a subunits are themselves guanine nucleotide binding proteins which possess intrinsic GTPase activity. Upon G-protein activation by ligated cell surface receptors, a subunits disassociate from the β-γ complex. Dissociation results from receptor-dependent conformational changes within the guanine nucleotide binding site of the a subunit, resulting in the release of GDP and its replacement by GTP, which is prevalent in the cytosol of resting cells. Complexed with GTP, liberated a subunits interact with cellular targets. Hydrolysis of bound GTP by the intrinsic GTPase returns the subunit to its inactive (GDP-bound) state, resulting in the reformation of the heterotrimeric G-protein complex.

In general, targets of activated G-proteins are dictated by the α subunit liberated, which, in turn, depends on the nature of the activating receptor, the conditions of activation and the G-protein composition of the cellular membrane. Different α subunits, when complexed to GTP, activate (or inhibit) different targets, including phospholipases, adenylate cyclase, phosphodiesterases and ion channels. Recent evidence indicates that liberated β-γ subunits also activate critical targets, including phospholipase C, **phosphatidylinositol 3'kinase (PI3K)** and a novel protein tyrosine kinase that activates the adaptor protein, **Shc**. Activation of Shc by activated G-proteins provides a mechanism to link G-proteins receptors to the tyrosine kinase-activated MAP kinase system (see below).

Receptors that activate G-proteins have seven transmembrane domains flanked by an N-terminus and a C-terminus and separated by cytoplasmic loops of varying lengths. G-proteins activated by these receptors are grouped into four families based on the amino acid sequence of their a subunit, G_s, $G_{i/o}$, G_q and G_{12}. Subunits from the G_q family possess the ability to stimulate the hydrolysis of the membrane phospholipid, **phosphatidylinositol 4,5-bisphosphate (PIP$_2$)** by activating **phosphoinositide-specific**

phospholipase C. The products of PIP_2 hydrolysis, diacylglycerol and inositol trisphosphate, continue the signalling pathway by activating protein kinase C and effecting the mobilization of intracellular stored Ca^{++}.

Since high β-γ subunit concentrations are required to activate cellular targets, the physiological relevance of this effect is not clear. However, a function for β-γ subunit signalling has been implicated under conditions in which agonist-induced inositide-specific PLC activation is inhibited by prior treatment of cells with pertussis toxin, which inhibits responses conveyed by the $G_{i/o}$, but not the G_q, family of G-proteins. This implication derives from failure to show activation of phosphoinositide-specific phospholipase C by $G_{i/o}$ a subunits. There is now extensive support for the concept, first put forth by Gierschik and associates (10), that the β-γ complex mediates the effects of $G_{i/o}$ proteins on phosphoinositide-specific phospholipase C, and thereby accounts for pertussis toxin-sensitive PIP_2 hydrolysis in agonist-treated cells.

Phosphoinositide hydrolysis is an early event in neutrophil activation by several classes of agonists. Pioneering studies by Ralph Snyderman and his associates using intact and disrupted neutrophils helped clarify the role of G-proteins in phosphoinositide hydrolysis and cellular activation (11–12). These investigators demonstrated that certain chemoattractant receptors were coupled to an inositide-specific phospholipase C through a pertussis toxin-sensitive G-protein and proposed that these receptors transmitted signals resulting in intracellular Ca^{++} mobilization by stimulating phosphoinositide hydrolysis. Studies using a cell free system indicated that this receptor-coupled G-protein exerted its influence by reducing the Ca^{++} requirement for expression of PLC activity to levels found in resting cells. This response has been linked to a novel G protein found in neutrophilic leukocytes.

3.1.1 Neutrophil migration

The cellular mechanisms linking G-protein receptor ligation to cellular movement have not been elucidated. In fact, mechanisms involved in the induction of cellular movement remain unresolved in many well studied systems, including embryonic cells during differentiation, re-aggregating slime mold and even motile bacteria. Based on results with inhibitors and fluorescent probes, directed migration in neutrophils is thought to involve assembly of actin-based cytoskeletal proteins and the anchoring of these proteins at pivotal membrane sites. Reversible adherence by advancing psuedopods may anchor the bow the migrating cell to the supporting matrix, while the actin cytoskeleton pulls the stern forward (see Fig. 1.5).

How these processes localize in certain areas of cells in response to a chemoattractant gradient is not known. Localized Ca^{++} fluxes and regional areas of kinase activation are probably necessary components, but not the sole

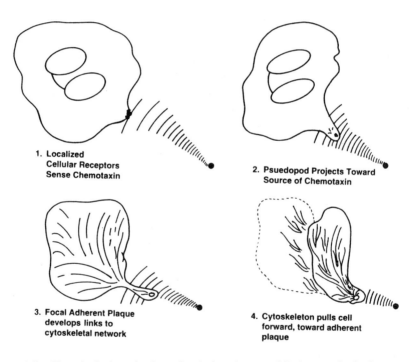

1. Localized
   Cellular Receptors
   Sense Chemotaxin

2. Psuedopod Projects Toward
   Source of Chemotaxin

3. Focal Adherent Plaque
   develops links to
   cytoskeletal network

4. Cytoskeleton pulls cell
   forward, toward adherent
   plaque

Figure 1.5. Hypothetical mechanism of actin based neutrophil chemotaxis. In the proposed scheme, neutrophils extend a pseudopod toward the source of the chemoattractant, in response to chemoattractant receptor occupation at the leading edge of the cell. This pseudopod adheres to the substratum and develops links to the cytoskeletal network which function to pull the cell forward, toward the anchored adherent plaque and the source of the attractant. How localized receptor occupation results in pseudopod extension remains to be determined.

determinants, of the process. As stated above, G-protein subunits are now known to activate additional effectors, including PI3K and a variety of proteins with **pleckstrin homology (PH)** domains. These effectors may link G-proteins to actin binding proteins and other determinants of cellular migration. Defining how regional activation and desensitization of G-protein coupled receptors by concentration gradients of chemoattractants leads to cellular migration in response to chemotaxin gradients promises to be a fruitful field of investigation in the years ahead.

3.2 *Tyrosine phosphorylation and neutrophil activation*

In addition to chemotaxis, pertussis toxin treatment inhibits other cellular responses to chemotactic agonists, including induction of aggregation and adherence, degranulation and initiation of oxidative metabolism. Thus, all of these responses probably share a common starting point; a distinct, pertussis toxin sensitive G-protein linked to individual chemoattractant receptors. Another response to chemotactic agonists is activation of **tyrosine kinases**, resulting in the **tyrosine phosphorylation** of multiple intracellular substrates. Like other functional and biochemical responses, tyrosine phosphorylation in FMLP and C5a-treated neutrophils is inhibited by pretreatment of cells with pertussis toxin, suggesting that tyrosine kinase activation is a downstream consequence of G-protein receptor ligation in these cells. It is not clear how this occurs, and the role of tyrosine phosphorylation in migration induced by these G-protein coupled receptors has recently been questioned. Thus, we have described conditions under which certain inhibitors blunted tyrosine phosphorylation induced by these chemoattractants, but had little influence on migration (see below). In any case, there is now an enormous amount of interest in pathways by which G-protein coupled receptors lead to activation of intracellular tyrosine kinases, ultimately linking the G-protein pathway to the MAP-kinase pathway of signal transduction. The interested reader is referred to the recent review by Sugden and Clerk for an in-depth discussion of this important subject (13). Briefly G-protein coupled receptors may activate receptor or non-receptor tyrosine kinases directly or exert their effects through

G protein activated serine/thyronine kinases, such as novel isoforms of protein kinase C. The latter pathway likely involves activation or translocation of **c-Raf** (possibly as a result of PKC-dependent PLD activation). The former probably results in the activation of an "**adaptor**" protein, such as **Shc** or **Grb2**, which initiates Ras activation and consequent induction of the MAP kinase pathway. Neutrophils present an ideal model for further definition of the pathways linking G-protein coupled receptors to tyrosine kinases.

In many cells, ligand activation of receptors with intrinsic tyrosine kinase activity is the initial step in induction of functional responses (14). These receptors exert their effects by attracting and activating key cytosolic proteins, including members of the Src family of tyrosine kinases, phospholipase Cγ, PI3K and regulators of critical downstream effectors. The initial step in activation of tyrosine kinase receptors involves autophosphorylation of specific tyrosine residues in their cytoplasmic domains as a result of ligand-dependent dimerization of their extracellular domains. Phosphorylated intracellular domains provide a docking site for other signalling mediators, which are activated as result of their own tyrosine phosphorylation after translocation. Ligands which induce effects by binding tyrosine kinase receptors include epidermal growth factor, transforming growth factor α, hepatocyte growth factor and CSF-1.

Receptors with inherent tyrosine kinase activity do not appear to play a major role in neutrophil activation. However, several agonists exert their influence on neutrophils by binding receptors that activate or rearrange intracellular tyrosine kinases. Ligand binding to certain cytokine receptors, known as the cytokine receptor superfamily, rapidly leads to tyrosine phosphorylation of multiple intracellular substrates in neutrophils (15). This process leads to functional activation. The identity of the tyrosine kinases involved in this response are, for the most part, unknown. In other cells, members of this receptor family recruit members of the **Janus** family of cytoplasmic tyrosine kinases (including the **JAK** kinases, **JAK-1**, **JAK-2** and **JAK-3**) to their cytoplasmic domains, where they interact with and activate other cytoplasmic proteins, such as the STAT family of signalling molecules (16). Tyrosine phosphorylation appears necessary to get JAK activated and on the receptor; tyrosine phosphatases presumably play a role in getting the JAK off.

Although JAK kinases are expressed in neutrophils, it is not clear if the JAK-STAT pathway plays a role in neutrophil activation induced by cytokine receptor agonists, such as G-CSF. Recent studies by Brian Druker and associates suggest an alternative pathway for cytokine receptor signalling, wherein the intracellular kinases **Lyn** and **Syk** exert effects in neutrophils similar to those mediated by JAK family members in other cells (17). As discussed below, Lyn and Syk mediate critical tyrosine kinase-dependent functions in activated platelets and B-lymphocytes, and their involvement in neutrophil functional activation is beginning to emerge. A role for Lyn in activation of PI3K in cytokine activated neutrophils has recently been proposed by Naccache and coworkers (18). However, how any of these enzymes mediate functional responses remains unclear.

3.2.1 Tyrosine-kinase dependent chemotactic responses

The role of tyrosine kinase activation in actin polymerization, focal adhesions and stress fiber formation in fibroblasts and other cells is beginning to become apparent (19–20). The ability of tyrosine kinase receptor agonists such as platelet derived growth factor, hepatocyte growth factor and epidermal growth factor to induce migration of other types of cells has recently been documented (21–23). These responses appear to involve activation of PI3K and are regulated by complex interactions involving multiple tyrosine phosphorylated substrates. The role of MAP kinase activation in tyrosine kinase - dependent chemotaxis in these cells is not yet clear. More importantly, the relevance of these results to mechanisms involved in neutrophil migration is unknown, as similar pathways have not yet been described. However, the possibility that agonists that bind tyrosine kinase receptors induce neutrophil chemotaxis in much the same way remains open.

As stated above, the involvement of intracellular tyrosine kinases in the migratory response induced by activation of neutrophils with FMLP and other G-protein coupled receptor agonists is not clear. Tyrosine kinase activation may not, in fact, be a critical component of all signalling pathways leading to cell movement. However, tyrosine kinases may play critical roles in neutrophil migratory responses induced by other physiologically relevant agonists. Research conducted in the laboratories of Silvani Sozzani described the chemotactic effects of dispersions of phosphatidic acid, a biologically active lipid previously investigated for its role as an intracellular second messenger (23). Subsequent work from our laboratory documented the striking sensitivity of phosphatidic acid-induced chemotaxis to tyrosine kinase inhibitors (24). This inhibition was found to be associated with blockage of the tyrosine phosphorylation of three substrates with approximate molecular sizes of 52, 72 and 85 kDa. They have been preliminarily identified as Lyn, Syk and the 85 kDa regulatory subunit if PI3K. Inhibition of phosphorylation of these substrates by the tyrosine kinase inhibitor herbimycin had no influence on chemotaxis to other chemoattractants, including C5a, FMLP and casein. Phosphorylation of these substrates in phosphatidic acid-treated neutrophils was found to be an essential step in a novel signalling cascade leading to Ca^{++} mobilization and ultimately actin polymerization. This study provides the first demonstration of tyrosine kinase-dependent actin polymerization in stimulated neutrophils and sets the stage for further definition of steps leading to chemotactic migration.

Lysophosphatidic acid induces metabolic responses in fibroblasts, neurons and other cell types by ligating a heptahelical G-protein coupled receptor (25). Many cellular responses to lysophosphatidic are inhibited by pertussis toxin treatment, but in some systems a pertussis toxin-resistant G-protein may be involved. The responses induced by lysophosphatidic acid include mitogenesis, morphological alterations and, of great interest to neutrophilologists, directed migration. While lysophosphatidic acid has little effect on neutrophils, it is possible that phosphatidic acid induces its effects on neutrophil migration by ligating a receptor analogous to the lysophosphatidate receptor. Our preliminary data show dramatic, but not complete inhibition of phosphatidate-induced migration by pertussis toxin pretreatment. In addition, chemotactic responses to phosphatidic acid were inhibited by inclusion of the PI3K inhibitor, wortmannin (unpublished observations). If these result are confirmed, they will further define the novel aspects of the PA/LPA signalling system, linking a functional G-protein coupled receptor to activation of key tyrosine kinases involved in cell migration. The relation of this pathway to the PI3K-dependent pathway activated by IL-8 (7) remains to be explored, but studies are in progress to compare the two systems. In other cells, Syk and Lyn (molecular size 72 kDa nd 52 kDa respectively) mediate tyrosine kinase dependent Ca^{++} mobilization by a unique mechanism leading to functional activation (26). These kinases may similarly mediate PA-induced Ca^{++} mobilization. If they do, clarification of their activation, relation to PI3K and distribution in regions of cells exposed to concentration gradients of chemoattractants may yield new insights into how G-protein coupled receptors are linked to directed migration.

3.3 *PIP₃ and the role of PI3 kinase*

The novel phospholipid, **phosphatidylinositol-3, 4, 5-trisphosphate (PIP₃)** was first described in neutrophilic leukocytes by Alexis Traynor-Kaplan and associates (27). PIP₃ is generated from PIP₂ by the action of PI3K. There is now quite a bit of interest in the role of this enzyme in cellular activation. As discussed above, PI3K plays an important role in neutrophil migration induced by certain agonists. However, its mechanism or mechanisms of action in promoting migration in neutrophils and in other cells is unclear. Recent studies indicate that the novel enzyme may facilitate cross talk between two important signalling pathways. Neutrophils are known to possess two types of PI3K. The conventional heterotrimeric form is activated by tyrosine phosphorylation while a recently identified form is directly stimulated by G-protein β-γ subunits. Although the latter form may be activated by chemoattractant-receptor G proteins, tyrosine kinase - dependent activation of PI3K may lead to functional activation under some circumstances. Bokoch and colleagues demonstrated the activation of Lyn in chemoattractant-stimulated neutrophils (28). This activation apparently results in the binding of Lyn to the Shc adaptor protein, which also becomes tyrosine phosphorylated in chemoattractant-stimulated neutrophils. Importantly, the Lyn-Shc complex then formed a complex with previously inactive PI3K, resulting in its activation. How this process leads to migration is not known, but may involve the interaction of newly formed plasma membrane phospholipids with actin binding proteins.

Since Shc adaptor proteins are known to interact with upstream effectors of the Ras/MAP kinase cascade, PI3K activation in chemoattractant- stimulated neutrophils may exert its effects via this important pathway. However, attempts to link migratory responses to MAP kinase activation in neutrophils have consistently failed. Recent studies suggest an alternative link between PI3K activation and cytoskeletal organization. Recent work by Karlund and associates demonstrate the tight association of PIP3 with the cytoskeletal protein cytohesin-1 (29), an association brokered by the protein's **pleckstrin homology** **(PH) domain**. Thus, proteins with pleckstrin homology domains potentially play a role in PI3K-dependent migration, by targeting cytoskeletal structures to specific membrane locations. The role of this process in chemoattractant stimulated migration is not yet known, but important clues may be derived from recent work by Sergio Grinstein and associates (30). These investigators studied the expression and distribution of **pleckstrin**, a major substrate of protein kinase C, in neutrophils. The pleckstrin molecule consists of two copies of the PH domain bridged by a short region including the PKC phosphorylation site. While the function of pleckstrin is unknown, it may be an important intracellular adaptor, targeting PH domain-associated molecules to subcellular compartments or plasma membrane binding sites. Since pleckstrin possesses two PH domains, phosphorylated pleckstrin potentially targets proteins which associate with PH domains to lipids generated on the inner surface of the cell's plasma membrane, such as PIP3. In this scheme, pleckstrin phosphorylation is a key event leading to cytoskeletal reorganization. Grinstein and colleagues demonstrated that pleckstrin phosphorylation in stimulated neutrophils resulted from the activity of a non-conventional PKC isoform, an isoform activated by phosphatidic acid rather than diacylglycerol. This pathway thus links pathways that end in phosphatidate generation to those that begin with PI3K activation. Further work is underway to delineate the involvement of pleckstrin in stimulated neutrophil migration.

3.4 *Role of PLD in stimulated Neutrophils*

Early reports documented a rapid increase in phosphatidate in plasma membranes of neutrophils stimulated with chemoattractants and other metabolic agonists. While some of the phosphatidate generated in stimulated neutrophils is derived from products of PLC — mediated phospholipid hydrolysis, it is now known that a substantial portion of the phospholipid is generated by the action of phospholipase D (PLD). The presence of PLD in mammalian cells was discovered only a few years ago, and many of the first studies of the role of this enzyme in cell signalling were carried out with neutrophils (see ref. 31). These studies immediately led to the recognition of the second messenger function of the enzyme's product, phosphatidic acid, in pathways leading to migration, oxidative activation, exocytosis and other cellular functions. They also led to an immediate recognition of the potential role of phosphatidate phosphohydrolase, an enzyme that converts phosphatidic acid to diacylglycerol, in the regulation of functional activation.

In early studies, various phosphatidate phosphohydrolase inhibitors were used in attempts to define the role of phosphatidic acid in neutrophil activation. Propranolol was found to be well suited for this purpose, since it a water soluble compound that is relatively non-toxic at high concentrations. The ability of propranolol to affect other signalling system was no deterrent to these early workers, who linked most effects of the drug — such as potentiation of FMLP induced oxidative activation- to potentiation of phosphatidic acid levels. Another early approach involved treating neutrophils with certain primary alcohols, which reduce PLD-dependent phosphatidic acid generation by providing substrates for the transphosphatidylation reaction. As could be expected, this approach generally resulted in inhibition of agonist-dependent functional activation, consistent with the view that functional activation resulted from the accumulation of phosphatidate in the membranes of stimulated cells. While this conclusion appears generally to remain valid, the manner by which phosphatidate exerts its effect remains unknown.

3.4.1 Phosphatidic acid and oxidative activation

Compelling evidence has linked the generation of phosphatidic acid to activation the neutrophils' oxygen-based antimicrobial system. Dormant in resting cells, this system provides substrates for potent bactericidal and cytocidal mechanisms when the cells are activated. Activation of this system has been studied extensively in a cell-free system, and the emerging data demonstrate that activation is a dynamic process resulting from the interaction of several cytosolic components with a dormant membrane associated enzyme, the NADPH oxidase. This interaction may be promoted by phosphatidic acid.

Early studies of the neutrophil superoxide generating system demonstrated that plasma membranes derived from activated cells effectively mediated the generation of the superoxide free radical in the presence of oxygen and NADPH, an effect ascribed to the presence of an active NADPH oxidase. Little or no activity was present in membranes of resting neutrophils, indicating that stable activation of the enzyme resulted from cellular stimulation. For many years, attempts at activating the enzyme in a cell free system met with limited success, until Heyneman and Vercauteren demonstrated its activation in membranes of resting horse neutrophils upon exposure to cytosol in the presence of certain fatty acids (32). Similar activation was quickly documented in Guinea pig and human neutrophils. Bellavite and colleagues demonstrated that phosphatidate could replace both fatty acid and cytosol in the activation of this enzyme in plasma membranes of pig neutrophils (33). Subsequently, Agwu et al demonstrated that phosphatidate was an effective, albeit weak, activator of the human neutrophil enzyme when used with cytosol (34). Subsequent studies by Linda McPhail and colleagues demonstrated that this property was markedly enhanced in the presence of low concentrations of diglycerides (35). Thus, phosphatidic acid generated by the action of phospholipase D in the presence of diacylglycerol generated by phosphatidate phosphohydrolase-mediated dephosphorylation of its substrate may play an important role in the activation of the neutrophil superoxide generating enzyme.

The nature of the cytosolic involvement in NADPH oxidase activation has proven quite complex. Several cytosolic and granule-derived components appear to impinge upon a flavocytochrome in the cellular membrane, resulting in the assembly of a functional superoxide generating enzyme (36). An important component of this process is the translocation of the small molecular weight G-protein, Rac2. Rac2 is active in its GTP-bound form. Post-translational isoprenylation facilitates its interaction with regulatory proteins that stimulate the exchange of GTP for GDP. In resting neutrophils, Rac2 is exclusively confined to the cytosol in a complex with GDP dissociation inhibitor

(GDI). When cells are activated, this complex is disrupted, allowing Rac to translocate to the plasma membrane and participate in NADPH oxidase activation. Phosphatidic acid effectively disrupts the Rac-GDI complex (37), which may explain the role of the phospholipid in neutrophil activation (see Fig. 1.6).

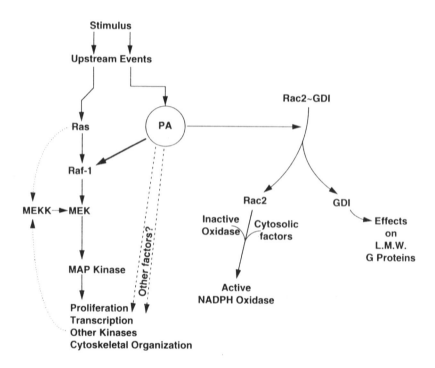

Figure 1.6. Downstream effects of phosphatidic acid. Phosphatidic acid generated during the initial phases of cellular signalling may induce cell function by activating the Raf 1- MEK cascade. Dissociation of Rac2-GDI promoted by phosphatidic acid results in activation of the neutrophil NADPH oxidase. GDI released during this process may have other important effects on cellular activation, including contributing to the activation of Rho and consequent actin polymerization. Thus, phosphatidic acid generated by the action of phospholipase D may play an important role in many aspects of neutrophil activation, in addition to its activity as an extracellular inflammatory mediator. (Reprinted with permission: from D. English, "Phosphatidic acid: A lipid messenger involved in intracellular and extracellular signalling", Cell. Signal., 8, 341–447, 1996, Elsevier Science Inc.).

As attractive as this hypothesis at first appears, further investigation will be necessary to substantiate its validity, since the physiologic relevance of NADPH oxidase activation by phosphatidic acid in comparison to other potential activators is not clear. In addition, it is not known if the ability of the phospholipid or other agents to activate the oxidase in the presence of cytosol derives exclusively from disruption of Rac-GDI or if other factors are involved. However, if phosphatidate — promoted Rac-GDI complex disassociation is involved in neutrophil oxidase activation in intact cells, similar processes may govern second messenger functions of phosphatidic acid in other systems as well.

Candidates to explain the role of phosphatidic acid in activation of cellular functions include novel **phosphatidate-dependent kinases**. As discussed above, one such kinase, a non-conventional PKC isoform, may mediate pleckstrin phosphorylation, and thus its intracellular distribution. Another kinase potentially activated by phosphatidic acid is **Raf-1** kinase, an oncogene product ubiquitously expressed in mammalian cells. Robert Bell and associates have shown that this serine/threonine kinase possesses distinct binding domains for phosphatidate which target it to specific plasma membrane docking sites where it may function to activate downstream mediators of cellular function (38). Finally, McPhail and colleagues have identified a novel phosphatidic acid-dependent kinase that phosphorylates the 47 kDa oxidase component, p47-*phox*, and may thereby facilitate activation of the NADPH oxidase (39). In this respect, it is noteworthy that oxidative activation of intact cells exposed to metabolic agonists correlates with p47-*phox* phosphorylation (40). Phosphorylation seems to elicit conformational changes and alter charges within the molecule, enabling its association with a binding site in another oxidase component, p-67-*phox*, which then translocates to the plasma membrane, completing assembly of the active oxidase.

4. Activation of PLD

In recent years, it has become clear that phospholipase D plays a key role in cell signalling in a variety of cells. The phospholipase D system is now regarded as a universally applicable signalling pathway which plays a major role in many cell functions, including actin polymerization, cellular migration, mitogenesis, neurotransmission, differentiation and responses to hormones, eicosanoids, growth factors and other agonists (9). As noted above, many of the initial studies defining a role for phospholipase D in signal transduction were carried out in neutrophilic leukocytes. More importantly, studies with neutrophils were instrumental in confirming the existence of this enzyme in mammalian cells and the importance of its product in metabolic activation. More recently, studies with neutrophils have yielded valuable insights related to the unique pathways involved in the activation of this enzyme in stimulated cells.

Unlike G-protein coupled phospholipase C, phospholipase D appears to be activated by mechanisms which are not directly linked to cell surface receptors. Pioneering studies by the team of McIntyre, Prescott and Zimmerman at the University of Utah demonstrated three distinct mechanisms of phospholipase D activation in neutrophilic leukocytes (41). Each of these now appears to be applicable in other mammalian cells. Phospholipase D can be activated as a result of the action of protein kinase C, as a consequence of Ca^{++} mobilization and as a result of protein tyrosine kinase activation. Although considerable attention has been directed to clarify the details of these activation systems, a unified picture is only now beginning to emerge (Fig. 1.7).

In studies with permeabilized granulocytes, the laboratories of Cockcroft and Sternweis simultaneously demonstrated the requirement for a cytosolic factor in the activation of phospholipase D effected by the G-protein agonist, GTP-γ-S (42, 43). This factor was identified as ADP ribosylation factor or ARF, which was known to mediate the ADP ribosylation of G proteins effected by cholera toxin. Using a unique cell-free activation system developed from neutrophilic leukocytes, David Lambeth and associates have studied this activation system in detail and provided answers to some very important and long unresolved questions. First, these investigators demonstrated the requirement of a 50 kDa cytosolic protein in the ARF-dependent activation of phospholipase D (44). These studies led to the identification of members of the Rho family of small G proteins as participants in the activation of PLD. This development was somewhat surprising, since Rho is known to play a

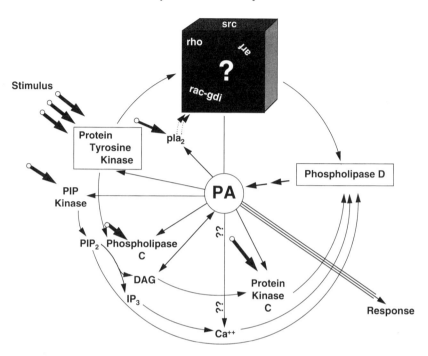

Figure 1.7.   Interaction between signalling pathways leading to the activation of phospholipase D. In neutrophils as in other cells, phospholipase D can be activated as a result of pathways mediated by protein kinase C, increased cellular free Ca^{++} and protein tyrosine kinases. Some of the effects of tyrosine kinases have been recently attributed to the activation of small molecular weight G-proteins which, after phosphorylation, regulate the function of upstream effectors of phospholipase D activation, as represented by the black box. Studies with neutrophils are beginning to provide a unified picture, wherein many aspects of these otherwise distinct activation pathways overlap and interact with one another in an orchestrated and highly efficient manner. (Reprinted with permission: from D. English, "Phosphatidic acid: A lipid messenger involved in intracellular and extracellular signalling", Cell. Signal., 8, 341–447, 1996, Elsevier Science Inc.).

major role in regulation of the cytoskeleton, controlling the formation of stress fibers and focal adhesions. Bowman and Lambeth went on to show that Rho acts in concert with protein factors in both the cytosol and plasma membrane, and is itself regulated by GDI (45, 46). Since, as discussed above, GDI itself may be regulated by phosphatidic acid, the product of PLD activated in the initial stages of neutrophil activation may potentiate subsequent responses, and thereby perpetuate the inflammatory response. Many questions pertaining to the activation, function and regulation of phospholipase D await further investigation. It is likely that some of the answers will derive from further studies with neutrophilic leukocytes.

5. Concluding Remarks: Joining Upstream and Downstream Processes

The cell free systems for investigating biochemical events involved in several aspects of neutrophil activation have thus resulted in a clear picture of the downstream processes that activate key cellular functions. The terminal events in few other cellular activation systems have been so thoroughly defined. However, the manner by which these activation processes are set in motion after cells are stimulated remains unclear. Similarly, mediators and processes linking the terminal events involved in phagocytosis, chemotaxis, adherence and exocytosis to initial events in cellular activation are not understood. The neutrophil provides a unique model to investigate this linkage and clarify key aspects of universally applicable signalling systems. Future studies with this dynamic cell promise to yield many of Nature's best kept secrets of cellular activation.

6. References

1. Siddiqui, R., English, D and Garcia, J.G., *J. Lab. Clin. Med.* **125** (1995), 18–25.
2. Chanock, S.J., el Benna, J., Smith, R.M. and Babior, B.M., *J. Biol. Chem.* **269** (1994), 24519–24522.
3. Ding, C., *et al.*, *Blood* **88** (1996), 1834–1840.
4. English, D., Rizzo, M.T., Tricot, G. and Hoffman, R., *J. Immunol.* **143** (1989), 1685–1691.
5. Olson S.C., Tyagi, S.R. and Lambeth, J.D., *FEBS Lett.* **272** (1990), 19–24.
6. English, D., Taylor, G. and Garcia, J.G. *Blood* **77** (1991), 2746–2756.
7. Knall, C., Worthen, G.S. and Johnson, G.L., *Proc. Natl. Acad. Sci. USA* **94** (1997), 3052–3057.

8. Santana, C., Noris, G., Espinoza, B. and Ortega, E., *J. Leuko. Biol.* **60** (1996), 433–440.
9. Exton, J.H. *Eur. J. Biochem.* **243** (1997), 10–20.
10. Camps, M, et al., *Eur. J. Biochem.* **206** (1992), 821–831.
11. Smith, C.D., Cox, C.C. and Snyderman, R., *Science* **232** (1986), 97–100.
12. Verghese M.W., Smith, C.D. and Snyderman, R. *Biochem. Biophys. Res. Comm.* **127** (1985), 450–457.
13. Sugden P.H. and Clerk, A., *Cell. Signal.* **9** (1997), 337–351.
14. Fantl, W.J., Johnson, D.E. and Williams, L.T. *Ann. Rev. Biochem.* **62** (1993), 453–481.
15. Mufson, R.A., *FASEB J.* **11** (1997), 37–44.
16. Ihle, J.N., *Adv. Cancer Res.* **68** (1996), 23–65.
17. Avalos, B.R., *et al.*, *Exptl. Hematol.* **25** (1997), 160–168.
18. Al-Shami, A., Bourgoin, S.G. and Naccache, P.H., *Blood* **89** (1997), 1036–1044.
19. Ridley, A.J. and Hall, A., *EMBO J.* **13** (1994), 2600–2610.
20. Cross M.J. *et al.*, *Curr. Biol.* **6** (1996), 588–597.
21. Shimokado, K., *et al.*, *Ann. New York Acad. Sci.* **748** (1995), 171–175.
22. Kundra, V., Soker, S. and Zetter, B.R., *Oncogene* **9** (1994), 1429–1435.
23. Zhou, D., *et al.*, *J. Biol. Chem.* **270** (1995), 25549–25556.
24. *Siddiqui, R.A. and English, D.*, Biochem. Biophys. Acta **1349** (1997), 82–96.
25. Moolenaar, W.H., *J. Biol. Chem.* **270** (1995), 12949–12952.
26. Qin, S., *et al.*, *Eur. J. Biochem.* **236** (1996), 443–449.
27. Traynor-Kaplan, A.E., *et al.*, *J. Biol. Chem.* **264** (1989), 15668–15673.
28. Ptasznik, A., Traynor-Kaplan, A. and Bokoch, G.M. *J. Biol. Chem.* **270** (1995), 19969–19973.
29. Karlund, J.K. *et al.*, *Science* **275** (1997), 1927–1930.
30. Brumell, J.H. *et al.*, *J. Immunol.* **158** (1997), 4862–4871.
31. English, D., Cui, Y., Siddiqui, R.A., *Chem. Phys. Lipids* **80** (1996), 117–132.
32. Heyneman, R.A. and Vercauteren, R.F., *J. Leuko. Biol.* **36** (1984), 751–755.
33. Bellavite, P., *et al.*, *J. Biol. Chem.* **263** (1988), 8210–8214.
34. Agwu, D.E., *et al.*, *J. Clin. Invest.* **88** (1991), 531–539.
35. Qualliotine-Mann, D., *et al.*, *J. Biol. Chem.* **268** (1993), 23843–23849.
36. DeLeo, F.R. and Quinn, M.T., *J. Leukoc. Biol.* **60** (1996) 677–691.
37. Chuang, T.H., Bohl, B.P. and Bokoch, G.M., *J. Biol. Chem.* **268** (1993), 26206–26211.
38. Ghosh, S., *et al.*, *J. Biol. Chem.* **271** (1996), 8472–8480.

39. Waite, K.A., Wallin, R., Qualliotine-Mann, D. and McPhail, L.C., *J. Biol. Chem.* **272** (1997), 15569–15578.
40. El Benna, J., Faust, L.P. and Babior, B.M. *J. Biol. Chem.* **271** (1996), 6374–6378.
41. Reinhold, S.L., Prescott, S.M., Zimmerman, G.A. and McIntyre T.M. *FEBS Lett.* **272** (1990), 19–24.
42. Cockcroft, S., *et al.*, *Science* **263** (1994), 523–526.
43. Brown, H.A., *et. al.*, *Cell* **75** (1993), 1137–1144.
44. Lambeth, J.D., *et al.*, *J. Biol. Chem.* **270** (1995), 3172–3178.
45. Bowman, E.P., Uhlinger, D.J., and Lambeth, J.D., *J. Biol. Chem.* **268** (1993), 21509–21512.
46. Kwak, J.-Y., *et al.*, *J. Biol. Chem.* **270** (1995), 27093–27098.

CHAPTER 2

THE RESPIRATORY BURST OF NEUTROPHILS: OXIDATIVE PATHWAYS FOR THE INITIATION OF TISSUE DAMAGE AT SITES OF INFLAMMATION

Jay W. Heinecke[1]

1. Introduction

The respiratory burst makes a critical contribution to the phagocytic response to infection (1–8). This sudden cyanide-resistant increase in oxygen consumption depends on the activation of the NADPH oxidase, a membrane-associated electron transport chain. The product of the oxidase is superoxide, which dismutates to hydrogen peroxide. Activated phagocytes use the peroxide as an oxidizing substrate for the heme protein myeloperoxidase, which they also secrete. The enzyme greatly amplifies the toxic potential of the peroxide, generating potent microbicidal and cytotoxic oxidants.

The key role of the NADPH oxidase system in host defenses against microbial pathogens is illustrated by chronic granulomatous disease (7,8). In this genetic disorder, defects in specific components of the oxidase impair superoxide production, and recurrent bacterial and fungal infections result. Thus, superoxide and hydrogen peroxide are critical for killing pathogenic organisms.

[1]Correspondence to: Jay W. Heinecke, Division of Atherosclerosis, Nutrition and Lipid Research, Box 8046, 660 S. Euclid Ave., St. Louis MO 63110, USA. Fax: 314-362-0811, E-mail heinecke@im.wustl.edu

Phagocytes' ability to generate oxidants has a deleterious side, however, because reactive species can damage tissue at sites of inflammation (9–12). Indeed, many lines of evidence implicate this process in the pathogenesis of diseases ranging from atherosclerosis to ischemia-reperfusion injury to cancer (13–16). This chapter summarizes the pathways by which phagocytes harness the respiratory burst to generate oxidants. It focuses on recent studies implicating myeloperoxidase as one agent for LDL oxidation and tissue damage in atherosclerosis (14,16).

2. Respiratory Burst Oxidase

The use of potentially lethal oxidants by professional phagocytes — neutrophils, monocytes, macrophages and eosinophils — suggests that the generation of superoxide and other oxidants must be carefully controlled. The mechanisms that regulate oxidant production can be studied in neutrophils, which are readily isolated in large quantities from blood.

Circulating neutrophils are quiescent, but they are quickly and synchronously activated by a wide array of agonists (2). One important agonist *in vivo* is a component of opsonized bacteria that binds to receptors on the neutrophil membrane. The binding leads to the activation of NADPH oxidase; it also triggers phagocytosis of the particulate bacterium (1–3). Superoxide ($O_2^{\bullet-}$) and myeloperoxidase are secreted into the phagolysosome containing the bacterium, bathing the microbe in high local concentrations of hydrogen peroxide (H_2O_2) and myeloperoxidase-derived oxidants (Fig. 1). Neutrophil granules containing an array of microbicidal proteins also are secreted into the phagocytic vacuole, further enhancing its toxic environment (1–6). Moreover, phagocytosis also stimulates neutrophils to secrete $O_2^{\bullet-}$, H_2O_2 and myeloperoxidase into the extracellular milieu, as do soluble agonists that trigger oxidant production.

The major electron transport element of the neutrophil NADPH oxidase is a membrane-bound b-type cytochrome, b_{558} (4,5,8,17,18). It contains two heme groups and a non-covalently associated flavin group (19,20). Flavocytochrome b_{558} is composed of a large β subunit, gp91-*phox*, and a small α subunit, p22-*phox* (gp for glycoprotein, p for protein, and *phox* for *ph*agocyte *ox*idase;

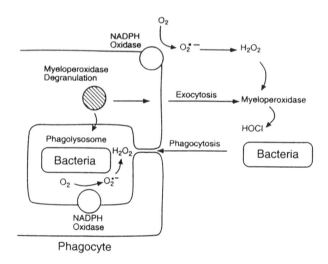

Figure 2.1. Activation of the respiratory burst oxidase by phagocytosis. Binding of a bacterium or other particulate material to the plasma membrane of a phagocyte triggers $O_2^{\bullet-}$ production by the NADPH oxidase as well as the secretion of myeloperoxidase and other neutrophil granule proteins (defensins, proteases) into the phagolysosome. Dismutation of $O_2^{\bullet-}$ yields H_2O_2, which myeloperoxidase uses to generate the potent microbicidal oxidant HOCl.

ref. 4,5,8,21–23). The two subunits are probably present at a 1:1 stoichiometry, but the exact number of heme groups and flavins in flavocytochrome b558 is unknown. There is some evidence that gp91-*phox* contains one heme group; a second may be interposed between the heavy and light subunits of the flavocytochrome (20).

The NADPH oxidase catalyzes the direct reduction of molecular oxygen to $O_2^{\bullet-}$ (24). It uses NADPH, but not NADH, as a co-factor (2,3):

$$NADPH + 2\,O_2 \rightarrow 2\,O_2^{\bullet-} + NADP^+ + H^+ \qquad \text{(Eq. 2.1)}$$

A wide variety of both soluble and particulate agents activate the oxidase (1–3). Commonly used soluble activators include phorbol ester, calcium ionophore, complement peptide C5a, tumor necrosis factor and N-formylated peptides (such as fMetLeuPhe) that mimic bacterial cell wall proteins. Particulate material such as opsonized bacteria and yeast cell wall preparations are also potent agonists.

Active NADPH oxidase is assembled from both membrane and cytosolic components (Fig. 2.2). It requires translocation of an activation complex from the cytosol to membrane-bound flavocytochrome b_{558} (4–6,8). Genetic studies have identified two critical cytosolic components, p47-*phox*, and p67-*phox* (25–30).

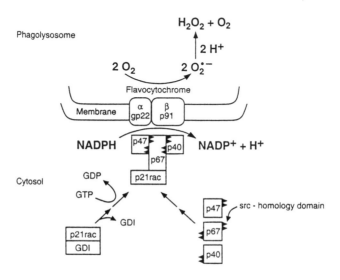

Figure 2.2.   Assembly of active NADPH oxidase in phagocytes. Stimulation of the cells causes p47-*phox*, p40-*phox* and p67-*phox* to assemble into an activation complex, which then translocates to the plasma membrane. Oxidase activity and $O_2^{\cdot-}$ production are triggered by the interactions of membrane-associated flavocytochrome b_{558} with the activation complex and p21*rac*-GTP.

Biochemical studies indicate that a third component, p40-*phox*, is associated with the other cytosolic components (31), but this protein is not required for oxidase activity (8). p47-*phox*, p40-*phox* and p67-*phox* each contain proline-rich regions and *src*-homology 3 domains (32) that are likely to mediate the interactions of the proteins (33,34). Genetic, biochemical and modeling studies implicate specific structural elements in the association of the different components as well as in the interaction of the activation complex with flavocytochrome b_{558} (4–6,8).

A small cytosolic GTP-binding protein, p21*rac*, is also likely to be required for activation of the oxidase (35–38). In quiescent neutrophils, p21*rac* is thought to be complexed in an inactive form with GDI, a GDP-dissociation protein. Neutrophil activation causes dissociation of p21*rac*-GDI, followed by association of p21*rac* with GTP to form an active complex (4–6,8). Binding of p21*rac*-GTP to p67-*phox* may be critical to assembly of the activation complex. Genetic defects in p21*rac* have not yet been identified, probably because this protein plays a critical role in cellular processes required for a viable organism.

$O_2{}^{\bullet-}$ production begins within 30 to 60 seconds after activation of the cell. Though the biochemical mechanisms for activation of the NADPH oxidase are understood in exquisite molecular detail, the signal transduction events (e.g. G proteins, protein kinases and phosphatases) that lie upstream of the oxidase operate by a complex, incompletely understood set of pathways (4–6,8,39 and Chapter 1). Cell stimulation with a variety of agonists is accompanied by phosphorylation of p47-*phox* and p67-*phox*, which likely plays an important role in regulation of oxidase activation. The details of the events that promote phosphorylation of oxidase components have not yet been elucidated, however.

The factors that shut down $O_2{}^{\bullet-}$ generation by the NADPH oxidase are poorly understood. Possible pathways may involve dephosphorylation of components of the activation complex and dissociation of p21*rac* from p67-*phox* bound to flavocytochrome b_{558}. Oxidants generated by myeloperoxidase also contribute to inactivation of the NADPH oxidase; both $O_2{}^{\bullet-}$ and H_2O_2 production are increased in neutrophils isolated from myeloperoxidase deficient patients and in the presence of myeloperoxidase inhibitors (1,40).

3. Oxidative Killing Mechanisms

Activated phagocytes use a battery of oxygen-dependent and -independent mechanisms to kill invading bacterial, viruses and fungi (1–8). Oxygen-dependent mechanisms are clearly of critical importance in this armamentarium because individuals with chronic granulomatous disease suffer recurrent, potentially life-threatening deep tissue infections (41). The role of oxygen-independent mechanisms is less clear, though the defensins — small, cysteine-rich proteins found in azurophilic granules — exhibit potent antimicrobial properties in vitro (42,43).

3.1 *Superoxide*

Despite the key role of the NADPH oxidase in microbial killing, it is far from clear why $O_2^{\bullet-}$ is necessary for microbicidal activity. $O_2^{\bullet-}$ itself is relatively impotent and kills bacteria poorly in vitro (44–46). However, it is possible that $O_2^{\bullet-}$ is cytotoxic at the high concentrations reached in the phagolysosome. Although neutrophil preparations that lack cytoplasmic granules will still phagocytose bacteria and generate a normal respiratory burst, these "cytoplasts" fail to kill staphylococci (47), indicating that cytoplasmic granules are of critical importance in bacterial killing.

Activation of the NADPH oxidase results in an initial increase in the pH of the phagolysosome (43), and alkalization is required for optimal bacterial killing by certain neutrophil granule proteins (42,43). For example, defensins are inactive within phagolysosomes that fail to undergo alkalinization, such as those of patients suffering from chronic granulomatous disease.

It is important to note that $O_2^{\bullet-}$ is a good reducing agent (48), and that it possesses the ability to scavenge many potential oxidants. It inhibits tyrosyl radical formation, for example. Bacteria that overexpress superoxide dismutase, which converts $O_2^{\bullet-}$ to H_2O_2, exhibit increased susceptibility to killing by ionizing radiation (49). A potential explanation is that superoxide dismutase increases the production of H_2O_2. Alternatively, $O_2^{\bullet-}$ might scavenge hydroxyl radical generated by ionizing radiation. These observations suggest that $O_2^{\bullet-}$ may serve as an antioxidant for certain types of reactions.

3.2 *Hydrogen peroxide*

The spontaneous or enzymatically catalyzed dismutation of $O_2^{\bullet-}$ yields oxygen and hydrogen peroxide (50):

$$2 \, O_2^{\bullet-} + 2 \, H^+ \rightarrow H_2O_2 + O_2 \qquad \text{(Eq. 2.2)}$$

H_2O_2 is cytotoxic, but its bactericidal properties are greatly increased by myeloperoxidase (2,3,43). Moreover, many bacteria produce catalase, which renders the peroxide harmless by converting it to oxygen and water (50):

$$2 \, H_2O_2 \rightarrow O_2 + 2 \, H_2O \qquad \text{(Eq. 2.3)}$$

However, certain bacteria lack catalase and even generate their own extracellular H_2O_2 (51). Myeloperoxidase can use this bacterial-generated peroxide as well as that generated by NADPH oxidase to enhance bacterial killing. Catalase-positive organisms (*Staphylococcus aureus*, *Aspergillus* and gram negative enteric bacilli), which fail to produce extracellular H_2O_2, cause many of the infections in patients suffering from chronic granulomatous disease (1,6–8).

3.3 *Myeloperoxidase-hydrogen peroxide-chloride system*

The heme protein myeloperoxidase is found in the azurophilic granules of neutrophils and monocytes, where it constitutes about 3% and 1% of total cell protein, respectively (1). This enzyme can use Cl^-, Br^- or I^- as a reducing substrate to produce hypohalous acid (2,3,52,53).

In plasma, where Cl^- is present at ~100 mM, the major reaction is thought to be the two- electron oxidation of Cl^- to hypochlorous acid (HOCl).

$$Cl^- + H_2O_2 + H^+ \rightarrow HOCl + H_2O \qquad \text{(Eq. 2.4)}$$

HOCl is an extremely potent cytotoxin for bacteria, viruses, fungi, mycoplasmas and cultured mammalian cells (2,3). In vitro studies confirm that it plays a key role in bacterial and viral killing by phagocytes (2,3,43) as originally proposed by Klebanoff (54–56). Reconstitution of the enzyme into cytoplasts, which lack neutrophil granule proteins, restores the ability of the cell preparation to kill staphylococci (43,47). However, myeloperoxidase does not appear essential for microbicidal activity in normal humans, presumably due to compensatory bacterial killing mechanisms (110). In contrast to healthy subjects, diabetic patients with complete deficiency of the enzyme suffer from an increased risk of infection with *Candida* species (110,111).

3.4 *Hydroxyl radical*

Reduction of H_2O_2 by $O_2^{\bullet-}$ generates hydroxyl radical ($HO^\bullet$), an extremely potent oxidant that reacts at a diffusion-controlled rate with a wide variety of biological molecules (50,57).

$$H_2O_2 + O_2^{\bullet-} \rightarrow HO^\bullet + HO^- + O_2 \qquad \text{(Eq. 2.5)}$$

The uncatalyzed rate of this reaction, originally described by Haber and Weiss, is extraordinarily slow and unlikely to be physiologically relevant (50,58). However, the reaction is facile in the presence of certain redox-active transition metal ions such as iron or copper (50,58). The reaction involves the initial reduction of the metal ion by $O_2^{\bullet-}$; the reduced metal then reacts with H_2O_2 to generate $HO^\bullet$.

$$O_2^{\bullet-} + Fe^{3+} \rightarrow O_2 + Fe^{2+} \qquad \text{(Eq. 2.6)}$$

$$Fe^{2+} + H_2O_2 \rightarrow Fe^{3+} + HO^- + HO^\bullet \qquad \text{(Eq. 2.7)}$$

Inhibition of oxidation reactions by superoxide dismutase (a scavenger of $O_2^{\bullet-}$), catalase (a scavenger of H_2O_2) and metal chelators is often interpreted to indicate the involvement of $HO^\bullet$ (50,58). It is noteworthy, however, that certain chelators such as EDTA actually promote $HO^\bullet$ formation in vitro (59), while other chelators such as DTPA and desferrioxamine are inhibitory (58).

In model systems, $HO^\bullet$ is a potent microbicidal oxidant (60). However, it is uncertain the free or low-molecular weight complexes of iron or copper required for metal-catalyzed hydroxyl radical formation exist in vivo (61). Despite extensive investigation, a biologically relevant catalyst of the Haber-Weiss reaction has not been identified. This may reflect the intricate mechanisms the body has developed for chelating metals and rendering them redox inactive (15,16,61,62).

3.5 *Singlet oxygen*

Oxygen in its ground state has two unpaired electrons with parallel spins (63). Excitation of oxygen by a variety of mechanisms inverts the spin of one of the electrons, generating singlet oxygen (9,63,64). Singlet oxygen is an extremely reactive electrophile that reacts with electron-dense regions of molecules, including carbon-carbon double bonds. Some studies suggest that singlet oxygen might be an important oxidant generated by neutrophils (64), but other studies suggest that this is a minor reaction pathway (15,65–67).

3.6 *Reactive nitrogen species*

Nitric oxide (NO) is a relatively stable free radical that plays a central role in the regulation of vasomotor tone as a product of endothelial nitric oxide synthase (68). Nitric oxide generated by inducible nitric oxide synthase contributes to inflammation, however (15,68).

In vitro, NO reacts with $O_2^{\bullet-}$ in vitro to form peroxynitrite (ONOO⁻), a reactive nitrogen species (69):

$$NO + O_2^{\bullet-} \rightarrow ONOO^- \qquad \text{(Eq. 2.8)}$$

In vitro studies demonstrate that ONOO⁻ promotes protein, nucleic acid and lipid oxidation and is a potent cytotoxin (70). Murine phagocytes generate high levels of NO, which reacts to form intermediates that appear to be important in certain types of microbicidal activity (70,71). However, it is controversial whether human phagocytes generate significant levels of NO (15,72).

Recent studies suggest that myeloperoxidase converts *nitrite* (NO_2^-), a decomposition product of NO, into reactive nitrogen species (73). For example, NO_2^- reacts with HOCl to form nitrating and chlorinating intermediates. It also may be oxidized by myeloperoxidase to nitrogen dioxide radical ($NO_2^{\bullet}$), a potent nitrating and oxidizing species.

4. Phagocytes, Myeloperoxidase and Oxidative Damage of Tissue

Although activated phagocytes play a key role in host defense, the oxidants they generate may also damage biomolecules at sites of inflammation. Indeed, oxidative damage is implicated in the pathogenesis of many diseases and in aging (13).

We have been interested in the hypothesis that oxidation of low density lipoprotein (LDL), the major carrier of blood cholesterol, is an important risk factor for atherosclerosis, the leading cause of death in industrialized societies. Although LDL fails to exert atherogenic effects in vitro, oxidation of its lipid and/or protein moieties renders it atherogenic (16,74,75).

A wealth of evidence indicates that oxidized LDL but not LDL itself promotes vascular disease (74,75). Immunohistochemical studies with monoclonal antibodies specific for protein-bound lipid oxidation products provide direct evidence for LDL oxidation in the artery wall (76). Moreover, LDL-like lipoproteins with indications of oxidative damage have been isolated from human and animal atherosclerotic lesions (77,78). Several chemically unrelated lipid-soluble antioxidants retard or inhibit atherosclerosis in animal models of hypercholesterolemia (79), and epidemiological studies suggest that a high dietary intake of antioxidants is associated with a decreased risk for coronary artery disease (80). Most significantly, vitamin E prevents acute coronary events in patients with known atherosclerotic vascular disease (81), suggesting that oxidative events are of central importance in atherogenesis.

The physiologically relevant mechanisms for oxidative damage to the artery wall have not been identified. However, phagocytes use oxidative chemistry to destroy invading pathogens, and lipid-laden macrophages are the cellular hallmark of the early atherosclerotic lesion (75). This suggests that activated phagocytes may generate substances that inadvertently damage LDL along with microbial targets.

Myeloperoxidase has been detected in human atherosclerotic plaques (82), where it co-localizes with macrophages and lipid oxidation products. Moreover, it is a potent catalyst for LDL oxidation in vitro, and products specific for its actions on proteins have been detected in human atherosclerotic tissue (16). Studies from our laboratory have outlined a number of mechanisms whereby myeloperoxidase could amplify the oxidative power released by the respiratory burst to oxidize LDL and damage tissues.

4.1 *Tyrosyl radical*

Myeloperoxidase cannot directly damage large macromolecules because its active site is buried in a hydrophobic cleft (3). Instead, myeloperoxidase relies on low-molecular weight intermediates to convey oxidizing equivalents from its heme group to the target for damage. One such intermediate is the long-lived tyrosyl radical (83,84), which the enzyme generates from the phenolic amino acid tyrosine (85). The productive interaction of two tyrosyl radicals yields o,o'-dityrosine, an intensely fluorescent compound (86).

(Eq. 2.9)

Myeloperoxidase rapidly converts tyrosine to dityrosine by a reaction requiring H_2O_2 (85). Neutrophils and macrophages stimulated by phorbol ester to produce H_2O_2 also generate dityrosine from tyrosine. This reaction is inhibited by catalase (a scavenger of H_2O_2) and heme poisons, indicating that myeloperoxidase operates in the cellular pathway. In contrast, superoxide dismutase stimulates dityrosine synthesis by cells, suggesting that the yield of H_2O_2 is increased, that $O_2^{\bullet-}$ inactivates myeloperoxidase or that $O_2^{\bullet-}$ acts as an antioxidant in this system. These results indicate that activated phagocytes use the myeloperoxidase-H_2O_2 system to generate tyrosyl radical. Because this reactive intermediate is an oxidant in other biological systems (84), it might oxidize lipoprotein in vivo.

4.2 *Human phagocytes use myeloperoxidase to generate a family of tyrosine oxidation products by a tyrosyl radical-dependent pathway*

The oxidation of tyrosine by myeloperoxidase (85) is strikingly similar to the production of phenoxyl radical (87). In both cases, a one-electron oxidation reaction generates a reactive intermediate that undergoes radical coupling to yield carbon-carbon cross-linked dimers. Because phenoxyl radical also forms carbon-oxygen cross-links as well as complex polymers (87), we investigated the possibility that myeloperoxidase can similarly convert tyrosine into other oxidation products.

When the myeloperoxidase-H_2O_2 system oxidized tyrosine, we saw three major fluorescent peaks during ion exchange chromatography (88). We purified each compound to apparent homogeneity by cation- and anion-exchange chromatography and identified them by mass spectrometry and high-resolution NMR spectroscopy. The products proved to be dityrosine, trityrosine and pulcherosine (Fig. 2.3). Kinetic studies demonstrated that dityrosine was a precursor to trityrosine. Searching for the precursor for pulcherosine, we identified isodityrosine, a nonfluorescent oxidation product.

Activated human phagocytes generated the same family of fluorescent tyrosine oxidation products (88). The cells had to be activated by phorbol ester to produce $O_2^{\bullet-}$ and H_2O_2, and they did not generate the oxidation products when exposed to catalase and heme poisons, indicating the involvement of myeloperoxidase.

These observations suggest that human phagocytes use the myeloperoxidase-H_2O_2 system to convert tyrosine to a family of oxidation products. These products are typical for a para-substituted phenoxyl radical, and they include compounds with both carbon-carbon bonds (dityrosine, trityrosine) and carbon-oxygen bonds (isodityrosine and pulcherosine). These tyrosine oxidation products are stable to acid hydrolysis, intensely fluorescent, and readily detected by mass spectrometry. Therefore they are attractive markers for studies of protein oxidation. Finding such tyrosine oxidation products in proteins isolated from sites of inflammation would strongly support the hypothesis that tyrosyl radical, perhaps generated by myeloperoxidase, contributes to oxidative damage in vivo.

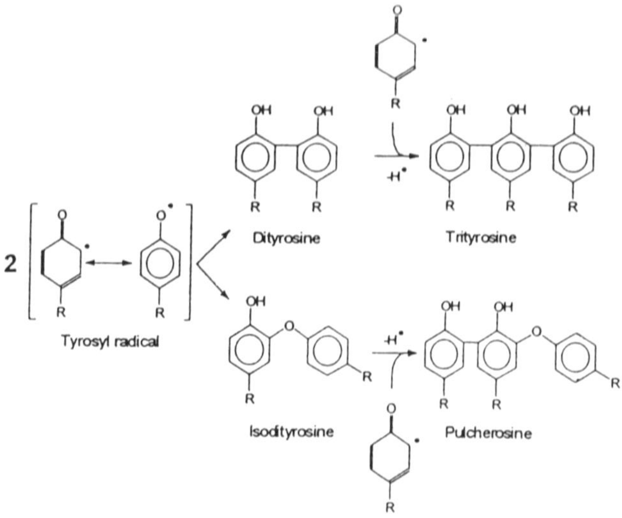

Figure 2.3.   Myeloperoxidase generates a family of tyrosyl radical addition products.

4.3 *Tyrosyl radical promotes the cross-linking of tyrosine residues in proteins*

Myeloperoxidase's ability to generate tyrosyl radical raises the possibility that proteins may be one target for phagocytic damage. We tested this idea by exposing albumin to the myeloperoxidase-H_2O_2 system and then analyzing the albumin for protein-bound dityrosine (89). In the absence of tyrosine, there was little modification of albumin. In its presence, there was a marked increase in dityrosine-like fluorescence. To confirm that this was in fact due to dityrosine, we reisolated and hydrolyzed the albumin and then subjected the amino acid hydrolysate to ion exchange chromatography. A single major fluorescent peak of material eluted from the column at the same ionic strength as dityrosine.

To conclusively identify the fluorescent oxidation product, we subjected the fluorescent amino acid isolated from the hydrolyzed protein to gas chromatography/mass spectrometry. The retention time and mass spectrum of the product were virtually identical to those of authentic dityrosine (89).

Synthesis of protein-bound dityrosine by myeloperoxidase required active enzyme, H_2O_2 and tyrosine; it was inhibited by heme poisons and catalase.

Activated neutrophils similarly modified albumin; again, the reaction required tyrosine and was inhibited by heme poisons and catalase, strongly implicating myeloperoxidase as the catalytic agent.

Collectively, these results indicate that human neutrophils use the myeloperoxidase-H_2O_2 system to oxidatively cross-link proteins by a reaction involving tyrosyl radical (89). The phenolic coupling reaction is independent of free metal ions but requires tyrosine, implying that tyrosyl radical is serving as a diffusible catalyst. The proposed intermediate in the reaction — protein-bound tyrosyl radical — might then undergo several subsequent reactions (89,90). First, it might cross-link with free tyrosyl radical to form a tyrosylated protein. Second, two protein-bound tyrosyl radicals might undergo intermolecular or intramolecular cross-linking. Third, protein-bound tyrosyl radical might interact with other protein or lipid moieties that are susceptible to oxidation.

4.4 *Tyrosyl radical peroxidizes lipid moieties of LDL*

Lipid peroxidation is thought to play a critical role in rendering LDL atherogenic (74). To test the potential role of myeloperoxidase in this process, we examined the ability of human neutrophils to stimulate LDL lipid peroxidation (91). LDL exposed to activated cells and tyrosine underwent extensive lipid peroxidation, monitored as the production of hydroxy fatty acids (after saponification and reduction) and cholesterol ester hydroperoxides. Lipid peroxidation required cell activation and tyrosine; it was inhibited by heme poisons and catalase. Other aromatic amino acids, including histidine and tryptophan, could not substitute for tyrosine in the oxidation reaction.

To further explore the role of myeloperoxidase in neutrophil-mediated lipid peroxidation, we incubated LDL with the enzyme and a system that generates H_2O_2 (91). Little LDL oxidation occurred in the absence of free tyrosine. Addition of tyrosine greatly stimulated LDL lipid peroxidation. Again, the reaction was blocked by heme poisons and catalase. Together with the neutrophil studies, these results indicate that myeloperoxidase stimulates lipid peroxidation by a pathway involving tyrosyl radical.

We have suggested that tyrosyl radical initiates lipid peroxidation by abstracting hydrogen atom from bis-allylic methylene groups of polyunsaturated fatty acids (92).

Alternatively, tyrosyl radical may oxidize other molecules, such as α-tocopherol, that can then promote lipid peroxidation of LDL (75). Indeed, chemical studies indicate that phenoxyl radical is unusually reactive with tocopherol and other substrates (92).

(Eq. 2.10)

In contrast to most other mechanisms for LDL oxidation (16,75), the tyrosyl radical-dependent reaction is independent of free metal ions, suggesting that it may stimulate LDL oxidation under physiological conditions.

4.5 *Myeloperoxidase converts tyrosine to a reactive aldehyde by an HOCl-dependent reaction*

When myeloperoxidase oxidizes chloride, dityrosine formation is suppressed (85). Therefore in plasma, where Cl^- concentrations are high, myeloperoxidase may convert tyrosine to products other than dityrosine. Indeed, indirect evidence has long suggested that amino acids are decarboxylated and deaminated to form compounds with reactive carbonyls (2).

To explore this possibility, we exposed tyrosine to myeloperoxidase, H_2O_2 and Cl^- and analyzed the reaction products by high performance liquid chromatography (93). In the presence of the complete system, a single major oxidation product appeared. Generation of the product was absolutely Cl^--dependent. Using mass spectrometry, Fourier transform infrared spectroscopy, and high resolution NMR spectroscopy, we identified the isolated product as a highly reactive aldehyde, *p*-hydroxyphenylacetaldehyde (*p*HA).

At plasma concentrations of Cl^- and tyrosine, pHA production consumed more than 80% of the H_2O_2 in the reaction mixture.

This reaction also proceeded readily in the presence of activated neutrophils; with optimal stimulation, pHA production consumed most of the cells' output of H_2O_2 (93). Reagent HOCl also converted tyrosine into pHA, strongly implicating HOCl in the cellular reaction pathway.

Recent studies indicate that myeloperoxidase converts virtually all of the common amino acids to reactive aldehydes (94,95). For example, threonine is converted into the potent cytotoxin acrolein (94). Using isotope dilution gas chromatography/mass spectrometry, we detected a covalent adduct of pHA and lysine in inflammatory tissues (96). This strongly suggests that myeloperoxidase generates reactive aldehydes in vivo.

Reactive aldehydes are thought to be of central importance in the genesis of vascular disease (74,75). Aldehydes derived from lipid peroxidation convert LDL to a ligand for the macrophage scavenger receptor (74), which plays a key role in the formation of foam cells, the cellular hallmark of atherosclerosis. Oxidation of proteins and lipids by glucose (an aldehyde in its open chain form) during chronic hyperglycemia may play a similar role in cross-linking arterial wall proteins with plasma components, an event that may accelerate the vascular disease of diabetes mellitus (97). Reactive aldehydes therefore may damage the vascular wall in both diabetes and atherosclerosis.

4.6 Myeloperoxidase generates chlorine gas

HOCl is in equilibrium with Cl_2 via a reaction that requires H^+ and Cl^- (ref. 98):

$$HOCl + Cl^- + H^+ = Cl_2 + H_2O \qquad \text{(Eq. 2.11)}$$

This suggested to us that Cl_2 might be a chlorinating intermediate in reactions catalyzed by myeloperoxidase, though Cl_2 was not known to be a metabolite in living organisms. Because molecular chlorine, the solvated form of Cl_2, is in equilibrium with Cl_2 gas, we analyzed the head space gas above the myeloperoxidase-H_2O_2-Cl^- reaction system (99). Electron impact mass spectrometric analysis revealed a gas with the expected mass-to-charge ratio of Cl_2. Both the retention time and isotopic distribution of the compound were identical to those of authentic Cl_2. These observations, together with previous studies of the formation of HOCl, provide unambiguous evidence that myeloperoxidase generates Cl_2 via a reaction pathway that involves HOCl as an intermediate.

Myeloperoxidase is the only human enzyme known to generate hypochlorous acid (HOCl), a potent oxidizing agent, at plasma concentrations of halide ion (52,53,100). Thus, the detection of chlorinated molecules in atherosclerotic lesions would constitute strong evidence that myeloperoxidase was one pathway for oxidative damage in vivo. Most oxidation products generated by HOCl are either non-specific or yield uninformative compounds (101). However, recent studies demonstrate that myeloperoxidase converts tyrosine into 3-chlorotyrosine (99,102), a stable product that may serve as a molecular fingerprint of the enzyme's action.

LDL exposed to the complete myeloperoxidase-hydrogen peroxide-Cl^- system underwent chlorination of its protein tyrosyl residues (103). Reagent HOCl chlorinated tyrosine similarly, implicating this oxidizing intermediate in the enzymatic pathway. 3-Chlorotyrosine was undetectable in LDL oxidized with hydroxyl radical, copper, iron, hemin, glucose, peroxynitrite, horseradish peroxidase, lactoperoxidase, or lipoxygenase, indicating it was specific marker of LDL oxidation by myeloperoxidase.

4.7 *Myeloperoxidase chlorinates cholesterol*

Activated phagocytes lyse phospholipid liposomes via a reaction that also requires halide and H_2O_2, implicating HOCl in the pathway (104). Reagent HOCl reacts with fatty acid acyl groups to form chlorohydrins (105), suggesting that polar chlorohydrins disrupt membrane structure. These electrophilic addition compounds appear stable and may therefore represent specific markers for myeloperoxidase-mediated damage.

Because chlorohydrins are oxygenated as well as chlorinated, and because oxygenated sterols have been isolated from human vascular lesions, we were interested in the idea that HOCl also might react with cholesterol, a major component of plasma membranes and circulating LDL. Therefore we exposed cholesterol incorporated into phospholipid liposomes to a myeloperoxidase-H_2O_2-Cl^- system and analyzed the reaction mixture by normal phase chromatography (106). Three major products were apparent. They were identified by gas chromatography/mass spectrometry as cholesterol α- and β-chlorohydrins, cholesterol α- and β-epoxides, and a novel cholesterol chlorohydrin. Cholesterol chlorination by myeloperoxidase was optimal under acidic conditions (106). This pH dependence was not due to enzymatic activity because the yield of cholesterol chlorohydrins with reagent HOCl also increased with increasing [H^+]. HOCl itself did not appear to be the chorinating intermediate because the pK_a for HOCl/ClO^- is ~ 7 (107).

HOCl is in equilibrium with Cl_2 via a reaction that requires H^+ and Cl^- (Eq. 2.11). To determine whether Cl_2 might be the chlorinating intermediate, we examined the reaction requirements for the oxidation of LDL cholesterol by HOCl (108). Generation of Cl_2 should require Cl^- (Eq. 2.11) and, indeed, reagent HOCl failed to chlorinate cholesterol in the absence of this halide. The reaction also was optimal under acidic conditions, consistent with a requirement for H^+. Finally, at neutral pH and in the absence of Cl^-, molecular chlorine readily generated cholesterol chlorohydrins in LDL. These results strongly suggest that Cl_2 — not HOCl — is the chlorinating intermediate when myeloperoxidase oxidizes cholesterol (108).

In our initial studies of cholesterol chlorination by myeloperoxidase, we identified an unknown oxidation product that migrated near the solvent front on thin layer chromatography (106). To determine whether this product was chlorinated, we isolated the compound from LDL that had been oxidized by the myeloperoxidase-H_2O_2-Cl^- system. Then we subjected it to electrospray mass spectrometric analysis. The positive ion mass spectrum revealed that the molecular mass of the compound and its isotopic distribution were as expected for a dichlorinated sterol (108). These results indicate that myeloperoxidase converts LDL cholesterol to a novel dichlorinated sterol, and they strongly support the hypothesis that Cl_2 is the reactive intermediate.

The oxidation of LDL cholesterol by myeloperoxidase exhibited another remarkable feature. At acidic pH, the yield of the reaction was high; nearly 50% of the H_2O_2 in the mixture was used for cholesterol chlorination (108).

Thus, cholesterol is targeted selectively for oxidation, perhaps because of its location at the interface between the aqueous and lipid phases. In marked contrast, only trace quantities of lipid oxidation products are formed at neutral pH by reagent HOCl, and the major targets for oxidation are amino acid residues (109). These findings indicate that HOCl and Cl_2 oxidize different reactive moieties of LDL.

Collectively, these results demonstrate that the myeloperoxidase-H_2O_2-Cl^- system converts LDL cholesterol into a family of chlorinated products at acidic pH by a reaction involving molecular chlorine. A number of acidic compartments may exist in vivo that favor such a reaction, including the closely juxtaposed membranes of adherent phagocytes and endothelium (or other target cells), as well as hypoxic tissues such as atherosclerotic lesions. Moreover, oxidation-specific epitopes are present in the lysosomal-like structures of the macrophages that congregate in atherosclerotic lesions (76), and these compartments ultimately become acidified during phagocytosis in vitro (3,43).

5. Active Myeloperoxidase is Present in Human Atherosclerotic Lesions

To test the hypothesis that myeloperoxidase represents one mechanism for oxidizing lipoproteins in vivo, we searched for evidence that the enzyme is expressed in human atherosclerotic tissue (82). A rabbit polyclonal antibody monospecific for myeloperoxidase recognized a single 56 kDa protein in detergent extracts of human atherosclerotic tissue. The protein co-migrated with authentic myeloperoxidase on Western blots, strongly suggesting the enzyme was present.

Because myeloperoxidase is mannosylated, it binds with high affinity to lectins (110). Immunoreactive material extracted from human lesions bound to a concanavalin A column and eluted with methyl mannoside; the reisolated protein and myeloperoxidase demonstrated the same molecular size on high-resolution non-denaturing size exclusion chromatography (82). The reisolated protein also generated HOCl (82). Moreover, atherosclerotic tissue but not normal tissue from the artery wall also showed this activity. Collectively, these results demonstrate that active myeloperoxidase is a component of human atherosclerotic tissue.

We localized myeloperoxidase in atherosclerotic lesions using a monoclonal antibody to the enzyme (82). In transitional lesions, immunoreactive material was predominantly localized to the highly cellular shoulder region. Cells in this region strongly reacted with an anti-macrophage antibody. Myeloperoxidase also was present in advanced lesions, where intense foci of staining appeared adjacent to cholesterol clefts. In macrophage-rich lesions from hypercholesterolemic animals, antibodies that react selectively with protein-bound lipid oxidation products bound mostly to cells (76). Material in the necrotic core of advanced lesions stained extensively, especially near lipid deposits.

In vitro studies with cultured human cells and mouse peritoneal macrophages suggest that myeloperoxidase normally disappears as monocytes differentiate into macrophages (110,111). In contrast, our observations suggest that myeloperoxidase is present in lipid-laden macrophages in human atherosclerotic tissue (82). Macrophages may therefore continue to express the enzyme in vivo under certain conditions, perhaps in response to cytokines or other stimulatory factors.

The striking similarity between the immunostaining patterns of myeloperoxidase in human lesions (82) and oxidized lipids in rabbit atherosclerotic lesions (76) suggests that myeloperoxidase catalyzes LDL oxidation in vivo. This hypothesis is strongly supported by the recent demonstration that an antibody that reacts with HOCl-modified LDL, but not with LDL oxidized by copper, exhibited similar reactivity in lesions (112). Moreover, the antibody also recognized LDL-like material isolated from vascular tissue but not LDL isolated from plasma.

6. Oxidation Products Generated by Myeloperoxidase are Present in Human Atherosclerotic Lesions

To explore the role of one myeloperoxidase product, tyrosyl radical, in promoting LDL oxidation in vivo, we used stable isotope dilution gas chromatography/mass spectrometry to quantify the level of dityrosine in lesion LDL and human atherosclerotic tissue (113). We detected a remarkable

100-fold increase in dityrosine levels in lesion LDL compared with those in circulating LDL. Analysis of fatty streaks revealed a similar pattern of oxidation products — compared with normal tissue, there was a 10-fold increase in dityrosine with no difference in either o-tyrosine or m-tyrosine. These results suggest that tyrosyl radical, perhaps generated in part by myeloperoxidase, is one agent for LDL oxidation in the human artery wall (113).

To obtain direct evidence that myeloperoxidase promotes oxidation reactions in vivo, we used isotope dilution gas chromatography/mass spectrometry to quantify levels of 3-chlorotyrosine in atherosclerotic lesions (103). In vascular tissue freshly harvested at surgery, the level of 3-chlorotyrosine was 6-fold higher in atherosclerotic lesions than in normal aortic tissue. Moreover, lesion LDL contained 30-times more 3-chlorotyrosine than circulating LDL. These results provide strong evidence that halogenation reactions catalyzed by myeloperoxidase constitute one pathway for protein oxidation in vivo (103). Moreover, they suggest that myeloperoxidase may play a critical role in rendering LDL atherogenic.

To explore the role of reactive nitrogen species in oxidative damage in vivo, we measured the level of 3-nitrotyrosine in LDL isolated from human atherosclerotic lesions (114). There was a striking 90-fold increase in the level of 3-nitrotyrosine in lesion LDL compared with circulating LDL. These observations raise the possibility that NO, by virtue of its ability to form reactive nitrogen species, may promote atherogenesis, countering the well-established anti-atherogenic effects of NO.

7. Conclusions

The oxidants that phagocytes produce play critical roles in killing invading pathogens, but they also may inadvertently damage tissue at sites of inflammation. A potential mechanism involves the phagocytic heme protein myeloperoxidase (Fig. 2.3). This enzyme promotes LDL oxidation in vitro by a variety of different pathways, and it is present and active in atherosclerotic lesions. One of its reactive products is tyrosyl radical, which initiates lipid peroxidation and cross-links protein tyrosine residues into dityrosine. Dityrosine

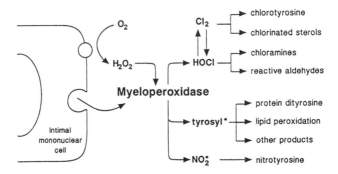

Figure 2.3.   Reaction pathways for the damage of biomolecules by myeloperoxidase.

levels are dramatically elevated in lesion LDL and in fatty streaks, suggesting that tyrosyl radical promotes LDL oxidation early in atherogenesis. Another product — generated exclusively by the myeloperoxidase system at plasma concentrations of halide — is 3-chlorotyrosine, a specific marker for oxidation by HOCl. Levels of 3-chlorotyrosine are increased in atherosclerotic lesions, strongly supporting the hypothesis that myeloperoxidase constitutes one mechanism for protein oxidation in the human artery wall.

NO decomposes into NO_2^-, which reacts with HOCl to form a chlorinating and nitrating intermediate. Myeloperoxidase also will convert NO_2^- into an $NO_2^\bullet$-like intermediate that nitrates the aromatic ring of tyrosine. We have detected elevated levels of 3-nitrotyrosine and 3-chlorotyrosine in LDL isolated from atherosclerotic lesions, suggesting that myeloperoxidase promotes both chlorination and nitration of proteins in the human artery wall.

Activated phagocytes have been implicated in tissue damage in diseases ranging from arthritis to inflammatory bowel disease to ischemia-reperfusion injury. It is unknown whether people or mice deficient in myeloperoxidase are protected against atherosclerosis and other inflammatory diseases. We speculate that reactive intermediates generated by myeloperoxidase play a role in the pathogenesis of many inflammatory disorders. Because this enzyme harnesses oxidative power that originally comes from the respiratory burst, inhibitors of phagocytic NAPH oxidase or of subsequent steps in oxidant production may have wide-ranging therapeutic potential.

8. References

1. Klebanoff S.J. and Clark R.A., *The neutrophil: Function and clinical disorders* (North Holland Publishing Co., Amsterdam, 1978).
2. Babior B.M., *N. Eng. J. Med.* **298** (1978), 659–663.
3. Hurst J.K. and Barrette W.C., *CRC Crit. Rev. Biochem. Mol. Biol.* **24** (1989), 271–328.
4. Shatwell K.P. and Segal A.W., *Int. J. Bioch. Cell Biol.* **28** (1996), 1191–1195.
5. DeLeo F.R. and Quinn M.T., *J. Leukocyte Biol.* **60** (1996), 677–691.
6. Leusen J.H., Verhoeven A.J. and Roos D., *J. Lab. Clin. Med.* **128** (1996), 461–476.
7. Lehrer R.I., Ganz T., Selsted M.E., Babior B.M. and Curnute J.T., *Ann. Int. Med.* **109** (1988), 127–142.
8. Roos D., *et al.*, *Blood* **87** (1996), 1663–1681.
9. Klebanoff S.J., *Ann. Intern. Med.* **93** (1980), 480–489.
10. Weiss S.J., *N. Eng. J. Med.* **320** (1989), 365–376.
11. Babior B.M., *Blood* **64** (1984), 959–966.
12. Malech H.L. and Gallin J.I., *N. Eng. J. Med.* **317** (1987), 687–694.
13. Ames B.N., Shigenaga M.K. and Hagen T.M. *Proc. Natl. Acad. Sci. U.S.A.* **90** (1993), 7915–7922.
14. Heinecke J.W., *Coron. Art. Dis.* **5** (1994), 205–210.
15. Miller R.A. and Britigan B.E., *J. Invest. Med.* **43** (1995), 39–49.
16. Heinecke J.W., *Cur. Opin. Lipid.* **8**, (1997), 268–274.
17. Segal A.W., *Nature* **326** (1987), 88–91.
18. Parkos C.A., Allen R.A., Chochrane C.G. and Jesaitis A.J., *J. Clin. Inv.* **80** (1987), 732–742.
19. Segal A.W., *et al.*, *Biochem. J.* **284** (1992), 781–788.
20. Quinn M.T., Mullen J.L. and Jesaitis A.J., *J. Biol. Chem.* **267** (1992), 7303–7309.
21. Dinauer M.C., Pierce E.A., Bruns G.A.P., Curnutte J.T. and Orkin S.H., *J. Clin. Inv.* **86** (1990), 1729–1737.
22. Dinauer M.C., Orkin S.H., Brown R., Jesaitis A.J. and Parkos C.A., *Nature* **327** (1987), 717–720.
23. Teahan C., Rowe P., Parker P., Totty N. and Segal A.W., *Nature* **327** (1987), 720–721.
24. Babior B.M., Kipnes R.S. and Curnutte J.T., *J. Clin. Inv.* **52** (1973), 741–744.
25. Segal A.W., Heyworth P.G., Cockroft S. and Barrowman M.M., *Nature* **316** (1985), 547–549.

26. Volpp B.D., Nauseef W.M., Clark R.A., *Science* **242** (1988), 1295–1297.
27. Clark R.A., *et al.*, *N. Eng. J. Med.* **321** (1989), 647–652.
28. Volpp B.D., Nauseef W.M., Donelson J.E., Moser D.R. and Clark R.A., *Proc. Natl. Acad. Sci. USA* **86** (1989), 7195–7199.
29. Lomax K.R., Leto T.L., Nunoi H., Gallin J.I. and Malech H.L., *Science* **245** (1989), 409–411.
30. Leto T.L., *et al.*, *Science* **248** (1990), 727–730.
31. Tsunawaki S., Mizunari H., Nagata M., Tatsuzawa O. and Kuratsuji T., *Biochem. Biophys. Res. Com.* **199** (1994), 1378–1387.
32. Ren R., Mayer B.J., Cicchetti, P. and Baltimore D., *Science* **259** (1993), 1157–1161.
33. Sumimoto H., *et al.*, *Proc. Natl. Acad. Sci. USA* **91** (1994), 5345–5349.
34. Leto T.L., Adams A.G. and DeMendez I., *Proc. Natl. Acad. Sci. USA* **91** (1994), 10650–10654.
35. Abo A., *et al.*, *Nature* **353** (1991), 668– 670.
36. Knaus U.G., Heyworth P.G., Evans T., Curnutte J.G. and Bokoch G.M., *Science* **254** (1991) 1512–1515.
37. Quinn M.T., Evans T., Loetterle L.R., Jesaitis A.J. and Bokoch G.M., *J. Biol. Chem.* **268** (1993), 20983–20987.
38. Heyworth P.G., Bohl B.P., Bokoch G.M. and Curnutte J.T., *J. Biol. Chem.* **269** (1994), 30749–30752.
39. Thelen M., Dewald B. and Baggiolini M., *Physiol. Rev.* **73** (1993), 797–821.
40. Jandl R.C., *et al.*, *J. Clin. Invest.* **61** (1978), 1176–1185.
41. Quie P.G., White J.G., Holmes P.G. and Good R.A., *J. Clin. Inv.* **46** (1967), 668–679.
42. Lehr R.I., Ganz T. and Selsted M.E., *Cell* **64** (1991), 229–230.
43. Segal A.W., *J. Clin. Invest.* **83** (1989), 1785–1793.
44. Babior B.M., Curnutte J.T. and Kipnes R.S., *J. Lab. Clin. Med.* **85** (1975), 235–244.
45. Mandell G.L., *J. Clin. Inv.* **55** (1975), 561–566.
46. Gregory E.M. and Fridovich I., *J. Bacteriol.* **117** (1974), 166–169.
47. Odell E.W. and Segal A.W., *Biochim. Biophys Acta* **971** (1988), 266–274.
48. Sawyer D.T. and Valentine J.S., *Acc. Chem. Res.* **14** (1981), 393–400.
49. Scott M. D., Meshnick S.R. and Eaton J.W., *J. Biol. Chem.* **264** (1989), 2498–2501.
50. Fridovich I., *Science* **201** (1978), 875–880.
51. McRipley R.J. and Sbarra, A.J., *J. Bacteriol.* **94** (1967), 1425–1430.

52. Harrison J.E. and Schultz J., *J. Biol. Chem.* **251** (1976), 1371–1374.
53. Foote C. S., Goyne T.E. and Lehrer R.I., *Nature* **301** (1981), 715–716.
54. Klebanoff S.J., *J. Exp. Med.* **126** (1967), 1063–1078.
55. Klebanoff S.J., *J. Bacteriol.* **95** (1968), 2131–2138.
56. Klebanoff S.J., *J. Clin. Inv.* **46** (1967), 1078–1086.
57. Haber F. and Weiss J., *Proc. Royal Soc. London: Math. Phys. Soc.* **147** (1934), 332–351.
58. Cohen G., in *CRC Handbook of Methods for Oxygen Radical Research*, ed. Greenwald R.A. (CRC Press, Inc., Boca Raton, FL. 1985), 55–64.
59. McCord J.M. and Day E.D., *FEBS Lett.* **86** (1978), 139–141.
60. Klebanoff S.J., *Biochem.* **21** (1982), 4110–4116.
61. Ramos C.L., Pou S., Britigan B.E., Cohen M.S. and Rosen G.M., *J. Biol. Chem.* **267** (1992), 8307–8312.
62. Halliwell B. and Gutteridge J.M.C., *Arch. Biochem. Biophys.* **246** (1986), 246–501.
63. Kearns D.R., *Chem. Rev.* **71** (1971), 395–427.
64. Steinbeck M.J., Khan A.U., Karnovsky M.J. and Hegg G.G., *J. Biol. Chem.* **267** (1992), 13425–13433.
65. Dahl T.A., Midden W.R. and Hartman P.E., *Photochem. Photobiol.* **46** (1987), 345–352.
66. Dahl T.A., Midden W.R. and Hartman P.E., *J. Bacteriol.* **171** (1989), 2188–2194.
67. Wagner J.R., Motchnik P.A., Stocker R., Sies H. and Ames B.N., *J. Biol. Chem.* **268** (1993), 18502–18506.
68. Moncada S. and Higgs A., *N. Eng. J. Med.* **329** (1993), 2002–2012.
69. Beckman J.S., Beckman T.W., Chen J., Marshall P.A. and Freeman, B.A., *Proc. Natl. Acad. Sci. USA* **87** (1990), 1620–1624.
70. Koppenol W.H., *et al.*, *Chem. Res. Toxicol.* **5** (1992), 834–842.
71. Granger D.L., Hibbs J.B. Jr., Perfect J.R. and Durack D.T., *J. Clin.Invest.* **81** (1988), 1129–1136.
72. Murray H.W. and Teitelbaum R.F., *J. Infect. Dis.* **165** (1992), 513–517.
73. Van der Vliet A., Eiserich J.P., Halliwell B. and Cross C.E. *J. Biol. Chem.* **272** (1997), 7617–7625.
74. Witztum J.L. and Steinber D., *J. Clin. Invest.* **88** (1991),1785–1792.
75. Berliner J.A. and Heinecke J.W. (1996) *Free Rad. Biol. Med.* **20** (1996), 707–727.
76. Rosenfeld M.E., Palinski W., Yla-Herttuala S., Butler S. and Witztum J.L., *Arterioscler.* **10** (1990), 336–349.

77. Daugherty A., Zweifel B.S., Sobel B.E. and Schonfeld, G., *Arterioscler.* **8** (1988), 768–777.
78. Yla-Herttuala S., *et al.*, *J. Clin. Invest.* **84** (1989), 1086–1095.
79. Steinberg D., *Lancet* **346** (1995), 36–38.
80. Jha P., Flather M., Lonn E., Farkouh M. and Yusuf S., *Ann. Intern. Med.* **123** (1995), 860–872.
81. Stephens N. G., *et al.*, *Lancet* **347** (1996), 781–786.
82. Daugherty A., Dunn J.L., Rateri D.L. and Heinecke J.W., *J. Clin. Inv.* **94** (1994), 437–444.
83. Sealy R.C., Harman L., West P.R. and Mason R.P., *J. Amer. Chem. Soc.* **107** (1985), 3401–3406.
84. Prince R.C., *Trends Biochem. Sci.* **13** (1988), 286–288.
85. Heinecke J.W., Li W., Daehnke H. L. and Goldstein J.A., *J. Biol. Chem.* **268** (1993), 4069–4077.
86. Anderson S.O., *Acta. Physiol. Scand.* **66** (1996), 1–81.
87. Joschek H I. and Miller S I., *J. Am. Chem. Soc.* **88** (1966), 3273–3281.
88. Jacob J.S., *et al.*, *J. Biol. Chem.* **271** (1996), 19950–19956.
89. Heinecke J.W., Li W., Francis G.A. and Goldstein J.A., *J. Clin. Inv.* **91** (1993), 2866–2872.
90. Francis G.A., Mendez A.J., Bierman E L. and Heinecke J.W., *Proc. Natl. Acad. Sci.* **90** (1993), 6631–6635.
91. Savenkova M.I., Mueller D.M. and Heinecke J.W., *J. Biol. Chem.* **269** (1994), 20394–20400.
92. Foti M., Ingold K.U. and Lusztyk J. *J. Am. Chem. Soc.* **116** (1994), 9440–9447.
93. Hazen S.L., Hsu F.F. and Heinecke J.W., *J. Biol. Chem.* **271** (1996), 1861–1867.
94. Anderson, M.M., Hazen S.L., Hsu F.F. and Heinecke J.W. (1997) *J. Clin. Invest.* **99**, 424–432.
95. Hazen, S.L., d'Avignon, A., Anderson M.M., Hsu F.F. and Heinecke, J.W. (1997) *J. Biol. Chem.*, In press.
96. Hazen, S.L., Gaut, J.P., Hsu, F.F., Crowley, J.R., d'Avignon, A. and Heinecke, J.W. (1997) *J. Biol. Chem.* **272**, 16990–16998.
97. Baynes J.W., *Diabetes* **40** (1991), 405–412.
98. White G.C., in *Handbook of Chlorination.* (Van Nostrand Reinhold, New York, 1972), 182–227.
99. Hazen S.L., Hsu F.F., Mueller D.M., Crowley J.R. and Heinecke J.W., *J. Clin. Invest.* **98** (1996), 1283–1289.

100. Weiss S.J., Test S.T., Eckmann C.M., Ross D. and Regiani S., *Science* **234** (1986), 200–203.

101. Thomas E.L. and Grisham M.B., *Meth. Enzymol.* **132** (1986), 569–585.

102. Domigan N.M., Charlton T.S., Duncan M.W., Winterbourn C.C. and Kettle A.J., *J. Biol. Chem.* **270** (1995), 16542–16548.

103. Hazen S.L. and Heinecke J.W. *J. Clin. Invest.* **99** (1997), 2075–2081.

104. Sepe S.M. and Clark R.A., *J. Immunol.* **134** (1985), 1896–1901.

105. Van den Berg J.J.M., Winterbourn C.C. and Kuypers F. A., *J. Lipid Res.* **34** (1993), 2005–2012.

106. Heinecke J.W., Li W., Mueller D.M., Bohrer A. and Turk J., *Biochem.* **33** (1994), 10127–10136.

107. Morris J.C., *J. Phys. Chem.* **70** (1966), 3798–3805.

108. Hazen S.L., Hsu F.F., Duffin K. and Heinecke J.W., *J. Biol. Chem.* **271** (1996), 23080–23088.

109. Hazell L.J., van den Berg J.J.M. and Stocker R., *Biochem. J.* **302** (1994), 297–304.

110. Nauseef W.M., *Hematology/Oncology Clinics of North America* **2** (1988), 135–158.

111. Tobler A. and Koeffler H.P., *Blood Cell Biochemistry* Vol. 3; *Lymphocytes and Granulocytes* (1991), 255–288.

112. Hazell L.J., *et al.*, *J. Clin. Inv.* **97** (1996), 1535–1544.

113. Leeuwenburgh C., *et al.*, *J. Biol. Chem.* **272** (1997), 3520–3526.

114. Leeuwenburgh C., *et al.*, *J. Biol. Chem.* **272** (1997), 1433–1436.

CHAPTER 3

MECHANISM OF LEUKOCYTE ACCUMULATION IN POSTISCHEMIC TISSUES: ROLE OF OXYGEN FREE RADICALS

Jay L. Zweier[1]

1. Introduction

While timely reperfusion of ischemic tissues such as the heart can reduce the amount of cell death, there is evidence that reperfusion, can cause further damage to jeopardized cells [1,2]. The generation of reactive oxygen free radicals has been shown to be an important mechanism of this myocardial reperfusion injury [3,4]. Studies demonstrating reduced infarct size and increased functional recovery in hearts treated with antioxidant enzymes have provided indirect evidence of free radical mediated reperfusion injury. In addition electron paramagnetic resonance (EPR) measurements have directly demonstrated a burst of oxygen free radical generation with the generation of superoxide, hydrogen peroxide, and hydroxyl free radicals during the early minutes of reperfusion [5]. In the presence of leukocytes the magnitude and duration of this free radical generation is greatly increased [6].

Postischemic inflammation with influx of polymorphonuclear leukocytes, PMNs, has been demonstrated to be of great importance in the process of

---

[1]Address for correspondence: Dr. Jay L. Zweier, Johns Hopkins University, Division of Cardiology and EPR Center, 5501 Hopkins Bayview Circle, Baltimore, MD 21224. Phone: (410) 550-0339. Fax: (410) 550-2448.

reperfusion injury. It has been suggested that leukocytes mediate reperfusion injury by chemotaxis and activation with the generation of oxygen free radicals and the release of proteolytic enzymes and other toxic products. In addition they also release various inflammatory and chemotactic mediators which can result in a cycle of further cellular chemotaxis and injury [7]. Within reperfused myocardial tissue there is extensive margination of leukocytes as well as capillary plugging of the coronary microvasculature which subsequently leads to extensive myocardial damage [8–10]. Several studies have demonstrated that leukocyte depletion can decrease infarct size [11].

It has been shown that superoxide and hydroxyl radicals are generated in reoxygenated vascular endothelial cells in sufficient concentrations to cause cellular injury and death [12]. There is evidence indicating that this endothelial radical generation promotes both recruitment of PMNs as well as activation and subsequent endothelial cell-PMN adherence [13,14]. An adhesion molecule constitutively expressed on the PMN membrane, the CD18 glycoprotein complex, has been identified as one of the main mediators of PMN adherence to vascular endothelium as it rapidly alters its number or functional state in response to specific stimuli [15,16]. Once activated, PMNs adhere to endothelial cells and then diapedese through the endothelium to the myocardial parenchyma. The PMNs then adhere to myocytes and release free radicals and other pro-inflammatory mediators. These factors amplify reperfusion injury in situ due to the short diffusion distance to the myocyte from the adherent PMN [16].

Studies [17–19] have shown that postischemic myocardial dysfunction and cell death can be attenuated by administration of the antioxidative enzymes, superoxide dismutase, SOD, or catalase. Since SOD and catalase are specific enzymes that function to dismutate $^\bullet O_2{}^-$ to H_2O_2 and to reduce H_2O_2 to H_2O, respectively, these data provide strong evidence that $^\bullet O_2{}^-$ and H_2O_2 play an important role in postischemic heart injury. A number of recent studies also have shown that similar beneficial effects can be seen with specific monoclonal antibodies to the PMN adhesion molecule CD18 [15,20].

An essential initiating step in the process of PMN-mediated injury involves the adhesion of circulating PMNs to the coronary endothelium [20]. This is followed by PMN activation, diapedesis, and extravascular migration into surrounding myocytes. PMNs, once activated, can degranulate secreting numerous potent proteolytic and lipolytic enzymes as well as toxic and vasoactive substances [21]. Moreover, PMN activation causes a respiratory burst, resulting in the production of large additional quantities of the superoxide free radical by the univalent reduction of O_2 by membrane-bound NADPH oxidase [22,23]. These superoxide radicals can then dismutate to form H_2O_2. Hydrogen peroxide, in turn, can be transformed to the powerful oxidant, hypochlorite anion ($HOCl^-$), by the PMN enzyme myeloperoxidase in the presence of chloride ions [23]. A respiratory burst is described in details in previous chapter. Hydrogen peroxide may also interact with redox cyclable iron within the myocardium, resulting in the formation of the highly reactive hydroxyl radical [24].

For PMN-endothelial cell adhesion to occur regulated expression of molecules on both the leukocyte and endothelial cell must occur. The leukocyte adherence glycoproteins are a family of heterodimeric structures consisting of distinct α chains and a common $\beta2$ chain (CD18), and are, in turn, members of the integrin family of adhesion molecules. Following leukocyte activation conformational changes in the $\beta2$ integrins occur along with rapid movement of additional pre-formed molecules to the cell surface. The importance of the adhesion molecule CD18 in PMN adherence to endothelial cells during reperfusion injury has been demonstrated by studies which observed that treatment with a monoclonal antibody against CD18 at the onset of reperfusion inhibits PMN accumulation and prevents PMN-mediated injury [15,20].

While activated PMNs give rise to a marked oxidant burst, questions have remained regarding the central role of oxidants and oxygen free radicals generated by the endothelium in triggering subsequent PMN adhesion and activation. In this chapter recent studies from our laboratory examining the role of oxidants and oxygen free radicals in triggering the process of PMN adhesion and activation in postischemic tissues will be reviewed.

2. Effects of Oxidants and Oxygen Free Radicals on PMN Adhesion Molecule Expression and Functional Adhesion

It has been demonstrated that oxygen-derived free radicals and non-paramagnetic oxidants including: superoxide, $.O_2^-$; and hydrogen peroxide,

H_2O_2, are generated in reoxygenated vascular endothelial cells [12,25,26]. This suggests that the endothelium may be a particularly important site of oxidant generation [25]. A link between the generation of oxidant species and leukocyte recruitment to the reperfusion site has been suggested from the observation that both superoxide dismutase, SOD, and the xanthine oxidase inhibitor, allopurinol, reduce PMN infiltration in ischemic-reperfused tissues [27]. By intravital microscopy it has been demonstrated that the reperfusion-induced leukocyte adherence to the endothelial wall is decreased by various anti-oxidative enzymes or compounds that either scavenge or prevent the formation of free radicals and other oxidants [14,28]. Therefore it is important to determine the effect of oxidant molecules and oxygen free radicals including: $.O_2^-$, and H_2O_2 on the expression of integrin and selectin adhesion molecules on the surface of PMNs and to determine the functional effect of these alterations on PMN adhesion to the endothelium.

Flow cytometry experiments on PMNs exposed to H_2O_2 demonstrate, up-regulation of the adhesion molecules CD18 and CD11b with a clear shift to the right seen in the flow cytometry histograms from these cells. Down-regulation of L-selectin is seen in these cells with a marked shift to the left in the histogram (Figure 3.1). Increasing concentrations of H_2O_2 resulted in a concentration dependent increase in CD11b and CD18 on the surface of PMNs, while the expression of L-selectin is decreased (Figure 3.2). When compared to control, the lowest dose tested (0.1 mM) demonstrated small but statistically significant changes in CD18 ($6.2 \pm 3.6\%$) and L-selectin expression ($12.0 \pm 2.6\%$). For CD11b expression, the threshold dose for a significant effect was 0.5 mM. At the highest dose tested (10 mM), H_2O_2 completely abolished L-selectin expression (0.19 ± 0.07), while CD18 and CD11b expressions were increased by 73.1 ± 11.8 and 60.8 ± 18.1, respectively.

To determine if the superoxide free radical also induces changes in PMN adhesion molecule expression, experiments were performed exposing PMNs to a specific superoxide generating system consisting of xanthine and xanthine oxidase in the presence of catalase and deferoxamine. EPR experiments in the presence of the spin trap DMPO, 50 mM, showed that PMNs alone did not give rise to significant radical generation, while in the presence of xanthine and xanthine oxidase a prominent signal was observed. This signal was primarily due to the DMPO-OOH adduct of trapped superoxide with hyperfine

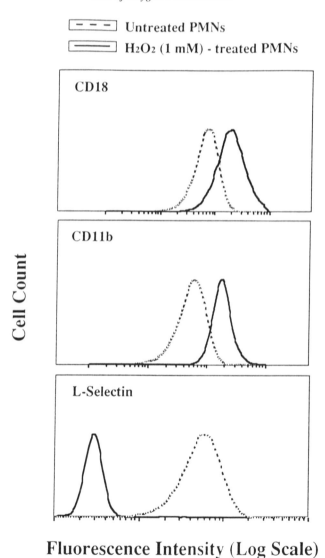

Figure 3.1. Flow cytometry histograms from PMNs, stimulated for 30 min with 1.0 mM H_2O_2, or from untreated PMNs. On the top panel, upregulation of CD18 is seen in H_2O_2 treated PMNs with a rightward shift of the fluorescence intensity histogram. On the center panel, a similar response is seen for CD11b surface expression. On the lower panel, a down-regulation of L-selectin expression is noted.

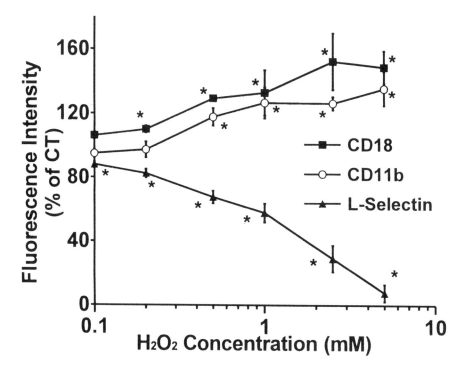

Figure 3.2.   Effect of varying concentrations of H2O2 on PMN adhesion molecule expression. Values are expressed in % of mode fluorescence intensity of control (CT), untreated PMNs. Data are plotted as mean ± SEM of 6 experiments and are compared by two-way analysis of variance. *P < 0.05: untreated versus treated PMNs.

couplings aN = 14.2 G aH = 11.4 G aHí = 1.2 G. SOD, 100 U/ml, totally quenched this radical generation (Figure 3.3). After exposure to this superoxide generating system, clear upregulation of CD11b and CD18 was observed with a loss of L-selectin (Figure 3.4). These effects were dose dependent as shown by experiments in which the concentration of xanthine was varied. In matched control experiments performed exposing PMNs to this superoxide generating system in the presence of SOD, 100 U/ml, these effects were abolished and no significant change in CD18, CD11b, or L-selectin expression from basal levels was seen. Thus, the observed alterations in adhesion molecule expression were due to superoxide.

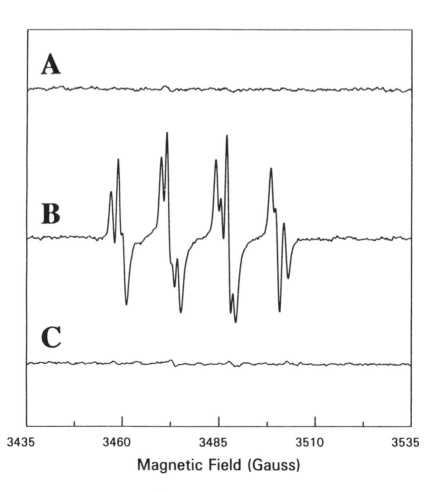

Figure 3.3.   EPR spectra of 1×10^6 PMNs/ml in the presence of 50 mM DMPO. A, PMNs in the presence of DMPO alone. B, with addition of xanthine oxidase 40 mU/ml and xanthine 0.4 mM, C, as in B but with the addition of 200 U/ml of superoxide dismutase. Each spectrum consists of the sum of 4, 1 min acquisitions. In the presence of DMPO alone no radical generation is seen while in the presence of xanthine oxidase and xanthine a prominent signal is seen consisting largely of the DMPO-OH adduct, DMPO-OOH, with a small component of DMPO-OH.

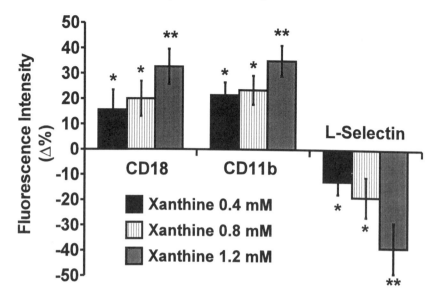

Figure 3.4.   Effect of superoxide on PMN adhesion molecule expression. PMNs were exposed to varying magnitude of superoxide generation by varying the concentration of the substrate xanthine. CD18, CD11b, and L-selectin surface expression responded to superoxide stimulation in a dose-dependent manner. Values are expressed in percent changes of mode fluorescence intensity of control, untreated PMNs. Data are plotted as mean ± SEM of 4 experiments and are compared by Student's T-test. P* < 0.05, ** < 0.01: untreated versus treated PMNs.

In order to determine if oxidant mediated alterations in PMN adhesion molecule expression were sufficient to influence the functional adhesion of these cells, endothelial adhesion assays were performed and the ability of H_2O_2 to alter the adhesiveness of PMNs to vascular endothelium was tested. Untreated and H_2O_2-treated, PMNs were washed and added to monolayers of human aortic endothelial cells, HAECs, for a static adhesion assay. Pretreatment with 5 mM H_2O_2 resulted in a 76.4 ± 3.3% increase in adherence (P < 0.0001 vs control) (Figure 3.5).

Treatment of PMNs with the known activator C5a (500 ng/ml) prior to the adhesion assay, induced a similar 84.4 ± 7.6% increase in the number of PMNs binding to unstimulated HAECs as that seen with H_2O_2 (P < 0.0001 vs control). In the presence of the monoclonal antibody R15.7 (20 μg/ml), the increase in

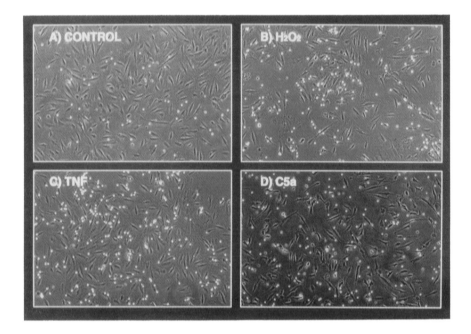

Figure 3.5. Photomicrographs of PMN-endothelial adhesion assays. Unstimulated PMNs and unstimulated monolayers of human aortic endothelial cells (CONTROL), hydrogen peroxide (5.0 mM)-stimulated PMNs and unstimulated endothelial cells (H_2O_2), complement 5a (500 ng/ml)-stimulated PMNs and unstimulated endothelial cells (C5a), and tumor necrosis factor-α (10 ng/ml)-stimulated endothelial cells and unstimulated PMNs (TNFα). When the PMNs were stimulated with H_2O_2, a marked increase in the number of adherent PMNs occured compared to unstimulated PMNs. This increase in PMN adhesion is similar to that observed with the PMN activator C5a or when the endothelial cells were stimulated with TNFα.

PMN adhesion seen with either H_2O_2 or C5a treated cells was totally blocked. When the endothelial monolayers were pre-incubated with TNFα (10 ng/ml), which stimulates the expression of endothelial adhesion molecules including ICAM-1, H_2O_2 further increased PMN adhesion to cultured endothelial cells from 379.5 ± 54.3 to $647.6 \pm 20.5\%$ of basal values ($P < 0.05$).

In view of the relatively high concentrations of H_2O_2 required to produce upregulation of Mac-1 expression, the physiological relevance of the effect might be questioned. High local concentrations of H_2O_2, however, may be generated at the site of reoxygenated endothelium or by activated granulocytes [12,23,25]. In addition, the effect of a given concentration of H_2O_2 may be further potentiated by the presence of other oxidants and oxygen free radicals that are also generated. We observed that superoxide generated from xanthine and xanthine oxidase also exhibited similar effects with clear dose dependent upregulation of CD18 and CD11b observed. The concentrations of xanthine and xanthine oxidase utilized to generate superoxide in these experiments were on the same order of magnitude as those which have been shown to occur in the ischemic rat heart [29]. Therefore, the H_2O_2 and superoxide dependent effects observed in these invitro studies could also occur within postischemic cells and tissues. In addition to being triggered by endothelial derived radical generation, these changes could be further triggered by the high levels of levels of oxidants which can be generated by the NADPH oxidase of the PMN itself after PMN activation by other chemotactic factors. This phenomenon may represent a feedback amplification loop where by activated PMNs further trigger recruitment, adhesion, and activation of other PMNs, that would in turn result in further oxidant formation.

Thus, oxidants and oxygen-derived free radicals can directly modulate the expression of the adhesion molecules CD11b, CD18, and L-selectin on the surface of human PMNs. These changes are accompanied by increased adhesion to resting and cytokine-stimulated human endothelial cells. This phenomenon could have a pathophysiologic role in the injury that occurs in reperfused tissues, where an endothelial derived oxidant burst is followed by leukocyte chemotaxis and activation [30]. It could also be of great importance in a variety of other inflammatory disease processes in which initial leukocyte activation occurs resulting in oxidant formation which could in turn trigger further leukocyte chemotaxis, adhesion, and activation.

3. Effects of Oxidants and Oxygen Free Radicals on CD18 Mediated PMN Adhesion in the Postischemic Heart

A burst of endothelial derived oxidants including hydrogen peroxide (H_2O_2) and superoxide ($^\bullet O_2^-$) occurs on reperfusion of ischemic tissues that directly causes injury; however, it was unknown if this also triggers further injury due to subsequent leukocyte adhesion and adhesion molecule expression. To address this question, we performed studies in an isolated heart model developed to enable study of the role of isolated cellular and humoral factors in the mechanism of postischemic injury. Isolated rat hearts were subjected to 20 min of 37°C-global ischemia followed by reperfusion with polymorphonuclear leukocytes (PMNs) and plasma in the presence or absence of superoxide dismutase (SOD), 200 U/ml, or catalase, 500 U/ml. Measurements of contractile function, coronary flow, high-energy phosphates, free radical generation, and PMN accumulation were performed.

After equilibration, baseline left ventricular pressures, coronary flow, and heart rate were measured. Hearts were then subjected to a 1-min preischemic control infusion of PMNs (0.5 million PMNs per ml of perfusate, 10 million total) and rat plasma (5% volume with respect to perfusate), to verify that the human PMNs and rat plasma did not cause injury before ischemia. Re-equilibration with perfusate alone was then performed for 5 min. Subsequently, the hearts were similarly infused with PMNs and plasma during the 30-sec just prior to the onset of ischemia. At the onset of ischemia, the intraventricular balloon was deflated, and after the 20 min period of ischemia, at the time of reperfusion it was reinflated with the same volume. During the first 5 min of reperfusion, the hearts were again subjected to infusion of PMNs (50×10^6) and plasma (5% volume), after which reperfusion was continued with perfusate alone for 40 min.

To evaluate the role of superoxide and hydrogen peroxide on PMN-mediated contractile dysfunction in this model, three experimental groups were studied: an untreated group of 12 hearts, an SOD treated group of 7 hearts treated with 200 units/ml dissolved in plasma and a catalase treated group consisting of 7 hearts treated, 500 units/ml dissolved in plasma. Plasma with or without the SOD or catalase was infused during the 30-sec preischemic and 5 min reperfusion periods. The coronary effluent was collected during each PMN infusion to estimate PMN retention and CD18 expression.

Preischemic baseline values of developed pressure did not differ significantly among the three groups of hearts studied (111.7 ± 7.8 mmHg). After 15 min of reperfusion, untreated hearts recovered only $25.4 \pm 8.2\%$ of baseline developed pressure, increasing gradually to $31.3 \pm 10.0\%$ of baseline at 45 min of reperfusion (Figure 3.6A). SOD-treated hearts recovered $80.7 \pm 3.0\%$ of baseline developed pressure at 15 min and $96.1 \pm 3.0\%$ of baseline at 45 min (P < 0.01). Likewise, catalase-treated hearts recovered 83.3(9.7% of baseline developed pressure after 15 min and $88.3 \pm 7.5\%$ after 45 min of reperfusion (P < 0.01 versus untreated hearts and P = not significant, NS, versus SOD-treated hearts). Thus, both SOD-treated and catalase-treated hearts exhibited a much greater recovery of left ventricular developed pressure than untreated controls.

Untreated, SOD-treated, and catalase-treated hearts had similar end-diastolic pressures during the equilibration period, with values of 13.3 ± 1.5, 11.7 ± 1.8, and 12.9 ± 0.6 mmHg, respectively (Figure 3.6B). However, after reperfusion, higher end-diastolic pressures were observed in all three groups indicating impaired diastolic relaxation. After 15 min of reperfusion, end-diastolic pressures then declined slowly. The untreated and treated hearts exhibited clearly different values: 80.6 ± 8.0 (untreated hearts), 12.6 ± 3.1 (SOD-treated hearts), and 20.0 ± 4.9 (catalase-treated hearts) mmHg. Final end-diastolic pressures were 77.7 ± 7.8 mmHg for untreated hearts, 9.7 ± 3.3 mmHg for SOD-treated hearts (P < 0.01 versus untreated hearts), and 13.4 ± 3.8 mmHg for catalase-treated hearts (P < 0.01 versus untreated hearts and P = NS versus SOD-treated hearts). Thus, in the SOD- or catalase-treated hearts diastolic relaxation returned to normal with end-diastolic pressure returning to baseline values, while in the untreated hearts left ventricular end-diastolic pressure remained considerably elevated.

Mean coronary flows measured before the onset of global ischemia for the untreated, SOD-treated, and catalase-treated hearts were 19.9 ± 2.3, 20.0 ± 1.5, and 18.9 ± 0.5 ml/min, respectively. After 15 min of reperfusion, the coronary flows recovered $28.7 \pm 10.7\%$ for the untreated hearts, $92.7 \pm 7.2\%$ for the SOD-treated hearts, and $80.6 \pm 9.3\%$ for the catalase-treated hearts (Figure 3.6C). The final recoveries were $32.3 \pm 8.7\%$ for untreated hearts, $82.9 \pm 4.5\%$ for SOD-treated hearts (P < 0.01 versus untreated hearts), and $74.6 \pm 5.4\%$ for catalase-treated hearts (P < 0.03 versus untreated hearts and P = NS versus SOD-treated hearts). Thus, coronary flow also exhibited much greater recovery in the SOD- or catalase-treated hearts.

To determine whether PMN retention was effected by treating the hearts with SOD and catalase during ischemia and reperfusion, and thus to infer,

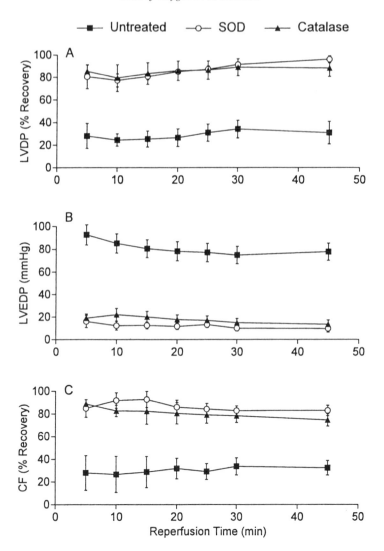

Figure 3.6. Graphs of the recovery of hemodynamic function upon reperfusion after 20 min global ischemia. A, left ventricular developed pressure; B, left ventricular end-diastolic pressure; and C, coronary flow. For A and C, values are expressed as percent of preschemic values. Data are plotted as mean ± SEM. Recovery of all parameters was markedly improved, both by SOD or catalase treatments, compared to untreated hearts.

whether this PMN retention might be influenced by the generation of $\cdot O_2^-$ or H_2O_2 within the heart, measurements of PMN retention were performed. PMN retention was calculated as the differential count between the amount of PMNs infused in the 1-min preischemic, 30-sec preischemic, and 5-min reperfusion periods and the total number of PMNs collected in the respective coronary effluents. The quantity of PMNs retained under preischemic conditions did not differ significantly between the untreated and treated hearts (Figure 3.7). However, SOD and catalase did decrease PMN retention during the first 5 min of reperfusion when compared to untreated hearts: $41.4 \pm 9.9\%$ for untreated hearts versus $25.4 \pm 6.7\%$ for SOD-treated hearts (P < 0.02) and $7.4 \pm 2.1\%$ for catalase-treated hearts (P < 0.01). Thus, SOD significantly decreased the retention of PMNs within the myocardium with almost a two-fold reduction while catalase markedly decreased PMN retention by almost six-fold.

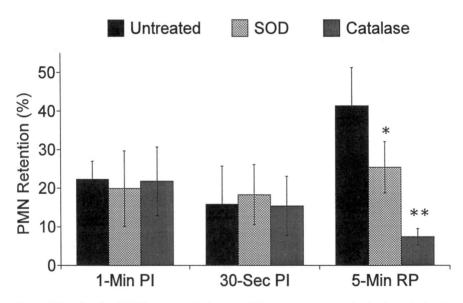

Figure 3.7.   Graph of PMN retention in the heart. Values shown are for the 1-min preischemic (1-min PI), the 30-sec infusion just prior to ischemia (30-sec PI), and the 5-min postischemic infusion (5-min RP). Data expressed as percentage of PMNs infused, are plotted as mean ± SEM, and are statistically analyzed by two-way analysis of variance. SOD (*P < 0.01) and catalase (**P < 0.02) significantly attenuated PMN retention during the first 5 min of reperfusion compared to untreated hearts.

Initial studies using flow cytometric techniques were performed to establish the basal PMN surface expression of CD18 in each group. Aliquots of freshly prepared PMNs were evaluated for CD18 expression before infusion. The PMNs used in the untreated, SOD-treated, and catalase-treated hearts were observed to have similar basal CD18 expression with mode fluorescence intensity of 65.6 ± 10.8, 73.8 ± 12.4, and 62.3 ± 11.3, respectively (Figure 3.8). CD18 expression of PMNs collected in the coronary effluent of the 1-min preischemic infusion also did not show significant differences among untreated, SOD-treated, and catalase-treated hearts with mode fluorescence intensity values of 70.1 ± 3.4, 83.5 ± 14.8, and 66.6 ± 15.6, respectively. Similar findings were observed for the 30-sec preischemic infusion: 71.3 ± 13.8, 85.6 ± 14.9, and 65.8 ± 9.8 for untreated, SOD-treated, and catalase-treated hearts, respectively. Thus, it was observed that PMN CD18 expression was not altered upon traversing the circulation of the preischemic heart. Measurements of the PMNs infused and collected during the 5-min postischemic infusion, however, demonstrated in untreated hearts that there was a marked increase in CD18 expression, with a value of 193.4 ± 3.9 ($P < 0.02$ versus respective 1-min preischemic CD18 expression). With the administration of SOD, CD18 expression was limited to 100.3 ± 6.2 ($P = NS$ versus respective 1-min preischemic CD18 expression and $P < 0.05$ versus untreated hearts) and with catalase, to 73.9 ± 5.5 ($P = NS$ versus respective 1-min preischemic CD18 expression, $P < 0.02$ versus untreated hearts, and $P = NS$ versus SOD-treated hearts) (Figure 3.8).

Histological experiments were performed to measure the presence and localization of PMNs within hearts from each of the three groups. In untreated hearts numerous PMNs were observed within myocardial arterioles, capillaries, and interstitial spaces that were associated with disrupted myofibrillar structure. While in the SOD- or catalase-treated hearts few PMNs were seen and myofibrillar structure appeared preserved. Thus, it was observed that either SOD or catalase treatment prevented the adhesion of PMNs to the endothelium of the microcirculatory vessels of the heart and this was associated with less myocyte injury.

These results demonstrate that superoxide and hydrogen peroxide are important mediators of the leukocyte-endothelial cell interactions observed

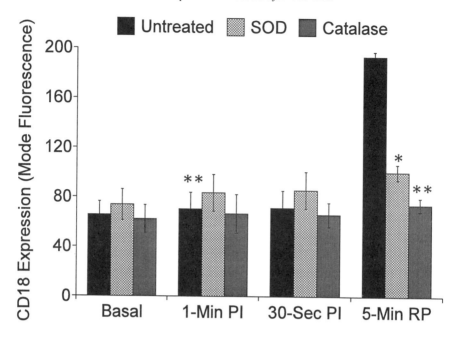

Figure 3.8.   Graph of the levels of PMN CD18 expression. Measured by fluorescence flow cytometry on basal PMNs and on PMNs collected from the 1-min preischemic (PI), 30-sec preischemic, and 5-min reperfusion (RP) infusions. Values expressed in mode fluorescence intensity, are plotted as mean ± SEM, and are compared by two-way analysis of variance. For untreated and treated hearts, CD18 surface expression on the PMNs collected after the 1-min and 30-sec preischemic infusions were similar to basal expressions. A marked upregulation of PMN CD18 expression occurred in the untreated hearts compared to 1-min preischemic values, **$P < 0.02$. This effect was decreased by either SOD or catalase treatment. *$P < 0.05$; **$P < 0.02$.

after reperfusion of the ischemic heart. In addition to triggering the upregulation of CD18 there are several other mechanisms by which $^{\bullet}O_2^-$ and $^{\bullet}O_2$ — derived radicals might trigger reperfusion-induced leukocyte adherence. It has been demonstrated that $^{\bullet}O_2^-$ reacts with the endothelial cell to produce and release humoral mediators, including leukotriene B4 and platelet activating factor, which in turn, then activate and promote the adherence of leukocytes [31]. Superoxide may also induce the formation and expression of endothelial adhesion molecules such as P-selectin or ICAM-1 [14]. Another possible mechanism by which $^{\bullet}O_2^-$ might further promote PMN adhesion is by inactivation of nitric oxide, an endothelial derived vasodilator which interferes with PMN adherence to microvascular endothelium [32].

Thus, in addition to their direct antioxidant effects, SOD and catalase can prevent PMN adhesion molecule expression, PMN accumulation, and PMN-mediated reperfusion injury. These data suggest that endothelial derived oxidants, including superoxide and hydrogen peroxide, are involved in triggering PMN adhesion and PMN-mediated injury in the postischemic heart.

4. Conclusion

The production of reactive oxidants and the recruitment of leukocytes are important mechanisms in the pathophysiology of a variety of inflammatory disease processes including the injury that occurs on reperfusion of postischemic tissues. As described above tissue-derived oxidants can increase the adhesiveness of circulating leukocytes in turn leading to PMN mediated injury [33,34]. Possible mechanisms for this oxidant-mediated adherence include: direct effects on the adhesive properties of the vascular endothelium; induction of inflammatory factors capable of activating PMNs; and direct effects on the adhesive properties of the PMNs [33]. It was observed that oxidants and oxygen free radicals can directly trigger increased CD18 and CD11b expression with L-selectin shedding on the surface of PMNs which in turn leads to PMN-endothelial adhesion. In the postischemic heart, it was shown that oxidants and oxygen free radicals trigger increased adhesion molecule expression on the surface of PMNs within the coronary circulation leading to PMN adhesion and PMN mediated reperfusion injury [34]. Thus, oxidants and oxygen free radicals have a central role in triggering the process of PMN mediated reperfusion injury.

5. References

1. Kloner, R.A., Ellis, S.G., Lange, R., and Braunwald, E., *Circulation* 68(suppl I) (1983), I8–I15.
2. DeWood, M.A., *et al.*, *Circulation* 68(suppl II) (1983), II8–II16.

3. Jolly, S.R., *et al.*, (1984) *Circ. Res.* **54** (1984), 277–285.

4. Manning, A.S., Flamigni, F., and Caldarera, C.M., *J. Mol. Cell. Cardiol.* **12** (1980), 797–781.

5. Zweier, J.L., *J. Biol. Chem.* **263** (1988), 1353–1357.

6. Shandelya, S.M.L., Kuppusamy, P., Weisfeldt, M.L., and Zweier, J.L., Circulation. **87** (1993), 536–546.

7. Rowe, G.T., Eaton, L.R., and Hess, M.L., *J. Mol. Cell. Cardiology* **16** (1984), 1075–1079.

8. Engler, R.L., Schmid-Schonbein G.W., and Pavalel, R.S., *Am. J. Pathology* **111** (1983), 98–111.

9. Engler, R, *Federation Proc* **46** (1978) 2407–2412.

10. Metha, J.L., Nichols W.W., Donnelly W.H., *et al.*, *Circulation Res* **65** (1989), 1283–1295.

11. Ramson, J.L., *et al.*, *Circulation Res* **67** (1983), 1016–1023.

12. Zweier, J.L., Kuppusamy, P., and Lutty, G.A., *Proc. Natl. Acad. Sci. USA.* **85** (1988), 4046–4050.

13. Petrone, W.F., English, D.K., Wong, K., and McCord, J.M., *Proc. Natl. Acad. Sci. USA.* **77** (1980), 1159–1163.

14. Suzuki, M., *et al.*, *Am. J. Physiol.* **257** (1989), H1740–H1745.

15. Ma, X., Tsao, P.S., and Lefer, A.M., *J. Clin. Invest.* **88** (1991), 1237–1243.

16. Entman, M.L., *et al.*, *J. Clin. Invest.* **90** (1992), 1335–1345.

17. Ambrosio G., *et al.*, *Circulation* 74 (1986), 1424–1433.

18. Gross, G.J., Farber, N.E., Hardman, H.F., and Warltier, D.C., *Am. J. Physiol.* **250** (1986), H372–H377.

19. Ambrosio, G., Weisfeldt, M.L., Jacobus, W.E., and Flaherty, J.T., *Circulation* **75** (1987), 282–291.

20. Lefer, D.J., Shandelya, S.M.L., Serrano Jr., C.V., Becker, L.C., Kuppusamy, P., and Zweier, J.L., *Circulation* **88** (1993), 1779–1787.

21. Smedley, L.A., *et al.*, *J. Clin. Invest.* **77** (1986), 1233–1243.

22. Babior, B.M., and Peters, W.A., *J. Biol. Chem.* **265** (1981), 2321–2326.

23. Klebanoff, S.J., Inflammation: Basic Principles and Clinical Correlates (Raven, New York, 1988).

24. Josephson, R.A., Silverman, H.S., Lakatta, E.G., Stern, M.D., and Zweier, J.L., *J. Biol. Chem.* **266** (1991), 2354–2361.

25. Zweier, J.L., Broderick, R., Kuppusamy, P., Thompson-Gorman, S., Lutty, G.A., (1994) *J. Biol. Chem.* **269** (1994), 24156–24162.

26. Ratych, R.E., Chuknyiska, R.S., and Bulkley, G.B., *Surgery* **102** (1987), 122–131.

27. Grisham, M.B., Hernandez, L.A., and Granger, D.N., *Am. J. Physiol.* **251** (1986), 567–574.
28. Granger, N.D. Benoit, J.N., Suzuki, M., and Grisham, M.B., *Am. J. Physiol.* **257** (1989), G683–689.
29. Thompson-Gorman, S.L., and Zweier, J.L., J. *Biol. Chem.* **265** (1990), 6656–6663.
30. Shandelya, S., Kuppusamy, P., and Zweier, J.L., *Circulation* **87** (1993), 536–546.
31. Patel, K.D., Zimmerman, G.A., Prescott, S.M., McIntyre, T.M., *J. Biol. Chem.* **266** (1991), 11104–11110.
32. Kubes, P., Suzuki, M., and Granger, D.N., *Proc. Natl. Acad. Sci. USA.* **88** (1991), 4651–4655.
33. Fraticelli, A., Serrano, C.V., Bochner, B.S., Capogrossi, M.C., and Zweier, J.L., *Biochem. Biophys. Acta* **1310** (1996), 251–259.
34. Serrano, C.V., Mikhail E.A., Wang P., Noble B, Kuppusamy P., Zweier, J.L., *Biochem. Biophys. Acta* **1316** (1996), 191–202.

CHAPTER 4

REGULATION OF NEUTROPHIL FUNCTIONS BY FATTY ACIDS

Antonio Ferrante[1], Charles S.T.Hii, Zhi H.Huang, and
Deborah A Rathjen

1. Introduction

Neutrophils play an important role in protecting against early invasion of tissues by bacteria and other pathogens. Experiments of nature are informative in this manner. Babies born with hereditary forms of neutropenia can die within a few days unless treated with antibiotics. In contrast a drastic reduction and dysfunction in T lymphocytes and B lymphocytes does not pose the same level of risk. Even where there are specific defects of the neutrophil functions, eg. in chronic granulomatous disease where there is an absence in ability to generate oxygen radicals, life threatening infections occur.

There are several key neutrophil functions which co-operate to contain and digest the invading microorganism. Marginated neutrophils transiently bind to the endothelium at sites close to the infection, they then roll and undergo transendothelial migration under the influence of a chemotactic gradient and accumulate at these sites of infection. Neutrophils then take on the active role of adhering to bacteria, phagocytosing the microrganism and releasing oxygen derived species and lysosomal enzymes to kill and digest the bacteria. Besides

---

[1]Address for correspondence Antonio Ferrante, Dept. Of Immunopathology, The Women's and Children's Hospital and the University of Adelaide, 72, King William Road, North Adelaide, SA 5006, Australia. Tel: 08-8204-6637; Fax: 08-8204-6046; aferrant@medicine.adelaide.edu.au

from this well-recognised beneficial effect, the cell is also known to be involved in causing serious damage to tissues when inflammation persists.

Besides their role in acute inflammations, recent evidence highlights the neutrophil as playing a significant role in chronic inflammation. This is particularly evident in rheumatoid arthritis where neutrophils become prominent during the exacerbated episodes of the disease. In addition they may influence the establishment of a chronic inflammatory response (cell-mediated immunity and resistance to intracellular parasites). Thus the cell may influence macrophage and T lymphocyte responses, through the release of mediators such as cytokines. Many of these cytokines act through stimulation of the activity of phospholipase A_2 and the release of AA (Fig. 4.1). Laboratory investigations of the regulation of these key functions of the neutrophil has enabled us to learn more about the role of biological mediators which form networks to regulate leukocyte accumulation in the inflammatory reaction. Amongst these mediators are polyunsaturated fatty acids (PUFA). Recent evidence has shown that polyunsaturated fatty acids such as arachidonic acid (AA, 20:4*n-6*) influence the process of neutrophil adhesion, chemotaxis, functional cell surface receptor expression, respiratory burst, degranulation and microbial killing. From a mechanistic perspective, mediators may act to not only induce each other's activity, but act synergistically on neutrophils to maximise responses.

Fatty acids are characterised by an alkyl chain and carboxyl group with the basic formula shown below:

$$CH_3—(CH_2)_n—COOH$$

The degree of unsaturation in the molecule is determined by the number of double bonds in the fatty acid backbone. Normally the double bonds are in a *cis* configuration and separated by a methylene group ($—CH_2—$). The position of the double bonds are numbered from the carboxyl group, with the carboxyl carbon atom as carbon 1. The *n-3* Polyunsaturated fatty acids have their first double bond between the 3rd and 4th carbon atom counting from the ω or methyl end of the chain, while the *n-6* Polyunsaturated fatty acids have their first double bond between the 6th and 7th carbon atom respectively. According to the number of carbon atoms in the fatty acid backbone, the fatty acids are

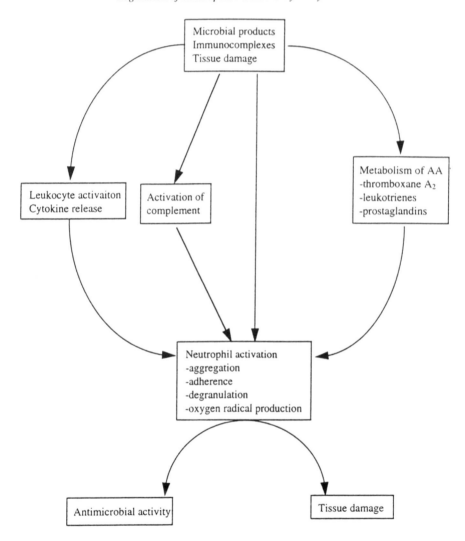

Figure 4.1.   A schematic and simplified representation of some of the inflammatory mediator network operating during an infection or autoimmune inflammation involving the neutrophil. Neutrophils become stimulated by both exogenously and endogenously generated mediators which include fatty acids (AA) and their metabolic products. These mediators attract neutrophil to sites of infection or tissue damage and stimulate their antimicrobial and tissue damaging properties.

divided into short chain (<6 carbon atoms), medium chain (6–12 carbon atoms), long chain (14–22 carbon atoms) and very long chain (>22 carbon atoms) fatty acids. The approved abbreviation of fatty acids involves firstly "the number of carbon atoms" followed by "the number of double bonds and the series number", eg. 20:4n-6 refers to a 20 carbon fatty acid with 4 double bonds of the n-6 series.

2. Sources of Arachidonic Acid and Other Fatty Acids

Fatty acids in the body can be obtained through *de novo* synthesis in tissues, through the diet or from the hydrolysis of membrane phospholipids Fig. 4.2).

2.1 *De novo synthesis*

Human beings can synthesize fatty acids up to 16:0 (palmitate) *de novo* from acetyl coenzyme A by a series of cycles of sequential condensation, reduction, dehydration and reduction. The chain is elongated by two carbon atoms per cycle. 16:0 is then elongated to 18:0 (stearate) and desaturated to yield 18:1n-9 (oleate). Alternatively, 16:0 is desaturated to 16:1n-9 (palmitoleate) and elongated to 18:1n-9. A variety of longer chain fatty acids can be derived from 18:1n-9 by a combination of elongation and desaturation reactions. However, mammalian cells are unable to perform these reactions because they do not express the enzymes, Δ12 and Δ15 desaturases to introduce double bonds at carbon atoms beyond C-9. Consequently, mammaliam cells cannot synthesise 18:2n-6 (linoleate) and 18:3n-3 (linolenate). These fatty acids, required by the animal but cannot be synthesised endogenously, are therefore considered as essential fatty acids and are obtained from the diet (Fig. 4.2). The essential fatty acids serve as starting points for the synthesis of longer chain fatty acids such as 20:4n-6.and the n-3 fatty acids 20:5n-3 (eicosapentaenoic acid, EPA) and 22:6n-3 (docosahexaenoic acid, DHA) by elongation and desaturation through the action of elongases and desaturases (e.g Δ6, Δ5 and Δ4). AA is derived from 18:2n-6 while EPA and DHA are derived from 18:3n-3.

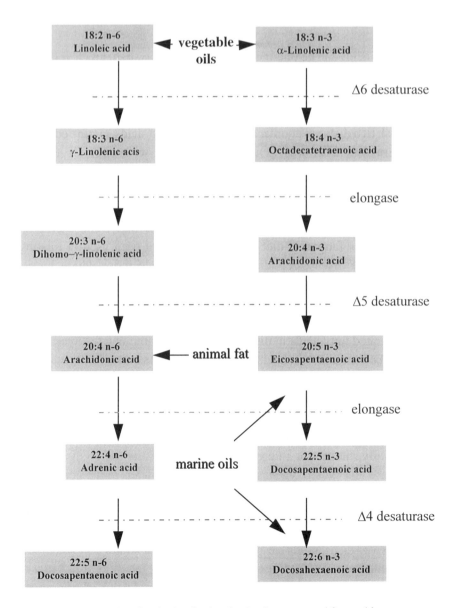

Figure 4.2.   Synthesis of *n*-6 and *n*-3 polyunsaturated fatty acids.

2.2 *Diet*

Dietary fatty acids can be obtained from animal meats, fish, green vegetables, and from oils derived from the above. They mainly occur as triacylglycerols. Essential fatty acids are found in abundance in green leafy vegetables and the seeds of most plants. The *n-3* fatty acids EPA and DHA are abundant in marine oils and fish rich diets are another source of these fatty acids. Grain-fed animals are rich in AA (Fig. 4.2) (1). Diets enriched with specific types of polyunsaturated fatty acids have been of interest because of their potential usefulness in treating a range of human diseases and conditions. In particular, it is well appreciated that increasing the ratio of *n-3* over *n-6* Polyunsaturated fatty acids in membrane phospholipids has some beneficial therapeutic effects (1). Thus fatty acid diet manipulations have been used in treating a wide variety of diseases/conditions. These include those which have an autoimmune and allergic base. While the mechanisms governing the beneficial effects of certain types of polyunsaturated fatty acids in different types of diseases is likely to vary, it is well appreciated that altering the types of polyunsaturated fatty acids in diets can modify the immune response. This is thought to be the major mechanism by which polyunsaturated fatty acids exert their protective effects in inflammatory and autoimmune disorders.

Some polyunsaturated fatty acids, such as AA, are an integral component of membrane phospholipids. Cell stimulation leads to the activation of phospholipase A_2 (PLA_2) and the release of AA from phospholipids (Fig. 4.3).

Classically, the major interest in AA has been its metabolism via the lipoxygenase and cyclooxygenase pathways which leads to the generation of some highly active eicosanoids and prostagnoids (Fig. 4.4). The ability of the lipoxygenase and cyclooxygenase systems to also generate fatty acid metabolites with substantially lower proinflammatory activity (<1000) than the AA-derived eicosanoids has provided the basis for strategies to manipulate the inflammatory reaction. For example, increasing the ratio of *n-3* to *n-6* in membrane phospholipids of leukocytes reduces the production of inflammatory eicosanoids in favour of metabolites with markedly reduced or those which lack proinflammatory activity. Thus diets which contain high levels of the *n-3* fatty acids, EPA and/or DHA as well as those which contain high levels of

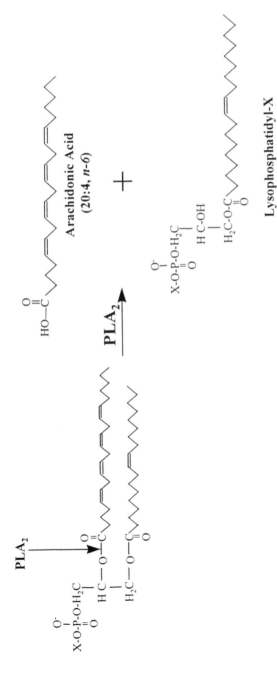

Figure 4.3. Stimulation of leukocytes and other cell types by a variety of mediators leads to activation of PLA$_2$. This enzyme liberates the fatty acid which is esterified at the sn-2 position of membrane phospholipids such as phosphatidylcholine (PC), phosphatidylethanolamine (PE), phosphatidylinositol (PI) and phosphatidylserine (PS) (The head groups are represented by X). 20:4n-6 is predominantly esterified at the sn-2 position of alkyl-PC and PI.

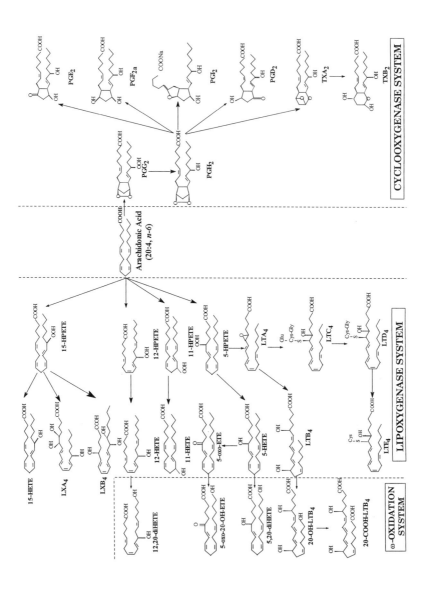

Figure 4.4.   The metabolism of AA via the lipoxygenase and cyclooxygenase systems is shown. Many of the lipoxygenase products are also metabolised by w-oxidation by the cytochrome P450 enzyme system. Abbreviations used HPETE, hydroperoxyeicosatetraenoic acid; HETE, hydroxyeicosatraenoic acid: LT, leukotriene; PG, prostaglandin; LX, lipoxin: TX, thromboxane.

their precursors have been used as ways of decreasing inflammatory reactions and relieving the symptoms of these diseases (1). (Fig. 4.4)

Clinical studies have shown that *n-3* fatty acids have beneficial effects in autoimmune and inflammatory diseases, such as ulcerative colitis, gingivitis, psoriasis, rheumatoid arthritis, systemic lupus erythematosus and asthma. A high *n-3* fatty acid intake for four months significantly increased the general score and sigmoidoscope score of active ulcerative colitis patients compared with a placebo diet (1,2). The effects were maintained for three months after the fatty acid treatment was discontinued. In a human gingival inflammation model, 28-day treatment with EPA and DHA (1.8 g/day) markedly reduced the gingival index in interdental papilla (3). Dietary supplementation with fish oil fatty acids rich in EPA and DHA in conjunction with conventional treatment (cyclosporin) in psoriasis patients has been shown to improve the skin lesions and decrease the nephrotoxicity of cyclosporin (1). In the treatment of rheumatoid arthritis, the beneficial effects of fish oil are pronounced and reproducible in both animal models and in human trials. It has been shown that feeding mice with *n-3* polyunsaturated fatty acids, EPA and DHA, reduces the incidence and severity of type II collagen-induced experimental arthritis (4). Dietary supplementation with *n-3* polyunsaturated fatty acids in rheumatoid arthritis patients shows significant relief of joint pain and swelling, duration of morning stiffness and has led to a reduction in requirement for nonsteroidal anti-inflammatory drugs (NSAIDs). Some patients were able to discontinue NSAIDs while receiving *n-3* PUFA treatment (5,6). A recent clinical study of γ-linolenic acid (GLA, $18:3n\text{-}6$) dietary manipulation in patients with rheumatoid arthritis also showed evidence of alleviation of disease severity (7).

Dietary supplementation of *n-3* Polyunsaturated fatty acids also decreases the symptoms of dysmenorrhoea, a prostaglandin-mediated condition in adolescents. After a two month treatment with fish oil, a significant reduction in the Cox Menstrual Symptom Scale was found compared with a placebo diet. This could be due to alteration of the prostanoid profile by the high *n-3* fatty acid intake (8,9). Essential fatty acids play an important role in brain and retinal development which mainly occurs during the latter half of pregnancy and the postnatal stage. The growth of fetal brain requires approximately

21 g/wk of DHA during the last trimester of pregnancy. Fatty acids are transported from maternal circulation across the placenta and fetal blood-brain barrier into the central nervous system. A deficiency of essential fatty acids during pregnancy leads to a reduced level of DHA in the newborn infants, which is related to a reduction in slow-wave sleep and impaired vision in these infants. Dietary supplementation of *n-3* fatty acids to pregnant women and increasing the amount of DHA in infant formula are beneficial for early neurological development and improve the visual recognition in preterm and term infants (10,11,12). It has also been shown that diets rich in *n-3* fatty acids can prevent premature labor and preeclampsia (13). Dietary *n-3* fatty acids also reduce the severity and frequency of relapses in patients suffering from multiple sclerosis (14). A significant improvement in schizophrenic symptoms has also been reported (15).

Many recent studies have shown that production of immunological/ inflammatory mediators can also be regulated by polyunsaturated fatty acids. Diets rich in *n-3* Polyunsaturated fatty acids significantly reduce the production of the pro-inflammatory cytokines, tumor necrosis factor (TNF), interleukin-1β (IL-1β) and IL-2, as well as the lipid mediator, platelet activating factor (PAF) (6,16,17).

However, in addition to downregulation of many leukocyte functions, which form the basis of their anti-inflammatory effects, polyunsaturated fatty acids of both the *n-6* and *n-3* types stimulate leukocyte function associated with proinflammatory activity and tissue damage. In particular, polyunsaturated fatty acids have been shown to stimulate neutrophils.

2.3 *Phospholipase A*

Fatty acids can also be derived from the hydrolysis of membrane phospholipids. Stimulation of cells by agonists interacting with specific receptors, such as growth factors, thrombin, bradykinin or f-met-leu-phe (fMLP), leads to activation of phospholipases, eg. phospholipase A$_2$ (PLA$_2$) and phospholipase C / diacylglycerol lipase which result in the liberation of fatty acids from the membrane phospholipids into the cytosol and plasma.

Several types of PLA_2 have been described. Besides the well characterised Groups I, II, III and IV, other forms of PLA_2 are being recognised and characterised (18). The PLA_2 which have been reported to participate in the generation of fatty acids from activated cells include the calcium-dependent, 85 kDa cytosolic PLA_2 ($cPLA_2$), and the secretory 14 kDa PLA_2 ($sPLA_2$) and a calcium-independent PLA_2 ($iPLA_2$) (18). $cPLA_2$, has a preference for 20:4n-6 in the sn-2 position of a phospholipid while $sPLA_2$ and $iPLA_2$ do not. $sPLA_2$, secreted from activated cells, and $iPLA_2$, therefore release 20:4n-6 and other fatty acids from membrane phospholipids. Recent studies in monocytic cells have suggested that activation of $sPLA_2$ may depend on the transient activation of $cPLA_2$ (19). n-3 fatty acids such as 20:5n-3 esterified at the sn-2 position of a phospholipid are released by $cPLA_2$ (20). Esterified fatty acids can also be liberated from phospholipids/lysophospholipids via the action of phospholipase A_1 and phospholipase B, the latter possessing both phospholipase A_1 and A_2 activity. While phospholipase A_1 and A_2 are generally thought to play major roles in phospholipids remodeling, there is some evidence that the activity of phospholipase A_1 may be regulated by receptor- mediated events (21) and hence may play a role in ligand-stimulated accumulation of non-esterified fatty acids. These free fatty acids (unesterified fatty acids) act as regulators of cellular responses and functions (Fig. 4.1). Non esterified fatty acids which are released by PLA_2 have been found to be cell-associated as well as being released into the extracellular space and many studies have monitored the release of radiolabelled 20:4n-6 in the incubation medium as a measure of PLA_2 activity. Consequently, nonesterified fatty acids which are released from an activated cell can exert paracrine and autocrine effects. It is well documented that the levels of nonesterified fatty acids are elevated at sites of inflammation. Cell-types which are likely to contribute to this pool of fatty acids include monocytes/macrophages, platelets, endothelial cells, chondrocytes, fibroblasts, mast cells, neutrophils and bacteria (22–35). Although mature T and B lymphocytes have been reported not to express $cPLA_2$ and that the T cell receptor/CD3 complex is not coupled to $cPLA_2$ (36), there is some evidence that activated T cells do release 20:4n-6. This is likely to be due to the action of diacylglycerol lipase and/or a CD28-mediated signalling event (37,38). There is also a substantial amount of evidence that some of the

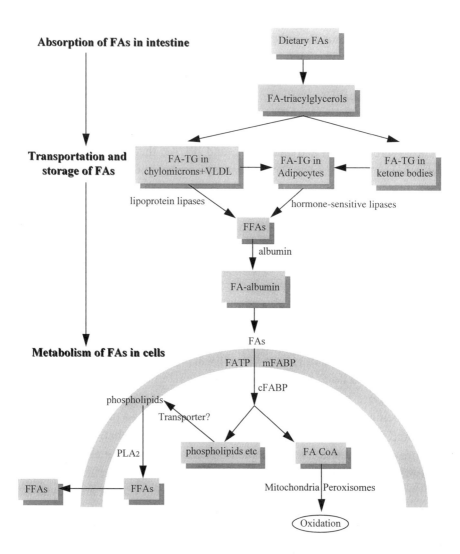

Figure 4.5.   Mechanisms of transportation and utilisation of fatty acids in the human body. FA: fatty acids. FFAs: free fatty acids. VLDL: very low density lipoprotein; TG: triacylglycerol; FATP: fatty acid transporting protein. FABP or cFABP: membrane or cytosolic fatty acid binding protein; FA CoA: fatty acyl coenzyme A.

above listed cell-types also release $sPLA_2$ upon activation (19,23,30,39,40). Indeed plasma of septic shock patients has been found to contain $sPLA_2$ which is active on monocytic cells, *E. coli* and synthetic phosphatidylethanolamine (32). Also, $sPLA_2$ isolated from human platelets has been reported to cause the formation of LTB_4 in human neutrophils (39). Consequently, neutrophils which infiltrate into sites of infection or inflammation will be exposed to non-esterified fatty acids in addition to agents such as chemoattractants and bacterial products. The newly recruited cells will, in turn, release more fatty acids and eicosanoids as they become activated. As the inflammatory cascade proceeds, recruitment of other cells and further release of nonesterified fatty acids will occur until the foreign body is eliminated or the inflammation is resolved.

Table 4.1 summarises the range of neutrophil agonists which have been shown to stimulate the activity of either PLA_2 and/or release of free 20:4*n-6* in neutrophils. Cytokines are a major group of molecules in the network of mediators which regulate physiological and pathophysiological processes. The cytokines which have been shown to stimulate the release of 20:4*n-6*; including TNF, GM-CSF, IL-8. Other mediators with this activity include, complement (C5a, complement coated zymosan, *E.coli*); Fc-γR receptor acting agents such as aggregated IgG or IgG-coated zymosan; classical neutrophil agonists, fMLP, PMA, Ca^{2+} ionophore (Table 4.1). Eicosanoids also have the ability to induce release of 20:4*n-6* and these include LTB_4, 5-oxo-ETE and 5-HETE. In addition, many of the above mediators also prime neutrophils for enhanced activation of PLA_2 in response to a second ligand. Thus pretreatment of neutrophils with TNF, IL8, GM-CSF, LPS, PMA or lipoxygenase products enhance the ability of a second ligand to stimulate the PLA_2 activity (33,34,41–44).

3. Transport and Uptake of Fatty Acids

After absorption by the intestine, the fatty acids are transported to tissues where they may be utilized immediately or stored (Fig. 4.5). Four types of vehicles have been shown to be involved in the transportation of fatty acids: (i) chylomicrons, where dietary triacylglycerol is carried in protein-coated lipid droplets and transported to the whole body from the intestine; (ii) ketone bodies

Table 4.1   Agonist induced PLA$_2$ activation/AA generation

Agonist	Details	Reference
C5a	Ca^{2+} independent PLA$_2$ activity stimulated	(59)
Complement-coated zymosan	Release of sPLA$_2$	(60)
Complement-coated *E.coli*	Activation of granule-associated group II PLA$_2$ (sPLA$_2$)	(35)
fMLP	Release of sPLA$_2$ AA release by cPLA$_2$	(40,61) (41,62)
LXA$_4$, LXB$_4$	Release of AA	(63)
Ca^{2+}/PAF	Measured in Ca^{2+} depleted human neutrophils AA release LTB$_4$ synthesis	 (64) (41)
TNF	Minimal AA release cPLA$_2$ phosphorylation Some AA release	(33) (65) (66)
5-oxo-ETE	cPLA$_2$ phosphorylation Small amount of AA release	(67)
LTB$_4$	Increase in cPLA$_2$ activity	(42)
5-HETE	Small increase in cPLA$_2$ activity	(42)
GM-CSF	 Phosphorylation of cPLA$_2$ Increase in activity of cPLA$_2$	(68) (42)
AA	 Release of AA	(69)

(acetoacetate and β-hydroxybutyrate) and (iii) very low density lipoprotein (VLDL), which are responsible for transporting fatty acids, processed by or synthesised in the liver, to either adipose tissue for storage, or to various tissues to be used for cell structure and metabolism; triacylglycerol in the blood is enzymatically hydrolysed by lipases, such as lipoprotein lipases, on the surface of endothelial cells. The released free fatty acids become bound to serum fatty acid binding protein eg. albumin, type IV fatty acid transporter, which carries the released fatty acids in the blood stream to appropriate tissue sites. The free fatty acids in the extracellular fluid continuously exchange with the intracellular fatty acids which are released by the action of phospholipase A_2 (Fig. 4.5) This process is called intracellular fatty acid turnover (45). How fatty acids are taken up by cells remains unclear. It has been proposed that fatty acids firstly become dissociated from albumin and then bind to a fatty acid transporter protein in the plasma membrane (Fig. 4.5). Thus, proteins with molecular weights of 40–43-kDa and 85-kDa have been reported in myocardial membrane, hepatocytes, adipocytes and jejunal enterocytes where they act as fatty acid carriers (46–49). Uptake via carrier-mediated systems was found to be saturable (47). A fatty acid translocase with homology to CD36 has also been reported to be involved in the transport of long chain fatty acids (50,51). There is some evidence in cardiac myocytes that fatty acids can also enter cells by diffusion (52,53). It has been proposed that fatty acid transfer across the plasma membrane by diffusion is influenced by a physicochemical equilibrium between the extracellular fatty acid/albumin complex, the membrane lipid phase, intracellular fatty acid binding proteins and the respective aqueous phases (53). In isolated cardiac myocyte cultures, uptake of ^{14}C-palmitate from a medium containing physiological interstitial concentration of albumin (2%) and varying palmitate/albumin ratios was found to be saturable, if the albumin concentration was kept constant (53). Uptake was rapid, so that intracellular ^{14}C-palmitate reached a plateau $\leq$30 sec. The initial rate of uptake was dependent on the palmitate/albumin ratio. At a constant ratio, there was a constant rate of uptake, even when the absolute concentration of palmitate was increased. Km of uptake was found to be dependent on the metabolic rate of the cells (54). Studies with ghost membrane vesicles demonstrated that the concentration of palmitate in membranes increased almost linearly with increasing palmitate/albumin ratios (54). These two proposed modes of fatty acid uptake need not be mutually exclusive. Once inside the cell, fatty acids are transported to various intracellular sites by the cytosolic fatty acid binding protein (FABP, 14–15 kDa) where they interact with appropriate proteins/ structures to evoke cellular responses (Fig. 4.5) (55,56). The precise mechanism by which fatty acids are taken up by neutrophils are still poorly defined. However, it has been demonstrated that the ability of a fatty acid to partition into the neutrophil plasma membrane is not sufficient to evoke superoxide production (57). Similarly, the observation that saturated fatty acids (lacking biological actions) have a greater ability to partition into the plasma membrane of cytotoxic T lymphocyte than *cis* unsaturated fatty acids is inconsistent with biological activity being totally caused by membrane partitioning of a fatty acid (58).

4. Metabolism of Arachidonic Acid and Other Fatty Acids

4.1 *General*

Nonesterified AA (n-6) can be metabolized via a number of pathways, including the lipoxygenase and cyclooxygenase pathways which produce a number of biologically active eicosanoids (Fig. 4.4). The products of AA metabolism via the cyclooxygenase pathway are the 2-series prostaglandins and thromboxanes. AA is first converted to PGH_2 which is followed by the formation of PGD_2, PGE_2, PGF_{2a} and PGI_2. The types of prostaglandins formed in different tissues varies depending on the type of prostaglandin synthases being expressed in tissues. For example PGI_2 is mainly found in the blood, PGE_2 and PGF_{2a} are generated in the kidney and spleen, while PGE_2 PGF_{2a} and PGI_2 are synthesised in the heart. The other product of the cyclooxygenase pathway is TXA_2, which is produced from PGH_2 by thromboxane A synthetase. TXA_2 is mainly synthesized in the lung and platelets. The generation of these eicosanoids is believed to play a major role in the inflammatory reaction in rheumatoid arthritis and psoriasis. The 2-series eicosanoids also increase sensitivity to pain, induce fever, platelet aggregation and thrombosis, and act as vasodilators to lower the systemic arterial blood pressure (1). The metabolism of AA via the lipoxygenase pathway is catalysed by three monoxygenases, 5-, 12- and 15-lipoxygenases which convert AA to either 5-, 12- or 15-monohydroperoxy-eicosatetraenoic acids (HPETE). These HPETE are the precursors of 5-, 12- or 15-hydroxyeicosatetraenoic acids (HETE). Leukotrienes are another important group of eicosanoids generated by this pathway (Fig. 4.4). Among the metabolites of AA, LTB_4 and 5-HETE stimulate neutrophil chemotaxis, degranulation, respiratory burst, adherence to endothelial cells and the transmigration of neutrophils across vascular barriers (70), (see section on "Regulation of neutrophil functions by metabolites of arachidonic acid"). The products also cause the contraction of smooth muscles in pulmonary airways and the gastrointestinal tract and in this manner promote inflammation and allergic reactions. These proinflammatory products of AA metabolism, along with other peptide inflammatory mediators, therefore form a network which modulates cell responses involved in various physiological responses (71,72).

The *n-3* fatty acids, EPA and DHA, can also be metabolised by the lipoxygenase pathway. However, the cyclooxygenase pathway preferentially metabolizes EPA (Fig. 4.6). In the presence of *n-3* fatty acids, less metabolites of AA are formed. In contrast to AA, the metabolism of *n-3* fatty acids, such as EPA, by the lipoxygenase and cyclooxygenase pathways give rise to products with different properties from those of AA-derived metabolites. Metabolism of EPA and DHA by the lipoxygenase and/or cyclooxygenase pathways results in the generation of less active metabolites, such as LTB_5, TXB_3, and 5-hydroxyeicosapentaenoic acid (5-HEPE) in the case of EPA and small amount of anti-inflammatory 7-hydroxydocosahexaenoic acid (7-HDHE) in the case of DHA in neutrophils and macrophages (1,73–75). The alteration of metabolic product profiles from proinflammatory to lower or negligible pro-inflammatory activity by EPA and DHA are shown to be beneficial in the prevention of disease progress and relieving the symptoms. This switch from the pro-inflammatory AA-derived metabolites to the less pro-inflammatory DHA or EPA-derived metabolites has been proposed as a mechanism by which *n-3* fatty acids exert their anti-inflammatory actions (1) (Fig. 4.6).

Dietary supplementation with *n-3* fish oil fatty acid also alter macrophage eicosanoid profile. It has been shown that EPA and/or DHA rich diets reduce the AA metabolites, such as LTB_4, 5-HETE, 11-HETE, 12-HETE, 15-HETE,

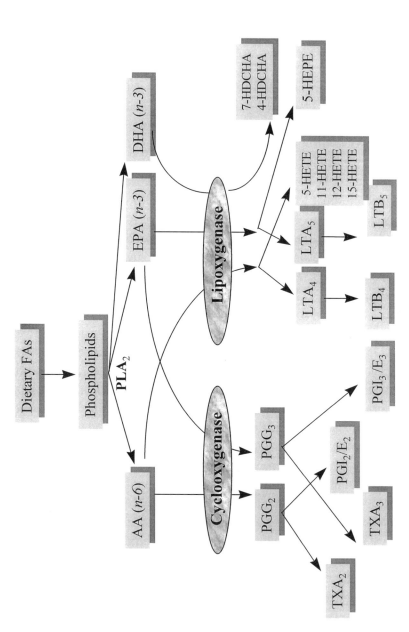

Figure 4.6.   Comparison of products formed from AA (*n*-6) and the *n*-3 fatty acids EPA and DHA when metabolised via the lipoxygenase and cyclooxygenase system. HDCHA: hydroxydocosahexaenoic acid; HEPE: hydroxyeicosapentaenoic acid. Other abbreviations as in Fig. 4.4.

PGI_2, PGE_2 and TXA_2, and increase the amount of LTB_5, 5-HEPE, PGI_3 6-keto-PGF_{1a} and PGE_3 being produced (73,76–84). Two plausible reasons for these changes are, an increase in serum *n-3* fatty acids by week two of feeding with MAX EPA (85) and to a reduction in the phospholipid AA:EPA ratio (49:1 being reduced to 8:1) (86). The ratio of DHA: AA in neutrophil phospholipids was not reduced until high doses of fish oil (15 capsules/day) were consumed (86). AA and other fatty acids are also metabolised by alternative routes including esterification into phospholipids and neutral lipids, β oxidation in the mitochondria, ω-oxidation and formation of epoxy eicosatrienoic acids by the cytochrome p450 enzyme systems.

4.2 *Metabolism in neutrophils*

It has been reported that neutrophils contain $100–2,200$ pmol/10^7 cells of AA (87). In neutrophils, AA is metabolised mainly via 2 routes: esterification into phospholipids or triglycerides (66) and conversion to various eicosanoids by 5-lipoxygenase (88). However, neutrophils have also been reported to metabolise AA via the 12- and 15-lipoxygenases and cyclooxygenase (89), albeit at very low levels compared to metabolism via 5-lipoxygenases. For example, stimulation of neutrophils with A23187 caused the formation of 3.51 ± 0.22 ng of LTB_4 and 0.81 ± 0.08 ng of $LTC_4/10^6$ cells compared to 0.144 ± 0.025 ng of TXB_2 and 0.15 ± 0.017 ng of PGE_2 ng/10^6 cells (89). In neutrophils, LTB_4 and related products are metabolised by w-oxidation (see below).

The 5 lipoxygenase of neutrophils, as in other cell-types can metabolise EPA. Thus, bovine and human neutrophils have been reported to metabolise EPA to 5-hydroxyeicosapentaenoic acid (5-HEPE) (79,90) as discussed above, metabolise DHA to give 7-hydroxydocosahexaenoic acid.

Acylation into phospholipids and triglycerides.

Fatty acids such as AA, taken up by cells are converted to fatty acyl coenzymeA (FACoA) by fatty acid CoA synthetase. FACoA can be then transported into the inner membrane of mitochondria to undergo β-oxidation. Alternatively, they are incorporated into phospholipids, glycosphingolipids, triglycerides, and cholesteryl esters which are involved in membrane biosynthesis, membrane replacement or energy storage. The exchange of intracellular and extracellular fatty acids is a continuous process essential for normal tissue function. This on-going turnover of cell lipids is regulated by both the intracellular and extracellular environment resulting in changing tissue functions through diet manipulation (Fig. 4.2) (55). As discussed in "Metabolism of AA and other fatty acid", an increase in EPA:AA ratio has been found in human neutrophils after diet supplementation with fish oil capsules for two weeks (85). Our studies have also demonstrated that fatty acids with different chain length are handled differently by neutrophils (see "Differences in metabolism of long chain and very long chain polyunsaturated fatty acids").

The incorporation of fatty acids into neutrophil phospholipids is regulated by a variety of ligands. LTB$_4$ has been reported to increase the incorporation of 20:4n-6 into phosphatidylinositol and acyl and alkyl phosphatidylcholine (91). This appeared to be due to increased acylation into lysophospholipids. Incorporation of 20:4n-6 into phosphatidylinositol was greater than into phosphatidylcholine (91). There is some specificity in fatty acid incorporation into neutrophil phospholipids. For example, [^{3}H] 20:4n-6 was found to be incorporated equally into both acyl and alkyl phosphatidylcholine at the sn-2 position (92). In resting neutrophils, 20:4n-6 was the only fatty acid that was incorporated into 1-O-alkyl-2-lyso-sn-glycero-3-phosphocholine (lyso-PAF) (93). 18:2n-6 (linoleate), on the other hand, was not found in alkyl phosphatidylcholine (92). Labelled saturated fatty acids were incorporated only into acyl phospholipids which contained 18:1n-9 or 18:2n-6 at the sn-2 position (92). The specificity in 20:4n-6 incorporation may be lost upon neutrophil activation. Thus, in neutrophil stimulated with A23187, the incorporation of 20:4n-6 into lyso PAF to form alkyl phosphatidylcholine was attenuated by up to 80% (93). A possible reason for the loss in specificity was found to be an accummulation of 1-O-alk-1'-enyl-2-lyso-sn-glycero-3-phosphoethanolamine which competed with lyso PAF (93). Neutrophils also incorporate metabolites of 20:4n-6 into their phospholipids. For example, endognously produced 5-HETE and exogenous 5-HETE are esterified into neutrophil phospholipids and triacylglycerol (94). While endogenously generated 5-HETE was esterified equally into phospholipids and triacylglycerol, exogenous 5-HETE was esterified predominantly into triacylglycerol. Similarly, 12-HETE has been found to be esterified into neutrophil phospholipids and triglycerides (95). Neutrophils also elongate fatty acids. For example, GLA has been reported to be elongated to dihomo-gamma-LA (DGLA) by neutrophils (96). Other examples of chain elongation in neutrophils (66) are discussed below.

4.2.1 5-lipoxygenase

In the neutrophils, there is some evidence that 5-lipoxygenase is secreted and the enzyme has been localised to the specific granules (97). Products of the 5-lipoxygenase which have been detected in neutrophils incubated with AA and A23187 include 5-HETE, 5-DiHETE, 5-HPETE, 5-oxoETE, LTA_4, LTC_4, LTD_4, LTB_4 and LXA_4 (Fig. 4.3). However, the conversion of AA to LTB_4 can be modulated by other fatty acids. For example, linoleic acid (LA) and dihomogammalinoleic acid (DGLA) were found to block LTB_4 formation and this was accompanied with the formation of 15-lipoxygenase products from LA (13-hydroxy-octadecadienoic acid; 13-HODE) and DGLA (15-hydroxy-eicosatrienoic acid; 15-HETrE) (98). Further studies revealed that 15-lipoxygenase products of LA, DGLA and AA directly blocked LTB_4 production (98), possibly via inhibition of 5-lipoxygenase. Further studies demonstrated that the inhibitory effect of 15-HETE was dependent on the degree of unsaturation. Thus, analogues with different degrees of unsaturation showed inhibition in the order of 3 double bonds > 4 double bonds > 2 double bond > 0 double bonds (99). 15-HPETE was four fold more effective than 15-HETE at inhibiting the 5 lipoxygenase (99). Diet supplementation with GLA or *n-3* fatty acids in healthy volunteers has also been reported to cause a reduction in the ability of their neutrophils to produce LTB_4 (86,100,101). The effect of GLA could be due to the formation of DGLA from GLA by chain elongation and subsequently leading to inhibition of LTB_4 synthesises by DGLA (see above). However, the effect observed with EPA has been reported to range from minor (86) to dramatic (101). Incubation of human neutrophils with EPA *in vitro* has also been found to inhibit LTB_4 formation (90), an observation which was in agreement with data obtained with neutrophils from volunteers whose diets had been supplemented with w3 fatty acids. Formation of 5-lipoxygenase products has been reported to be inhibited by pertussis toxin (102) and by ibuprofen, an inhibitor of cyclooxygenase. The 5-lipoxygenase was found to be six times less sensitive to ibuprofen compared to cyclooxygenase (103). Extracts from neutrophils, eosinophils and monocytes have recently been demonstrated to convert 5 HETE to 5-oxo-6, 8, 11, 14-eicosatetraenoic acid (5-oxo-ETE) by a highly specific microsomal dehydrogenase (104,105). The formation of 5-oxo-ETE has also been demonstrated in intact neutrophils and monocytes (105,106). In unstimulated neutrophils, the levels of 5-oxo-ETE is low and most of the 5-HETE is converted to 5-, 20-DiHETE (107,108). Upon stimulation with phorbol 12-myristate 13-acetate (PMA), the ratio of 5-oxo-ETE:5-,20-DiHETE has been found to increase from 0.7 to 1.85. PMA-stimulated neutrophils also produced 5-oxo-ETE from exogenous AA. In these studies, it was found that more 5-oxo-ETE than LTB_4 was formed under all conditions. The effect of PMA on the formation of 5-oxo-ETE required the activation of NADPH oxidase but was independent on the formation of superoxide (107, 108). Thus, phenazine methosulphate which converts NADPH to $NADP^+$, but not generation of superoxide by xanthine/xanthine oxidase, mimicked the actions of PMA on the synthesis of 5-oxo-ETE. Similarly, A23187 stimulated the formation of 5-oxo-ETE and with prolonged incubation with A23187, the amount of 5-oxo-ETE that was formed exceeded that of LTB_4 (107). These studies demonstrate that stimulated neutrophils have the capacity to synthesise a substantial amount of 5-oxo-ETE. The 5-oxo-ETE which accumulate in stimulated neutrophils is metabolised to 5-oxo-20-(OH) — 6E, 8Z, 11Z, 14Z — eicosatetraenoic acids by w-oxidation (106). However, monocytes have been reported not to form w-oxidised products of 5-oxoETE (105). When neutrophils were exposed to EPA and PMA or A23187, 5-hydroxy-6,8,11,14,17-eicosapentaenoic acid (5-HEPE), 5-oxoEPE and small amounts of LTB_5 and 20-OH-LTB_5 were formed (109), demonstrating that EPA, like AA, can be metabolised to form oxo-derivatives.

4.2.2 12-lipoxygenase

Compared to the 12-lipoxygenase in platelets, the 12-lipoxygenase in neutrophils is relatively inactive. Thus, products of 12-HETE were not formed in stimulated rat neutrophils (110). In fact, it has been suggested that 12-lipoxygenase metabolites, if detected in neutrophil preparations, could be produced by contaminating platelets (71). Nevertheless, studies with bovine neutrophils have demonstrated that while intact neutrophils did not metabolise AA via the 12-lipoxygenase, sonicates of bovine neutrophils readily converted AA and LA to their respective 12-lipoxygenase products (111). On the other hand, incubation of canine neutrophils wth AA has been reported to produce 12-HETE, 12,20-DiHETE and 12-hydroxyheptadecatrienoic acid (112). With human neutrophils, the production of 12-HETE in the 17,000 g supernatant of neutrophil homogenates and in intact cells incubated in the presence of A23187 have been reported (113,114). In both of these studies, indomethacin was found to be necessary for 12-HETE formation. However, this was not related to inhibition of cyclooxygenase since neither acetyl salicylic acid nor ibuprofen, inhibitors of cyclooxygenase, mimicked the action of indomethacin (114).

4.2.3 15-lipoxygenase

The 15-lipoxygenase in neutrophils is usually inactive, even in the presence of A23187 and AA. However, it has been reported that 5-, 12- and 15-HETE could stimulate the relatively inactive enzyme to metabolise AA in the presence of A23187 and nordihydroguaiaretic acid (115). The monohydroxy products of LA, 9- and 13-HODEs were found to be less active than the monohydroxy-derivatives of AA at stimulating 15-lipoxygenase (115). Similar results were obtained by Fogh et al (116). In this study, it was found that a number of 5-lipoxygenase inhibitors but not cyclooxygenase inhibitors, diverted the metabolism of AA via 5 lipoxygenase to the 15-lipoxygenase pathway and this was associated with a reduction in LTB_4 formation. On the other hand, ibuprofen (9 fold), indomethacin (2 fold) and aspirin (1.5 fold), have been reported to stimulate 15-lipoxygenase in human neutrophils (103). The stimulation of 15-lipoxygenase by ibuprofen was found to occur within 1 min of ibuprofen addition and was reversible.

4.2.4 Cyclooxygenase

In many cell types including neutrophils, cyclooxygenase (or prostaglandin endoperoxide synthase) has been localised to the lipid bodies (117). These are inducible cytoplasmic inclusions that develop in cells associated with inflammation. Lipid bodies act as repositories of arachidonyl phospholipids and have been proposed to play a role in the oxidative metabolism of AA to form eicosanoids. As discussed above, stimulated neutrophils produce some PGE_2 and TXB_2 (89). Production of PGE_2 was found to be agonist specific. Thus, exposure of human neutrophils to GM-CSF, G-CSF, LPS and fMLP was reported to stimulate PGE_2 production (118). Cytokine-induced PGE_2 production occur in 2 phases: an early phase (detectable at 20 min) and a late cycloheximide-sensitive phase (detected after 4 h). On the other hand, neutrophils were found to produce little or no PGE_2, TXA_2 or 6 keto PGF_{1a} in response to M-CSF, IL1 or IL3 (118,119). The amount of prostagnoids produced was dependent on gender. Hence, neutrophils obtained from women have been reported to produce 30% less TXB_2 and PGE_2 than those obtained from men (120). Production of PGE_2 by neutrophils obtained from alcoholics has also been reported to be lower than from neutrophils obtained from non-alcoholics (121).

4.2.5. ω-oxidation

ω-oxidation of LTB_4 by LTB_4-20-hydrolase of the cytochrome p450 enzyme family is the major route by which the catabolism of LTB_4 in human neutrophils proceeds (122). This pathway of LTB_4 catabolism was found to be exclusive to neutrophils since monocytes, lymphocytes or platelets were not able to produce ω-oxidised products of LTB_4. This enzyme system adds a hydroxyl moiety to C-20 (ω end) of LTB_4 to produce 20-OH-LTB_4. Catabolism of exogenous LTB_4 is rapid ($t_{1/2}$ of approximately 4 min at 37°C in reaction mixtures containing 1 mM LTB$_4$ and 2×10^7 neutrophils/ml). In addition to 20-OH-LTB$_4$, incubation of neutrophils with AA has widely been reported to result in the production of 20-COOH- LTB$_4$ (102,122,123), demonstrating that endogenously-derived LTB$_4$ is also ω-oxidised. Neutrophils can also metabolise 5-HETE, 5-oxo-ETE and 12 HETE by ω-oxidation (Fig. 4.4) (106,112,122,124).

5. Transcellular Metabolism

AA and eicosanoid metabolites released from one cell-type can be further metabolised by another cell-type (72). For example, in co-incubation experiments, the uptake and further metabolism of [^{3}H]-12-HETE, produced by prelabelled and activated platelets, to [^{3}H] 5-,12-DiHETE by activated neutrophils have been reported (72). However, with unstimulated neutrophils, platelet-derived 12-HETE was converted to 12-,20-DiHETE by the neutrophils (125). These studies imply that transcellular metabolism facilitates the formation of eicosanoids, which are formed at low levels or not formed by a single cell-type alone. In another set of co-incubation experiments, labelled AA which was released from aspirin-pretreated, calcium ionophore-stimulated platelets had been reported to be taken up by activated neutrophils, resulting in the formation of labelled 5-HETE and LTB$_4$ (72). Cell-cell interaction at the level of eicosanoid metabolism may alter the range and amount of eicosanoids formed at sites of inflammation.

6. Biological Properties of Arachidonic Acid

6.1 *Effects on neutrophil adhesion, cell migration and chemotaxis*

Human neutrophils treated with arachidonic acid showed increased adhesion to plasma coated surfaces (Table 4.2) Short term exposure of neutrophils to arachidonic acid alters the migration properties of the leukocyte (126). At physiologically attainable concentrations the ability of human neutrophils to migrate in a chemotactic gradient generated with the tripeptide f-met-leu-phe

Table 4.2   Effects of arachidonic acid on neutrophil functions

Function	Effect	Comment
Adherence	Increased	To plasma coated plastic surfaces
Migration	Decreased	Random migration and fMLP/complement-induced chemotaxis
Phagocytosis	Increased	Bacteria/parasites
Microbial killing	Increased	Bacteria/parasites
Tissue damage		endothelial cells
Increase in β_2 integrin expression	Increased	CR3 (CD11b/CD18) CR4 (CD11c/CD18)
Respiratory burst	Induced	Superoxide production
Degranulation	Induced	Of primary and secondary granules
Cytokine synthesis	Suppressed	TNF, IL-8

(fMLP) and complement (serum activated with yeast particles) was completely inhibited. However, the effect of AA was not specific for the chemotactic response of the cell. Random migration was inhibited concomitantly with the decrease seen in the chemotactic response. This suggests that the AA affects the elements involved in cell locomotion. The ability of fMLP to induce chemokinesis was also inhibited by AA. These results suggest that another characteristic of AA is to regulate the accumulation of neutrophils at inflammatory foci. The source of fatty acid may be the tissues, the bacteria and the infiltrating leukocytes.

6.2 *Activation of the NADPH oxidase*

Neutrophils interacting with various types of soluble agonists and particles undergo an oxygen-dependent respiratory burst which is associated with the phagocytosis of particles and leads to the release of toxic oxygen-derived reactive species (ODRS) such as superoxide, hydrogen peroxide, hydroxyl radical, singlet oxygen and hypochlorous acid. These are responsible for the killing of a range of microorganisms and tumor cells. Perturbation of the neutrophil membrane by either receptor ligation or non-specifically leads to the assembly of NADPH oxidase in the plasma membrane, which catalyses the reduction of molecular oxygen to superoxide (127–129). This oxidase consists of membrane components, cytochrome b558 and FAD, the cytosolic components, p47phox, p67phox, p40phox and a small GTP binding protein, rac2 (127–129).

AA induces the activation of the NADPH oxidase in neutrophils (Fig. 4.7) (130,131). The fatty acid has been shown to be a strong activator of the respiratory burst and the release of ODRS. At optimal agonist concentrations the response induced by AA was similar to that induced by the phorbol ester, PMA and both of these responses were significantly greater than that induced by fMLP (Fig. 4.7). The characteristics of the response was also examined. fMLP, as previously established, induces a weak to modest respiratory burst which is characterised by a very rapid release of superoxide which peaks within 30 seconds and returns to basal levels in the next one to two minutes (Fig. 4.7).

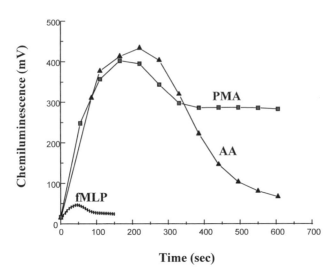

Time (sec)

Figure 4.7.   Comparisons of the characteristics of the lucigenin-dependent chemiluminescence response to fMLP, PMA and AA in human neutrophils. The agonists were used at optimal concentrations.

This is quite different to the response induced by PMA, which acts independently of a cell surface receptor and directly activates protein kinase C (132). At optimal concentrations, the PMA response is characterised by peak response at ≤ 2 min and is substantially greater than the fMLP response (Fig. 4.7). The activity of neutrophils stimulated with an optimal concentration of PMA returns to basal level within 30 minutes. The characteristics of the respiratory burst in response to AA is similar to but less persistent than that induced by PMA (Fig. 4.7).

AA also stimulates the production of superoxide in reconstituted systems. For this to occur, all the components of the active NADPH oxidase have to be present. (129,133). Compared with intact cells, the concentrations of AA which are needed to evoke these *in vitro* responses are 5–10 times more than those needed to produce the same response in intact neutrophils.

Interestingly, human monocytes and macrophages treated with polyunsaturated fatty acids showed very poor and often insignificant activation of the NADPH oxidase compared to neutrophils (Fig. 4.8) (134). However, pretreating these mononuclear phagocytes with AA, EPA and DHA or the simultaneous addition of fatty acids and either fMLP, PMA or A23187 gave rise to a major respiratory burst response (134).

6.3 *Stimulation of degranulation*

Extensive studies on the stimulation of degranulation by AA have been conducted (135,136). AA was found to be a complete secretagogue inducing the release of constituents from both the specific and azurophilic granules, shown by the release of vitamin B12 binding protein and β-glucuronidase, respectively. Similarly endogeously derived AA and other fatty acids have been demonstrated to regulate degranulation and degranulation-dependent receptor expression in intact neutrophils. Hence, neutrophils treated with inhibitors of phospholipase A_2 (137) released less secretory products from both the specific and azurophilic granules in response to A23187. The response to AA in terms of the vitamin B12 binding protein release was greater than that induced by FMLP and PMA (136). It has been proposed that AA acts by promoting the fusion between granules and plasma membrane (138).

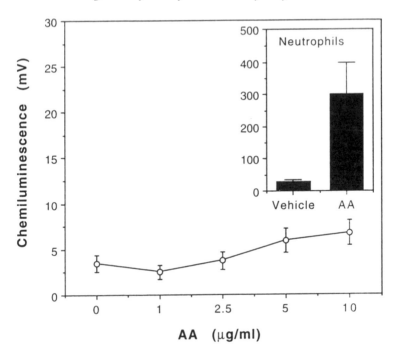

Figure 4.8.   Comparison of AA-induced lucigenin-dependent chemiluminescence response in human neutrophils (bar graph) and macrophages (open circles).

7. Effects of *n-3* Fatty Acids, Eicosapentaenoic and Docosahexaenoic Acid on Neutrophils

Over the last five years, extensive investigations in our laboratory on the effects of *n-3* polyunsaturated fatty acids on neutrophils have yielded some interesting results. Quite unexpectedly and against the perceived anti-inflammatory properties of these fatty acids, *n-3* polyunsaturated fatty acids have been shown to activate properties of neutrophils associated with the pro-inflammatory activity of the cell. This places a different perspective on the concepts held for the last two decades that *n-3* fatty acids eg. fish oils, can be used to depress the inflammatory reaction in allergic and autoimmune inflammatory diseases (7).

DHA was found to be particularly active compared with EPA in stimulating neutrophil adhesion (139). DHA was found to cause a rapid increase in neutrophil adherence which was always greater than that induced by AA (140). The other polyunsaturated *n-3* fatty acid, EPA was found to stimulate this property to a less extent than AA and DHA (140). In some cases DHA caused a substantial increase in this response which was also significantly greater than that induced by AA and EPA. The kinetics of this response induced by AA and the *n-3* polyunsaturated fatty acids showed that the response to DHA was greater than that induced by FMLP and PMA (140). The *n-3* polyunsaturated fatty acids were also found to induce marked degranulation of specific and azurophilic granules. It was again evident that on a molar basis DHA was much more active than either AA and EPA (136).

8. Regulation of Neutrophil Functions by Metabolites of Arachidonic Acid

Metabolism of AA via the lipoxygenase and cylooxygenase pathways leads to eicosanoids which regulate neutrophil functions (Table 4.3) Some products of the lipoxygenase such as LTB_4 have marked pro-inflammatory and neutrophil stimulating activity but others may show anti- and pro-inflammatory activity. In contrast cylooxygenase products such as PG_1 and PG_2 posses neutrophils suppressive actions.

8.1 *Products of the lipoxygenase pathway*

Products of the metabolism of AA via the lipoxygenase pathway have been shown to cause either potent activation of neutrophils, no effect or inhibit the ability of other agonists to induce a response. LTB_4 has been of major interest as a neutrophil activator. It has both chemotactic and chemokinesis properties (141–143), stimulates adhesion of neutrophils and release of lysosomal enzymes (144,145), and induces the generation of superoxide (146,147). Thus, this eicosanoid promotes all the steps of the inflammatory reaction with respect to the neutrophil behaviour in this response. LTC_4 and LTD_4 have also been shown to enhance neutrophil adherence properties (148).

Table 4.3   Effects of eicosanoids on neutrophil function

Lipoxygenase product	Neutrophil function			
	Chemotaxis	Adhesion	Superoxide production	Degranulation
LTB$_4$	+	+	+	+
LTC$_4$	−	+		
LTD$_4$	−	+		
5-HETE	+		−	−
12-HETE	+			
15-HPETE	−	−	−	−
15-HETE	−	−	−	−
5-oxo-ETE	+			+
5, 15 -oxo-diHETE	+			+
LXA$_4$	+	+	+	−

The + and − sign indicate the presence or absence of activity of the lipoxygenase product.

The hydroxy products, 5-HETE and 12-HETE are chemotactic, although higher concentrations than LTB$_4$ are needed (149,150). However 15-HETE has little stimulatory effects. The dehydrogenase product of 5-HETE and 5, 15-diHETE, namely 5-oxo-ETE, 5 (OH), 15-oxo-ETE and 5-oxo-15(OH)-ETE respectively, also stimulate stimulate neutrophil chemotaxis (151,152) degranulation (153) and adherence (154) are also stimulated by 5-oxo-ETE. The lipoxin A$_4$ (LXA$_4$) is chemotactic for neutrophils (63,155,156) and stimulates the respiratory burst (157) and adherence (158).

Administration of the 15-lipoxygenase product, 15-HETE, has been shown to reduce tissue injury associated with psoriasis vulgaris in humans (116) and carrageanan-induced experimental arthritis (159). This is possibly related to the finding that 15-HETE was a potent inhibitor of LTB$_4$-induced neutrophil migration and transmigration across endothelium (160). In addition, products of 15 lipoxygenase can also inhibit LTB$_4$ formation by inhibiting 5 lipoxygenase (98). It also blocked transmigration induced by C5a and fMLP. Interestingly 15-HETE was significantly more active than either 5-HETE or 12-HETE in inhibiting transmigration. While the 15-HPETE was found not to stimulate any of these neutrophil functions, 15-HPETE caused a marked suppression of cytokine production by neutrophils (unpublished) and macrophages (161). Evidence has also been presented that LXA_4 can inhibit neutrophil adhesion and transmigration (162). Nanomolar concentrations of a synthetic LTA_4 was shown to inhibit the above neutrophil functions (163).

8.2 *Products of the cylcooxygenase pathway*

The cyclooxygenase pathway of AA metabolism gives rise to products which modulate neutrophil responses and the inflammatory reaction. Products of the cyclooxygenase pathway contribute to the erythema, pain and fever of inflammation. They synergise with other mediators in producing these effects. The effects of the prostaglandins on neutrophil function is, by contrast, largely suppressive. For example, PGE_2 inhibits neutrophil aggregation induced by fMLP (164) and also fMLP stimulated chemotaxis by human neutrophils (165). PGE_1 similarly has been shown to inhibit the oxidative burst, chemotaxis and phagocytosis by human neutrophils (166). In addition, the prostacyclin produced by endothelial cells, PGI_2 has been shown to inhibit neutrophil adherence (167). The mechanism for the anti-inflammatory effects of some products of the cyclooxygenase pathway remains unclear, however, it may be related to their ability to increase intracellular cAMP levels (168), in inhibition of agonist-induced increases in Ca^{2+} (166), inhibition of phosphatidylinositol 3-kinase (164) or decreased receptor affinity for ligands such as fMLP (169).

In contrast to the anti-inflammatory properties of the prostaglandins and prostacyclins, thromboxane A_2, which is generated by stimulated neutrophils (170), enhances adherence of neutrophils to endothelial cells and thus may play a role in provoking some forms of vascular injury (171). Thromboxane A_2 generation and subsequent selective pulmonary sequestration of neutrophils is characteristic of several forms of the adult respiratory distress syndrome. Thromboxane B_2, the product of thromboxane A_2 metabolism (Fig. 4.3), has been reported to be increased in lung following challenge with proinflammatory stimuli such as lipopolysaccharide or cigarette smoke, and is accompanied by neutrophil influx into the lung (172). Dietary fish oil supplementation reduces thromboxane B_2 elicited following LPS challenge (173). Some evidence suggests that thromboxane-induced neutrophil adhesion to pulmonary microvascular and aortic endothelial cells requires activation of CD18 (174).

9. Relationship between Fatty Acid Structure and Biological Function

Fatty acids with different carbon chain length, degrees of unsaturation, position of double bonds have different physio-chemical properties. Accordingly, their uptake, incorporation, interaction with cellular proteins and metabolism may differ dramatically. Extensive studies on this question by our group has revealed that these impart different types and levels of biological activity on neutrophils. The data on this relationship has been summarised in Table 4.4.

Table 4.4   The relationship between fatty acid structural element and biological effect on neutrophils

Fatty acid	Adherence	Respiratory bursts	Degranulation		Migration inhibition
			Specific	Azurophilic	
18:0	±			±	
18:1n-9	+	+	+		−
18:2n-6	+ +	+ +	+ +	±	±
18:3n-6	+ + +		+ + +	+ + +	
18:3n-3	+ ±		+ ±	+ ±	+ ±
18:4n-3	+ + +		+	+	
20:4n-6	+ + + +	+ +	+ + + +	+ + + +	+ + + +
20:0		−			−
20:5n-3		+ + +			+ +
22:6n-3		+ + + +			+ + + +
24:6n-3		+ +			
26:6n-3		+			
28:6n-3		−			
30:6n-3		−			
32:4n-6					−
32:6n-3		−			
34:6n-3		−			

The + and − signs indicate the relative activity between each other for the various neutrophil functional tests. The − sign defines no activity.

Studies on neutrophil adhesion showed that there was a relationship between the carbon atom chain length, degree of unsaturation and position of double bonds with the biological activity of the fatty acid (135,139). The saturated 18:0 fatty acid failed to induce any significant increase in adherence. Increased adherence was seen following stimulation with all 18, 20 and 22 carbon polyunsaturated fatty acids; the order of activity was 20:4*n-6* > 18:4*n-3*, 18:3*n-6*, 18:2*n-6* > 18:3*n-3*, 18:1*n-9*. An examination of the three isomers of 20:3 (*n-6, n-3 and n-9*) revealed that they were as effective as 20:4*n-6* (135). Other studies demonstrated that 20:5*n-3* and 22:6*n-3* were less effective than 20:4*n-6* at stimulating adherence, with 20:5*n-3* being the least active (139).

The respiratory burst induced by polyunsaturated fatty acids is also dependent on the structure of the fatty acid (131,175,176) (Fig. 4.9). Poulos et al (131) demonstrated that the ability to stimulate superoxide production by neutrophils was highly dependent on fatty acid carbon chain length. At different concentrations of these fatty acids it was found that there was a steady decline in activity as the number of carbon atoms of the unsaturated fatty acids increased from 22 → 24 → 26, having almost no activity once 28 carbon atoms are reached. Further increases to 30 → 32 similarly failed to stimulate the respiratory burst (131,176) (Table 4.4).

To some extent, this trend was followed in relation to polyunsaturated fatty acid-induced inhibition of random and chemotactic migration (126). 18:1*n-9* lacked activity, while 18:2*n-6* and 18:3*n-3* showed partial and significant inhibition of neutrophil random and chemotactic migration. Marked inhibition of these responses were seen with 20:4*n-6*, 20:5*n-3* and 22:6*n-3*. However, the polyunsaturated very long chain fatty acid (32:4*n-6*) had no activity, illustrating how the carbon chain length of the fatty molecules affects its biological properties (Fig. 4.9).

The mono/polyunsaturated fatty acids behaved very similarly with respect to stimulation of degranulation as with the stimulation of adhesion (135,139). Most evident was their ability to stimulate release from specific granules (release of vitamin B_{12} binding protein). However, they also showed activity in inducing release from azurophilic granules (*β*-glucuronidase), making these complete secretagogues This was particularly evident with 20:4*n-6*, 22:6*n-3* and 18:3*n-6*. Comparisons between the different structures showed that the ability

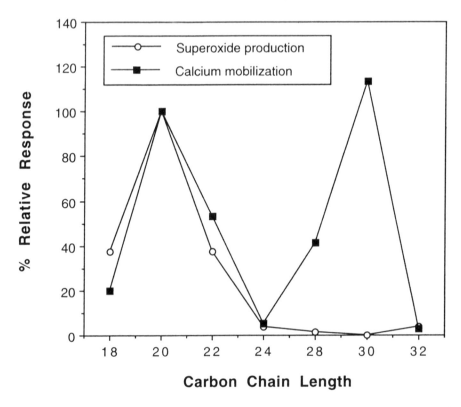

Figure 4.9. Relationship between calcium mobilisation and superoxide production induced by tetraenoic fatty acids with varying carbon chain length. The results are the mean ± sem of four experiments.

to induce degranulation of neutrophils was in the order of 22:6*n-3* > 20:4*n-6* > 20:3*n-6* > 20:5*n-3* > 18:2*n-6*, 18:4*n-3*, 18:1*n-9* (Table 4.4).

Evidence has been presented that most of the above activities of fatty acids are dependent on a free carboxyl group. Conversion of the fatty acids 20:4*n-6*, 20:5*n-3* and 20:6*n-3* to their methyl esters resulted in complete loss of neutrophil stimulating activity with respect to adherence (139), superoxide production (131), degranulation (135) and migration inhibition (126). Interestingly, the methyl esters are still capable of partitioning into neutrophil plasma membrane (57). This suggests that membrane perturbation is insufficient for biological activity.

10. Cytokine Induced Alteration in Neutrophil Responses to Polyunsaturated Fatty Acids

A variety of mediators are involved in regulating the different phases of the inflammatory reaction. While in many cases we have a comprehensive understanding of the effects of the individual mediators, the ability of these mediators to influence each other's activity remains ill-defined. Cytokines are another class of mediators which are generated during inflammation and it is of interest to know whether or not cytokines and polyunsaturated fatty acids act synergistically. This question was recently addressed by Li et al (175) in which the effects of pre-exposure of neutrophils to the pro-inflammatory cytokines, tumor neurosis factor (TNF), on fatty acid-induced superoxide productions were examined. Neutrophils pretreated with TNF showed a markedly increased response to a range of fatty acids; 18:1*n-9*, 18:2*n-6*, 18:3*n-3*, 20:4*n-6*, 20:5*n-3* and 22:6*n-3*. Neither the saturated fatty acid 20:0 nor the hydroperoxy-/hydroxyderivatives of 20:4*n-6* showed any interaction with TNF. A similar synergistic response was seen with LTB_4 and TNF. In contrast and as expected TNF-treated neutrophils showed no increase in response to PGE_2. In fact a reduction in the TNF response was observed. These findings illustrate that the combination of two quite different mediators leads to responses which are several fold higher than that achieved with an individual cytokine.

Although this network of interaction needs to be studied in more detail, it is evident that a synergistic response is also seen between granulocyte macrophage-colony stimulating factor and polyunsaturated fatty acids (Fig. 4.10). In addition, a synergistic superoxide response was also seen between polyunsaturated fatty acids and fMLP or PMA (131,177). Besides being evident for superoxide production, this network of interaction is likely to be relevant to other neutrophil responses. Indeed, this is demonstrated by our other finding that TNF and polyunsaturated fatty acids are synergistic with respect to degranulation (Li Y. & Ferrante A., unpublished). Synergistic responses between the lipoxygenase products, LTB_4 and 5-oxo-ETE, and TNF have been demonstrated in terms of superoxide production (175,153,154).

Robinson et al (178) found TNF specifically altered the metabolism of neutrophil phosphatidylinositol, phosphatidic acid, phosphatidylethanolamine

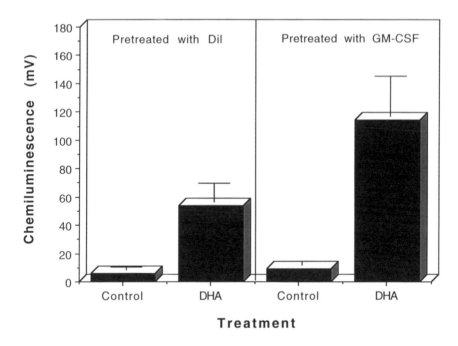

Figure 4.10.   Synergistic lucigenin-dependent chemiluminescence response induced by GM-CSF and DHA in human neutrophils. The results are the mean ± sem of three experiments and are presented as peak chemiluminescence response. The response of neutrophils treated with GMCSF and DHA simultaneously is greater than the sum of the responses observed with either compound alone ($p < 0.01$).

and phosphatidylcholine. TNF caused an increase in incorporation of radiolabelled AA into cellular phosphatidylinositol and phosphatidic acid but the incorporation into phosphatidylcholine and phosphatidylethanolamine was slower. AA was exclusively esterified at the sn-2 position of these phospholipids. There was no change in the labelling pattern of neutral lipids and eicosanoids and the cytokine showed no effect on the distribution of the radiolabel in 1-acyl, 1-akyl and 1-alk-1-enyl subclasses of phosphatidylcholine, phosphatidylethanolamine and triglyceride. TNF did not alter β-oxidation, chain elongation and desaturation of AA. Phospolipase D and C were not activated by TNF and it had no effect on the activity of the neutral and acidic sphingomyelinase.

11. Neutrophil Priming Properties of Fatty Acids

Many studies of microbicidal activity and target cell killing conducted *in vitro* usually use peripheral blood neutrophils which have not undergone the typical alterations induced by inflammatory mediators In reality, neutrophils come under the influence of a range of mediators which will regulate their antimicrobial activity. Over the past decade evidence has been presented that interactions of neutrophils with microbial, tumor and host tissue targets can be significantly modified by prior exposure of the leukocytes to various mediators. Particular interest has been paid to the role of cytokines in this neutrophil priming response. This priming results in an increase in the neutrophil response to a challenge agonist, observable as an increase in the binding of a ligand, biochemical responses elicited, phagocytosis and in microbial killing and tissue damage. It has been argued and evidence has been presented that both activated T lymphocytes and macrophages regulate these functions of the neutrophil through the release of cytokines (179,180).

Some of the most studied cytokines in relation to neutrophil priming for increased antimicrobial activity and tissue damage are TNFα, GM-CSF, IFN-γ and lymphotoxin (LT or TNFβ). For example TNF has been shown to play a critical role in immunity to infection (181). Pre exposure of neutrophils to TNF leads to increased phagocytosis and killing of bacteria and parasites (182,183). Many of these mediators also stimulate the release of 20:4*n-6* or alter the activity of PLA_2 (Table 4.1). The released fatty acids may act as second messengers, priming neutrophils for enhanced responses to other mediators.

11.1 *Alteration of responses to fMLP and PMA*

Our studies have demonstrated that pretreating neutrophils with polyunsaturated fatty acids enhances their capacity to respond to either fMLP or PMA, thereby producing more superoxide than when challenged with a compound alone (131,176), (Table 4.5). The simultaneous addition of a fatty acid and fMLP/ PMA also significantly enhances the response above that observed with one compound alone. On the other hand, a fatty acid *per se* is unable to stimulate

Table 4.5   Modulation of superoxide production by PUFAs in phagocytic cells

Effects/treatments	Neutrophils			Macrophages		
	AA	EPA	HDA	AA	EPA	HDA
FA alone	√	√	√	X	X	X
Synergisms						
with fMLP	√	√	√	√	√	√
with PMA	√	√	√	√	√	√
Priming for						
fMLP-induced CL	√	√	√	√	√	√

√: active; X: inactive/poor response; FA: fatty acids; CL: chemiluminescence

superoxide production in macrophages (134). Enhancement of superoxide production by macrophages is observed when macrophages are pretreated with a fatty acid or when a fatty acid is added simultaneously with fMLP or PMA. The reasons for the differences in the responses observed between macrophages and neutrophils are unclear. However, it could be related to the inability of fatty acids to stimulate the release of AA in macrophages (see "Activation of intracellular signals").

11.2 *Antimicrobial activity*

Neutrophils pre-exposed to polyunsaturated fatty acids show increased killing of intraerythocytic asexual stages of *Plasmodium falciparum* (182). This was seen both with respect to the antibody independent and antibody dependent killing of the parasite by neutrophils. Neutrophils pretreated with polyunsaturated fatty acids showed increased phagocytosis of the parasite and increased production of oxygen radicals. These fatty acids were also able to significantly reduce the parasitemia in murine malaria (184).

Extensive investigations show that the fatty acid structure plays a critical role in the ability of the fatty acid to enhance neutrophil parasite killing. Optimal stimulation was seen with polyunsaturated 20- 22- carbon fatty acids. The saturated fatty acids 18:0 and 20:0 had no effect and neither did 18:1*n-9*, 18:2*n-6*. As the carbon chain length was increased from 22 → 24 → 28 there was a gradual decrease in activity shown by comparing 20:4*n-6*, 24:4*n-6* and 28:4*n-6*. As previously seen with respect to their inability to induce responses in neutrophils, the methyl ester, 15-hydroperoxy- and 15-hydroxy derivatives of AA and DHA showed very little effect. It was evident from our studies that combined pre-exposure of neutrophils with TNF and polyunsaturated fatty acids led to a synergistic increase in neutrophil-mediated killing of the parasite (182). More recently we have demonstrated that these polyunsaturated fatty acids, 20:4*n-6* and 22:6*n-3* increase killing of the *Staphylococcus aureus,* non-typable *haemophilus influenza* and *Candida albicans* by neutrophils (unpublished).

11.3 *Tissue damage*

In exacerbated inflammation, the non-specific release of AA may lead to activation of neutrophils and damage to tissue. This is in addition to a cocktail of inflammatory mediators, including AA, which has been demonstrated to directly kill cells (185) We recently addressed this issue with respect to neutrophil mediated damage of the endothelium (140). The finding showed that 20:4*n-6* and 22:6*n-3* enhanced the neutrophil-mediated detachment of endothelial cell monolayers. Interestingly 20:5*n-3* was very poor in causing this damage. Correlating with effects on other neutrophil functions was the relationship between the type of fatty acid structure and ability to augment neutrophil-mediated damage to endothelial cells (135) (Table 4.6). Saturated fatty acids, methyl ester forms and hydroperoxy/hydroxy forms of polyunsaturated fatty acids were without effect. There was a slight but insignificant increase in this neutrophil function by 18:1*n-9*, 18:2*n-6*, 18:3*n-2* and 18:4*n-3*. For example 20:4*n-3* was 7–8 times more effective than 18:4*n-3* (135). It was also identified that the major mechanism by which polyunsaturated fatty acid-prime neutrophils for damage to endothelial cells is through the release of elastase (140).

Table 4.6   Effects of fatty acids on neutrophil-mediated microbial killing and tissue damage

Fatty acid	Parasite killing	Endothelial cell damage
18:0	–	–
18:1*n-9*	–	±
18:2*n-6*	–	+
18:3*n-6*	–	±
18:3*n-3*	–	+
18:4*n-3*	–	±
20:0	–	–
20:3*n-6*	+ +	
20:3*n-9*	+ + +	
20:4*n-6*	+ + + +	+ + + +
20:5*n-3*	+ + +	+
22:6*n-3*	+ + +	+ + ±
22:4*n-6*	+ + ±	
24:4*n-6*	+	
28:4*n-6*	–	
32:4*n-6*	–	

The number of + signs show the activity relative to each other. The – sign signifies no activity.

The above demonstrates that 20:4*n-6* and cytokines share many properties. Thus, both TNF and 20:4*n-6* enhance neutrophil microbial killing and phagocytosis, enhance the degranulation and respiratory burst response to fMLP, and inhibit migration of cells in a chemotactic gradient.

11.4 *Cell surface receptor expression*

As described above polyunsaturated fatty acids eg AA and their metabolic products eg LTB_4 alter the antimicrobial and tissue damaging properties of neutrophils. Some of the mechanisms responsible for this priming or enhancement have been partly defined. The basis of the fatty acid induced enhancement may relate to changes in the surface expression of functional receptors on neutrophils. Studies using long chain polyunsaturated fatty acids have shown that, while the saturated fatty acid 20:0 had no effect on the expression of β-2 integrin molecules, 20:4n-6, 20:5n-3 and 22:6n-3 significantly increased the expression of the complement receptor type 3 (CR3), CD11b/CD18 (139) (Table 4.7, Fig. 4.11). The fatty acids also caused a slight but insignificant increase in expression of CR4 (CD11c/CD18) and failed to alter the expression of the leucocyte adhesion functional antigen, LFA-1 (CD11a/CD18).

The CD11b/CD18 molecule is a receptor for the C3bi component of complement which is deposited on microorganisms and tissues, promoting neutrophil binding, phagocytosis and damage to these targets. This may explain, at least in part, the increase in bacterial and parasite damage seen with polyunsaturated fatty acid-primed neutrophils (182; Mogadhami N, Robinson B, Hii CST, Rathjen DA and Ferrante A, unpublished).

Table 4.7   Fatty acid induced changes to neutrophil β_2 integrins

Fatty acid	Receptor type		
	CD11a	CD11b	CD11c
20:0	–	–	–
20:4n-6	–	+ + + +	±
20:5n-3	–	+ + +	±
22:6n-3	–	+ + + +	+
LTB$_4$		+ + +	
5-oxo-ETE	–	+ +	–
5-HETE		+	
LTB$_3$		+ + +	
LTB$_5$		+	
LTC$_1$		+	
LTD$_4$		–	
5-HPETE		+	
LTC$_4$		±	

Number of + indicates degree of effectiveness. – indicates lack of effect.
± indicates intermediate effect.

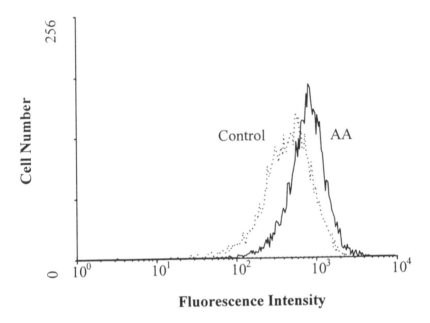

Figure 4.11. Increased expression of CD11b on human neutrophils stimulated with 20 μM AA. Neutrophils were treated with AA for 30 minutes at 37°C and then examined for expression of CD11b by flow cytometry analysis using phycoerythrin-labelled monoclonal antibodies to CD11b (Becton Dickinson, California).

The CD11b/CD18 molecules are also known to interact with fibrinogen, coagulation factor, bacterial lipopolysaccharide and ICAM-1 in endothelial cells. This may explain the increased adherence properties of neutrophils treated with these fatty acids (139,140) as well as their increase in endothelial cell damage (135). The increase in CD11b/CD18 expression is likely to be the result of increased degranulation caused by the polyunsaturated fatty acids (see "Stimulation of degranulation"). Ultrastructural and immunofluorescence studies have localised spare CD11b/CD18 to specific and secretory granules and recruitment of CD11b/CD18 have been tightly correlated with the release of specific granule content (186–188).

The effects of products of fatty acid metabolism on surface receptor expression of neutrophils has also been reported and is summarised in Table 4.7.

The lipoxygenase product LTB_4 is also a powerful stimulator of increased CR3 expression on neutrophils (189). Other eicosanoid with activity includes 5-oxo-ETE (154) which is much more active than 5-HETE. 5-oxo-ETE acts independently of LTB_4 and not via the same receptor (154). Although 5-oxo-ETE increases expression of CD11b it does not increase the expression of CD11a, CD11c, Fc(RII and Fc(RIII (154). LTB_3 is also highly active in increasing expression of CD11b (190,191).

12. Mechanisms of Fatty Acid-Induced Neutrophil Activation

12.1 *Polyunsaturated fatty acids stimulate neutrophils independently of lipoxygenase and cylooxygenase pathways*

Because AA gives rise to highly active eicosanoids, these products have been thought to be responsible for the stimulatory properties of AA on neutrophils. However, the effects of 20:4*n-6* are unlikely to be due to metabolism of 20:4*n-6*. In the first instance, the 20:5*n-3* which yields metabolites with lower proinflammatory activity than those derived from 20:4*n-6* was just as active as AA in stimulating neutrophil functions. Other evidence has also been provided. When neutrophils were pretreated with either lipoxygenase (caffeic acid or nordihydroguaiaretic acid — NDGA) or cycloxygenase (indomethacin) inhibitors, no effect on 20:4*n-6* induced adhesive properties of neutrophils or on the respiratory burst were observed (131,135).

Similar observations were made with the migration inhibition properties of polyunsaturated fatty acids (126). Pretreatment of neutrophils with either indomethacin or NDGA did not affect the fatty acid-induced inhibition of random and chemotactic migration (126). Under these conditions there was near complete inhibition of the cycloxygenase and lipoxygenase pathways.

Polyunsaturated fatty acid-induced increase in neutrophil-mediated damage to endothelial cells also occurs independently of the cycloxygenase and lipoxygenase pathways. Under conditions where indomethacin and NDGA inhibited these pathways, the enhancement of neutrophil-mediated endothelial cell damage by AA was not affected (140).

The effects of 20:4n-6 on intracelluar signalling molecules are also independent of the metabolism of 20:4n-6 by the lipoxygenases. Thus, we have demonstrated that stimulation of dual phosphorylation of p38 MAP kinase by 20:4n-6 in neutrophils was not affected by NDGA (unpublished data) On the other hand, some effects of 20:4n-6 in other cell-types are dependent on the formation of metabolites of 20:4n-6. For example, inhibition of gap junctional communication by 20:4n-6 in WB rat liver epithelial cells was prevented by NDGA (192).

12.2 Differences in metabolism of long chain and very long chain polyunsaturated fatty acids

Because the activity of the polyunsaturated fatty acids on neutrophils was highly dependent on structure, it has been of interest to know whether neutrophils handle the long and very long chain fatty acids differently. A study was undertaken by Robinson et al, (66) to compare the incorporation of two tetraenoic very long chain fatty acids, 34:4n-6 and 30:4n-6 with 20:4n-6 into neutral lipids and phospholipids of neutrophil and to examine their conversion into oxygenated derivatives. The findings showed that both 20:4n-6 and 24:4n-6 were readily taken up by human neutrophils. These were esterified into neutral lipids and phospholipids, and elongated by up to four carbon units. However 30:4n-6 was poorly incorporated and remained essentially in the original unesterified form. Both 24:4n-6 and 30:4n-6 were predominantly esterified into triacylglycerol. Neutrophils poorly β-oxidised and desaturated the three types of fatty acids. Activation of neutrophils with calcium ionophore, A23187, resulted in the generation of different oxygenated products. Metabolism of 20:4n-6 generated mainly 5-monohydroxy — 20:4n-6 and LTB$_4$, 24:4n-6 gave rise to monohydroxylated fatty acids, mainly the 9-hydroxy positional isomer, but not other lipoxygenase and cycloxygenase products. In contrast 30:4n-6 gave rise to negligible oxygenated fatty acids, suggesting that it is a poor substrate for neutrophil cylooxygenase and lipoxygenase enzymes.

12.3 Activation of intracellular signals

In order to understand how fatty acids induce neutrophil functional responses or alter the cell's response to a second agonist, there is a need to know which intracellular signals the fatty acids activate. Although polyunsaturated fatty acids have been found not to stimulate the activity of phospholipase C or D in neutrophils (177,193), various polyunsaturated fatty acids have been shown to activate a heterogenous group of intracellular signalling molecules (Table 4.8). These include the heterotrimeric G proteins, the neutral sphingomyelinase, protein kinase C (PKC) and the ERK and p38 MAP kinases. Fatty acids also stimulate calcium mobilisation, the release of rhoGDI from the rac2/rhoGDI complex and modulate ion channel conductance.

Table 4.8   Intracellular signals activated by polyunsaturated fatty acids

Fatty acid	Signalling molecules						
	Ca^{2+} mobilisation	ERK1 ERK2	p38	SMase	PKC	PLA$_2$	JNK
18:0	−			−			
18:1n-9				+			
18:2n-6				+		+	
18:4n-6							
20:0	−	−		−	−	−	
20:4n-6	+	+	+	+	+	+	+
20:5n-3	+	+		+	+	+	
22:4n-6	+						
22:6n-3	+	+		+	+	+	
24:4n-6	−						
28:4n-6	−			−			
30:4n-6	+						
32:4n-6	−						

The + sign and − sign indicate that the fatty acid is active or non-active in stimulating the respective function. Smase: sphingomyelinase; ERK: extracellular signal regulated protein kinase; PKC: protein kinase C; PLA$_2$: phospholipase A$_2$; JNK: c-jun N-terminal kinase.

12.4 *Mobilisation of intracellular calcium*

Ca^{2+} plays a central role in cell physiology. This second messenger regulates diverse functions such as secretion, muscle contraction, metabolism, neuronal excitability, cell proliferation and cell death. The cytosolic Ca^{2+} concentration is tightly regulated. In the resting cell, Ca^{2+} is maintained in the nM levels. Upon stimulation, intracellular Ca^{2+} concentrations can reach 1 mM (194,195). Ligand-stimulated increases in the intracellular Ca^{2+} concentration come mainly from 2 sources: release from intracellular stores such as the endoplasmic reticulum by inositol trisphosphate or from the sarcoplasmic reticulum.by cyclic ADP ribose, and influx via plasma membrane Ca^{2+} channels. The Ca^{2+} which is stored in the sarcoplasmic reticulum can also be released by ryanodine (196). Elevated intracellular Ca^{2+} concentrations are then returned to pre-stimulation levels by Ca^{2+} pumps which are located on the plasma membrane and membranes of the endoplasmic and sarcoplasmic reticulum.

In neutrophils, stimulation by agonists that bind to the G protein-coupled 7 transmembrane-type receptors such as the fMLP receptor, trigger increases in intracellular Ca^{2+}. Polyunsaturated fatty acids have been shown to cause an increase in intracellular Ca^{2+} concentrations in a variety of different cells, including neutrophils (193,197,198) (Fig. 4.12). Saturated fatty acids failed to mobilise Ca^{2+}. An examination of the Ca^{2+} mobilisation properties of polyunsaturated fatty acids with different structural elements was carried out by Hardy et al (193). The results showed that the ability to mobilise calcium was as follows: 20:4*n-6* > 30:4*n-6* > 22:4*n-6* > 18:4*n-6*. 28:4*n-6* > 24:4*n-6* > 32:4*n-6* (Table 4.8). While there is a general trend correlating the degree of Ca^{2+} mobilisation and ability to stimulate superoxide production it is evident that discrepancies exist (193) (Fig. 4.9). The most obvious is that 30:4*n-6* is a strong inducer of intracellular calcium mobilisation but induces no superoxide response (Fig. 4.9). It was also interesting that 20:4*n-6* releases intracellular Ca^{2+} via a thapsigargin-sensitive pool while 30:4*n-6* mobilises Ca^{2+} via a thapsigargin-insensitive pool in neutrophils (193).

20:4*n-6* derived products such as 5-oxo-ETE (152,153) and LTB_4 (199) also trigger calcium transients in neutrophils. LTB_4 effects occur via its binding to a receptor and it is believed that 5-oxo-ETE also acts via a specific receptor (106) and clearly independent of LTB_4 receptors. Other eicosanoids can also

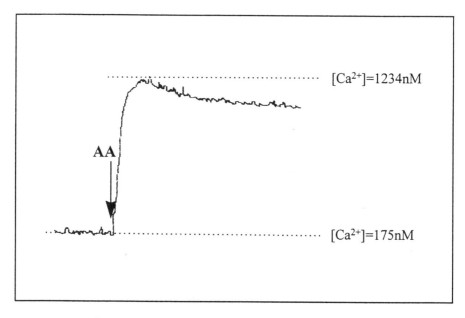

Figure 4.12. Ca^{2+} mobilisation response in human neutrophils stimulated with AA. Fura-2AM loaded neutrophils ($6 \times 10^6/2$ ml) were stimulated with 20 μM AA. The other polyunsaturated fatty acids gave essentially similar responses.

stimulate Ca^{2+} mobilisation. Thus, 12-HETE and 12-HPETE have been shown to stimulate the release of stored Ca^{2+} in neutrophils (200).

12.5 *Heterotrimeric G-proteins*

The heterotrimeric GTP-binding proteins are molecular switches which play crucial roles in transmembrane signalling. Composed of α, β and γ subunits, the G proteins couple the 7 transmembrane type receptors of hormones, growth factors, neurotransmitters and other bioactive molecules, including fMLP and PAF, to their intracellular signalling pathways. While the α submit is unique to a given G protein, the β and γ subunits of different G proteins are highly homologous. In the resting cell, the α subunit is bound by GDP. Receptor occupancy by a ligand causes a structural change in the receptor which then allows the receptor to interact with a G protein. This permits the exchange of GDP for GTP. The GTP-bound α subunit dissociates from the β and γ subunits and interacts with appropriate signalling molecules/structures such as adenylate cyclase, phospholipase Cb and phospholipase A_2. The α subunit also possessed an intrinsic GTPase activity which hydrolyses GTP. The resultant GDP-bound α subunit then reassociates with the β and γ subunits, thereby terminating effector activity.

The ability of AA to stimulate GDP/GTP exchange on the heterotrimeric G protein has previously been demonstrated in purified neutrophil membrane preparations (201). There was a positive correlation between the ability of fatty acid to increase [^{35}S] GTPγS binding and to elicit the respiratory burst. The order of effectiveness at causing GTP binding was 20:4*n-6* > 18:2*n-6* > 18:1*n-9*. The saturated fatty acids, 14:0 and 16:0 were ineffective. The ability of unsaturated fatty acids to stimulate nucleotide binding was blocked by pertussis toxin (201).

12.6 *Protein kinase C*

Protein kinase C (PKC, a family of serine/threonine protein kinases, is classified into three groups (i) classical PKC (α, βI, βII and γ), (ii) novel PKC (δ, ε, θ, η and μ) and (iii) atypical PKC (ζ, τ and λ). The classical PKC isozymes are activated by the combination of a phospholipid, calcium and diacylglycerol, and the novel PKC isozymes require phospholipid and diacylglycerol for activation. These forms can be activated in intact cells directly by PMA (132). The atypical forms require only a phospholipid and are not responsive to PMA (132).

Activation of PKC is required for a range of neutrophil activities such as the activation of the NADPH oxidase (202–205). *In vitro* studies using cell-free extracts/purified PKC have shown that many *cis*-fatty acids including 18:1*n-9*, 18:2*n-6*, 18:3*n-6*, 20:4*n-6*, 20:5*n-3* and 22:6*n-3* stimulate the activity of PKC α, β, γ, ε and ζ isozymes from rat brain in the presence of very low levels of Ca^{2+} and/or PS (206–208). Saturated fatty acids and *trans*-fatty acids failed to activate PKC. Hardy et al (209) demonstrated that while the very long chain polyunsaturated fatty acids 32:4*n-6* and 34:6*n-3* activated PKC *in* *vitro*, both failed to stimulate a respiratory burst in neutrophils (193). The ability of polyunsaturated fatty acids to stimulate PKC in whole cells has been documented (134,210). This is summarised in Table 4.9 for neutrophils and other cell types. In neutrophils polyunsaturated fatty acids stimulated the translocation of α, βI, βII to a particulate fraction. No increase in particulate fraction-associated PKCδ or ζ were detected (Hii C. S. T. et al. J. Biol. Chem. 1998; 273; 19277–19282). Similarly polyunsaturated fatty acids also stimulated the translocation of PKCα, βI, βII in macrophages (134) and of PKC α, δ and ε in WB cells (210) (Table 4.10).

12.7 *Activation of PLA$_2$ by 20:4n-6 and other fatty acids*

As shown in Table 4.1, neutrophils release radiolabelled 20:4*n-6* in response to a variety of external factors. This is due to the activation of PLA$_2$ (Fig. 4.3). It has been reported that neutrophils express at least three forms of PLA$_2$: sPLA$_2$, cPLA$_2$, iPLA$_2$ (40,60,211–213). A number of studies have demonstrated that exogenous 20:4*n-6* cause the release of radiolabelled 20:4*n-6* from prelabelled neutrophils (42,69).

This effect has been attributed to the formation of LTB$_4$ and the subsequent activation of cPLA$_2$ by LTB$_4$ binding to its receptor (42). However, our results argue against LTB$_4$ being a major cause for the fatty acid-stimulated activation of PLA$_2$. Thus, while 20:0 was inactive, 18:2*n-6*, 20:4*n-6*, 20:5*n-3* and 22:6*n-3* stimulated the release of 20:4*n-6* via both cPLA$_2$ and sPLA$_2$ (Robinson, Hii and Ferrante, Biochem. J. (in press)). The release of radiolabelled 20:4*n-6* and the production of superoxide caused by exogenous 20:4*n-6* or 22:6*n-3* were blocked by inhibitors of cPLA$_2$ or sPLA$_2$.

12.8 *Activation of the MAP kinases*

Mitogen-activated protein (MAP) kinases are proline-directed serine/threonine kinases which are activated by a wide variety of extracellular signals. Members of the MAP kinases include the extracellular signal-regulated kinases (ERK) 1 and 2, c-jun N terminal kinases (JNK) 1 and 2, and p38α, β, γ and δ. While

Table 4.9 Activation/translocation of PKC *in vitro* and *in vivo* by polyunsaturated fatty acids

Fatty acid	PKC activation		
	Cell free system	Neutrophils	Other cell types
18:1*n-9*	+		
18:2*n-6*	+		
18:3*n-6*	+		
20:0	−		
20:4*n-6*	+	+	+
20:5*n-3*	+		
22:6*n-3*	+		+
32:4*n-6*	+		
34:6*n-3*	−		
trans-fatty acids	−		

+: stimulate; −: no effect

Table 4.10 Activation/translocation of PKC isozymes by unsaturated fatty acids

		Activation in cell free system	Translocation in		
			neutrophils	macrophages	WB cells
cPKC					
	α	+	+	+	+
	βI	+	+	+	
	βII	+	+	+	
	γ	+			
nPKC					
	ε	+			+
	δ			+	+
aPKC					
	ζ	+		−	

cPKC: classical PKC; nPKC; novel PKC; aPKC: atypical PKC: +: stimulate/activate; −: no effect

ERK1 and ERK2 are activated by growth factors, serum and some cytokines, JNK1 and JNK2, and p38, also known as stress-activated protein kinases, are activated following the exposure of cells to inflammatory cytokines, bacterial toxins, hyperosmotic stress and UV irradiation. The MAP kinases are activated by MAP kinase kinases which phosphorylate the MAP kinases on threonine and tyrosine residues (Fig. 4.13). The MAP kinase kinases are, in turn, phosphorylated and activated by MAP kinase kinase kinases (Fig. 4.13). It is currently believed that the MAP kinase cascades form crucial links between the receptors at the plasma membrane and the nuclei since activated MAP kinases have been demonstrated to be present in the nuclei of activated cells (214–217).

We have previously demonstrated that AA, DHA and EPA stimulated the activity of ERK1 and ERK2 in rat liver epithelial WB cells (210). This effect was dependent on PKC since prolonged pretreatment of WB cells with PMA which resulted in the depletion of PMA-sensitive PKC isozymes, resulted in the complete abrogation of AA-induced ERK activation. Our recent studies have also demonstrated that AA also caused the activation and phosphorylation of the 42-kDa and 43-kDa forms of ERK in human neutrophils at concentrations which correlate well with stimulation of superoxide production (Hii C. S. T. et al. J. Biol. Chem. 1998; 273; 19277–19282). AA and DHA also stimulated the activity of ERK in human macrophages (Huang, Hii and Ferrante, unpublished). AA also stimulated the dual phosphorylation of p38 at concentrations which stimulate superoxide production. However, AA did not stimulate the activity of JNK in neutrophils although the fatty acid stimulated JNK activity in Jurkat T cells (unpublished data), proximal tubular epithelial cells (218) and stromal cells (219). Stimulation of JNK activity by AA in proximal tubule cells was dependent on the generation of superoxide (218). Given that AA stongly stimulates superoxide production in neutrophils, it is,therefore, surprising that AA did not stimulate JNK activity in neutrophils.

12.9 *Activation of sphingomyelinase*

A variety of extracellular agonists can trigger the activation of sphingomyelinase (Smase) which hydrolyses membrane sphingomyelin to generate the recently-

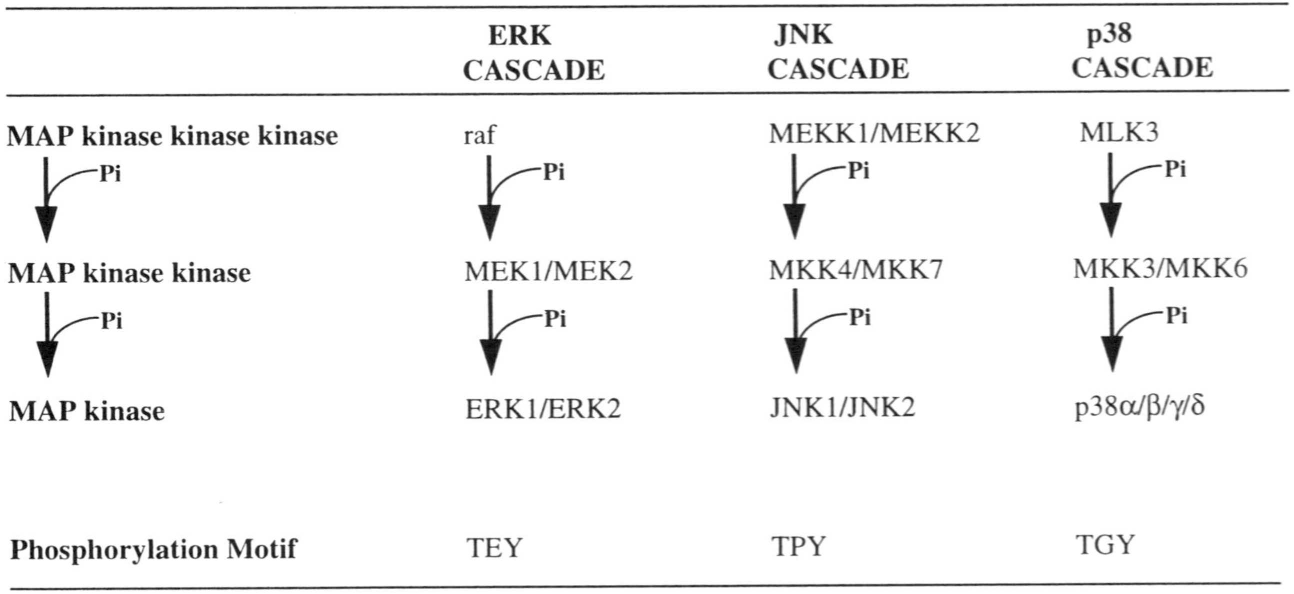

	ERK CASCADE	JNK CASCADE	p38 CASCADE
MAP kinase kinase kinase	raf →Pi	MEKK1/MEKK2 →Pi	MLK3 →Pi
MAP kinase kinase	MEK1/MEK2 →Pi	MKK4/MKK7 →Pi	MKK3/MKK6 →Pi
MAP kinase	ERK1/ERK2	JNK1/JNK2	p38α/β/γ/δ
Phosphorylation Motif	TEY	TPY	TGY

Figure 4.13. Components of the MAP Kinase cascades. The MAP Kinase cascades are involved in transmitting signals received at the plasma membrane into the nucleus. In haematopoietic cells, the ERK, JNK and p38 cascades have been reported to mediate cytokine synthesis, proliferation and survival/death. MAP kinase: Mitogen-Activated protein Kinase; ERK: Extracellular signal-Regulated protein Kinase; MEK: MAP ERK Kinase; MKK: MAP Kinase Kinase; MEKK: MEK kinase; MLK: Mixed Lineage Kinase; JNK: c-Jun N-terminal protein Kinase.

described second messenger molecule, ceramide (220). Several different types of sphingomyelinases have been described. These include a neutral, Mg^{2+}-dependent enzyme, localised in the outer leaflet of the plasma membrane; a neutral sphingomyelinase which shows no dependence on divalent cations, resident in the cytosol and an acidic sphingomyelinase which has no dependence on divalent cations, located in the endosomal/lysosomal compartments of the cell (221). Each enzyme appears to act on a distinct pool of sphingomyelin, releasing ceramide. Ceramide causes growth arrest, promotes cell differentiation, down-regulates *c-myc* proto-oncogene and induces apoptosis (220). 20:4*n-6* have been shown to stimulate the hydrolysis of sphingomyelin by the neutral sphingomyelinase in human neutrophils (222). This was associated with an accumulation of ceramide within the neutrophils. The activity of the acidic sphingomyelinase was not affected by the fatty acids (222). The effect of 20:4*n-6* on the activity of the neutral sphingomyelinase was transient, peaking at five minutes and returning to normal by 10 min after exposure. Significant increases in the activity of the enzyme was seen with 2.5 μM of 20:4*n-6*.

Other long chain mono/polyunsaturated fatty acids also caused the activation of sphingomyelinase in neutrophils (222). The fatty acids 18:1*n-9*, 18:2*n-6*, 20:5*n-3* and 22:6*n-3* were all active in this property. However, the saturated fatty acid 18:0 and 20:0, and the very long chain polyunsaturated fatty acids, 24:4*n-6* and 28:4*n-6* did not activate the enzyme system (222). Other alterations in the structure of 20:4*n-6*, such as derivatisation to the methyl ester, hydroxy- and hydroperoxy- forms lead to a loss of ability to stimulate sphingomyelinase activity (222).

12.10 *Ion channels*

Fatty acids, including AA, are implicated in the direct and indirect modulation of a number of voltage-gated ion channels. For example, in whole-cell patch-clamp experiments in rat pulmonary myocytes, external application of AA caused membrane depolarisation, accelerated the rate of rectifier K^+ current activation and a marked acceleration of current decay (223). The effects were not affected by indomethacin or NDGA, suggesting that AA *per se* was responsible for these effects. The actions of the fatty acids on K^+ current was dependent on the number of double bonds but was independent of carbon length between 14–22 carbons. An involvement of PKC in the actions of AA was suggested by inhibitor studies (223).

AA also alters the permeability of Na^+ channels. Thus, in skeletal muscle, AA can either inhibit or activate Na^+ channels (224) This effect was dependent on fatty acid structure and site of exposure. While cytoplasmic delivery of low concentrations of AA (5 μM) augmented voltage-activated Na^+ channel current, external application of the fatty acid inhibited Na^+ current (224). Similar effects were observed with 18:1n-9. Fatty acid-induced increase in Na^+ current was not dependent on PKC.

Effects of AA on ion channels in neutrophils have also been reported. The human neutrophil NADPH oxidase-associated H^+ channel acts as a charge compensator for the electrogenic generation of superoxide and it has been reported that a H^+-selective conductance is activated during the respiratory burst in neutrophils (225). Although the identity of this H^+ channel has not been clearly established, there is some evidence to suggest that the large subunit of the NADPH oxidase cytochrome b (gp91^{phox}) may act as a H^+ channel (225). Whole-cell patch-clamp studies of neutrophils have demonstrated that externally applied AA amplified a H^+-selective conductance (226). Thus, AA may also play a role in the respiratory burst by facilitating the dissipation of metabolically generated acid.

12.11 *Modulation of the activation status of small GTP binding proteins*

Fatty acids also alter the function of proteins which regulate the activation status of small GTP binding proteins. For example, AA has been found to inhibit the activity of p21^{ras} GTPase activating protein *in vitro* (227). This suggests that AA may prolong p21^{ras} function. Other *in vitro* studies have demonstrated that AA also cause the dissociation of rhoGDP Dissociation Inhibitor (rhoGDI) from rhoGDI-rac complex (228). This action can be mimicked by phosphatidic acid and phosphatidylinositol. In the resting neutrophil, all the cytosolic rac is complexed with rhoGDI (228). Current evidence suggests that rac has to be released from rhoGDI before rac can interact with GTP exchange factors and effectors. Given that rac is a component of the neutrophil NADPH oxidase and that only GTP-bound rac can interact with other components of the NADPH oxidase and stably translocate to the plasma membrane, it is possible that an important role for intracellular AA is to facilitate rac activation by causing the release of rac from rho GDI. However, this has yet to be demonstrated in intact neutrophils.

12.12 *Evidence for an involvement of PKC, ERK and p38 in AA-stimulated superoxide production*

The ability of AA and other polyunsaturated fatty acids to stimulate the translocation of a number of PKC isozymes and to stimulate the activity/ phosphorylation of ERK and p38 suggests that these kinases may be involved, at least in part, in mediating the effects of polyunsaturated fatty acids. It has previously been reported that PKC β can directly phosphorylate p47^{phox} in *in vitro* assays (229). Phosphorylation of p47^{phox} is currently believed to be a prerequisite for the translocation of p47^{phox} to the plasma membrane where it interacts with cytochrome b558. In activated neutrophils and in virally-transformed B lymphoblasts, p47^{phox} is phosphoylated on multiple serine residues. Phosphopeptide mapping revealed phosphorylation of serine 303/ 304, 315, 320,328, 345/348 and/or 359/370 (230–232). In *in vitro* phosphorylation experiments, it has been found that PKC phosphorylated all of the above serine residues except serine 345/348 while ERK and p38 phosphorylated serine 345/348 with similar rates (230-232). We have demonstrated that the ability of AA to stimulate superoxide production was partially blocked by GF109203X, PD98059 and SB203580, inhibitors of PKC, MEK and p38, respectively (unpublished data). Dose-inhibition curves showed that GF109203X, PD98059 and SB203580 maximally inhibited superoxide production by approximately 80, 60 and 55%, respectively. These inhibitors have been demonstrated to be very specific in their actions as demonstrated by *in vitro* kinase assays (233–235). For example, PD98059 has been demonstrated to inhibit MEK1 more than MEK2 and not to affect the activities of each of the 18 known kinases tested, including PKC and those in the JNK and p38 cascades (234). The IC_{50} of GF109203X for PKC is at least 100x lower than for other kinases (233).

The failure of each of the inhibitors to totally suppress AA-stimulated superoxide production suggests that activation of a number of kinases/ mechanisms are required for the assembly of an active NADPH oxidase and for optimal superoxide production. The effects of a combination of GF109203X, PD98059 and SB203580, at concentrations close to their IC_{50} in intact neutrophils, on AA-stimulated superoxide production were, therefore, determined. Simultaneous addition of these inhibitors suppressed superoxide production in an additive manner. However, total suppression of AA-stimulated superoxide production was still not observed, even when these inhibitors were used at twice their IC_{50} (unpublished data).

These data suggest that while PKC, ERK and p38 may play some roles in mediating the effects of AA on superoxide production, other mechanisms may also be involved in mediating the actions of polyunsaturated fatty acids on the respiratory burst. The active NADPH is a complex of a number of cytosolic proteins such as p47^{phox}, p67^{phox} and rac2 and components of the plasma membrane-bound cytochrome b558 (128,129). It is likely that signalling molecules in addition to PKC, ERK and p38 are also involved in regulating the translocation of these molecules to the plasma membrane. For example, rhoGDI has to be released from rac2 and the latter loaded with GTP before rac2 can translocate to the plasma membrane as has been proposed (228). There is currently no evidence that PKC, ERK or p38 is involved in facilitating these processes. Other signalling molecules such as phosphatidylinositol 3-kinase could also play a role in mediating the actions of polyunsaturated fatty acids on superoxide production since wortmannin, an inhibitor of phosphatidylinositol 3-kinase, has been demonstrated to inhibit fMLP-stimulated superoxide production. Another signalling molecule which may be involved in mediating, at least in part, the effects of AA on the NADPH oxidase is phospholipase A_2. It has been reported that incubation of neutrophils with radio-labelled AA resulted in the release of radio-labelled AA via the activation of PLA_2 (69; see Table 4.1). Inhibition of $cPLA_2$ with arachidonyltrifluoroketone inhibited fatty acid-stimulated release of radio-labelled AA and superoxide production (Robinson B., Hii C. S. T. and Ferrante, A. Biochem. J. (in press). This suggests that endogenously generated AA is involved in mediating the actions of exogenously added AA. It also suggests that exogenously added AA and endogenously generated AA may exist as two distinct pools of AA and each pool may regulate different processes in triggering superoxide production. In contrast to neutrophils, monocytes/macrophages do not release radio-labelled AA when exposed to exogenous AA (19), suggesting that AA does not stimulate the activity of PL A$_2$ in monocytes. This may provide a reason for the inability of polyunsaturated fatty acids *per se* to trigger a respiratory burst in monocytes/ macrophages.

On the other hand, other studies have questioned the role of PKC in the action of AA on neutrophil respiratory burst (236). Thus, inhibition of PKC by monochloramine which inhibited PMA-stimulated respiratory burst did not affect AA-stimulated response (236). Other observations which are not consistent with an involvement of PKC or other kinases in the action of AA include the direct stimulation of superoxide production by AA in reconstituted systems in the absence of ATP and Ca^{2+} (133,237). The ability of SDS to mimic the actions of AA on superoxide production in the cell-free system has led to the suggestion that AA acts in a detergent-like manner to stimulate superoxide production. However studies by Corey and Rosoff (238) have excluded a detergent-like action of polyunsaturated fatty acids as a primary mechanism by which fatty acids stimulate superoxide production. It is clear from cell-free studies that higher concentrations of AA are needed to stimulate superoxide production than from intact neutrophils. Thus, in intact neutrophils, AA-stimulated superoxide production was easily detectable at 5 μM or less (131) while at least 25 μM was needed to elicit a detectable response in cell-free systems (237). Hence, very high concentrations of AA (82–160 μM) were used in these *in vitro* studies (133,237). While the ability of AA to directly stimulate superoxide production in cell-free sytems cannot be denied, it is possible that the discrepancy between our results and those of Ogino et al (236) in intact neutrophils could be due to the amount of exogenous AA being used. It is unlikely that other physical parameters, such as the type of solvents and media that were used, could have caused the discrepancy since similar solvents and media were used. In our studies, we have used AA up to a maximum of 30 μM (usually 20 μM), a concentration which is within levels reported to prevail in stimulated cells (239) and in plasma of human malaria patients (240). The response observed at 30 μM (giving 10–20 fold stimulation above control) was still in the linear part of a dose-response curve. On the other hand, Ogino et al (236) used 100 μM AA to stimulate their neutrophils. At this higher concentration, the rate of AA uptake would be expected to be higher (see "Transport and uptake of fatty acids"), resulting in more AA being in the intracellular compartment at any given instance than at a lower exogenous AA concentration. Consequently, the higher amount of AA in the intracellular compartment could have created an environment which resembled that of a cell-free system, thereby, allowing AA to predominantly and directly stimulate superoxide production without the need to act via kinase such as PKC, ERK or p38. Although we cannot exclude the possibility that AA also interacts with components of the NADPH oxidase in neutrophils which are exposed to low concentrations of exogenous AA, it is unlikely that the stimulatory effect of AA on superoxide production in our studies is mediated entirely via a direct action of the fatty acid on components of the NADPH oxidase. In support of this, our results and those of Abramson et al (201) demonstrated that AA-stimulated responses could be inhibited by various kinase inhibitors and pertussis toxin. Futhermore AA-stimulated superoxide production could be inhibited by antagonists of calcium-binding proteins, and inhibitors and substrates of chymotrypsin-like proteases, thereby arguing against a detergent-like action of AA on the NADPH oxidase in intact neutrophils. (241).

Other biological actions of AA have also been reported to depend on PKC activation. These include effects of the fatty acid on K^+ conductance in arterial myocytes (222), on inhibition of gap junctional communication (192) and on the activity of ERK in WB cells and neutrophils (210 and unpublished data). On the other hand, the effects of AA on Na^+ channels in skeletal muscle are independent of PKC (224).

It is currently not clear how AA and other fatty acids stimulate the activity of cPLA$_2$. One possibility is via PKC, ERK and/or p38 since PKC, ERK and p38 have all been proposed to regulate the activity of cPLA$_2$ by phosphorylation (65,242). On the other hand, other studies have not found ERK or p38 to be responsible for regulating the activity of the cPLA$_2$ (23). This discrepancy may be due to cell-type differences. The intracellular signals employed by AA and other fatty acids to stimulate degranulation, adherence and enhance microbicidal activities have not been extensively studied, although the activation of cPLA$_2$ has been suggested to be required for degranulation (138).

13. Summary

The inflammatory response to infection and to auto-immune or allergic diseases is characterised by an accumulation of phagocytes at the sites of inflammation. These and other cell-types become activated by microbial products, opsonised particles and proinflammatory mediators. One of the consequences of cell stimulation is the activation of PLA$_2$ and release of AA and other fatty acids. During inflammation and infection, the concentrations of nonesterified fatty *acids in vivo* have been reported to be in the range which stimulate neutrophils *in vitro*. Essien (240) found that plasma free AA levels in human malaria patients were >100 μM and Yasuda *et al* (243) reported that the free AA levels in brain were 50 μM, rising to 500 μM under ischaemic conditions. Activated phagocytic cells *per se* produced 20–30 μM AA (244). Our studies and those of others have clearly demonstrated that polyunsaturated fatty acids such as AA stimulate and regulate a number of important functions of neutrophils, including adhesion, chemotaxis, activation of the respiratory burst and degranulation. These effects are specific, dependent on the activity of signalling molecules and are not due solely to the ability of a fatty acid to partition into the plasma membrane. Many of the biological properties of AA are retained by metabolites such as LTB$_4$ and 5-oxo-ETE.

Fatty acids and metabolites also modify the responses of neutrophils to other endogenous inflammatory mediators at sites of inflammation. Interaction between fatty acids and TNF or fMLP on neutrophil superoxide production have been demonstrated. Thus, AA ($\geq$3 μM) acted synergistically with fMLP to stimulate superoxide production. It needs to be appreciated that while *in vitro* studies on neutrophil functions have used a single fatty acid, in reality at sites of inflammation, a range of fatty acids and products will be found and hence the collective concentration of these lipids may be quite substantial. Consequently, the behaviour of neutrophils is likely to be influenced by AA and other lipid molecules *in vivo* and it is expected that the findings described in this Chapter deserve major consideration in events of acute and chronic inflammation.

Of particular importance is the demonstration that the biological actions of fatty acids on neutrophils can be dramatically altered by specific alterations to the structure of the fatty acids. These includes changes to carbon chain length, addition of hydroxy- or hydroperoxy- groups (and their position), degree of unsaturation and masking of the free carboxyl group. This has at least two implications. Firstly, it means that incorporation of different types of fatty acids into membrane phospholipids will result in a change in the composition of the phospholipids and an altered profile of lipid-based second messenger molecules (diacylglycerol, phosphatidic acid and fatty acids) being generated upon cell activation. This is likely to affect the activity of intracellular signalling molecules such as PKC. Secondly, because such alterations in fatty acid structure yields molecules which exhibit very specific actions (133,245) activity-dictated chemical engineering to produce novel fatty acids (246,247) offers potential therapeutic agents for treating a wide range of diseases.

The findings outlined in this Chapter are likely to have important implications in our understanding of the inflammatory reaction, during which inflammatory mediators, including lipids, generated from the surrounding cells, can interact with and prime neutrophils and monocytes/macrophages for enhanced respiratory burst. A likely scenario in which fatty acids can regulate the biological functions of neutrophils is proposed (Fig. 4.14). Stimulation of neutrophils and other cells-types such as monocytes, platelets and endothelial cells at sites of inflammation results in the activation PLA_2. This results in the liberation of non-esterified fatty acids such as AA from the sn-2 position of membrane phospholipids. While some of the liberated AA is released into the extracellular space, some is cell-associated. Cell-associated AA may play a direct second messenger role in regulating neutrophil biological responses. Although liberated AA can exist unmodified, some of it is metabolised by the lipoxygenases and cyclooxygenases to yield a number of biologically active products. Some of these metabolites such as LTB_4 are neutrophil

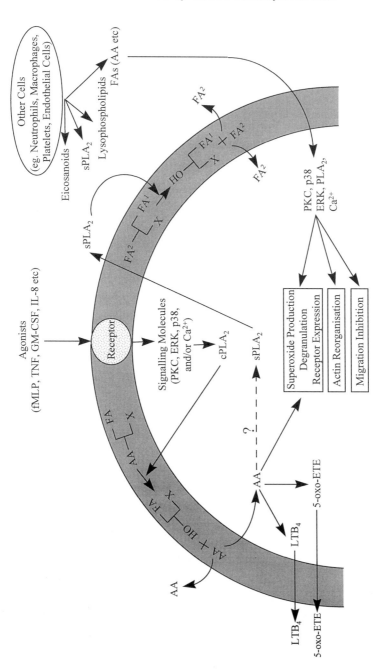

Figure 4.14.   Activated neutrophils and other cell types at sites of inflammation/tissue damage release non-esterified fatty acids and metabolites. These exert direct actions on the neutrophils and alter neutrophil responses to bacterial products, cytokines and other proinflammatory agents. The effects of the fatty acids are mediated by a number of intracellular signalling molecules. PKC: protein kinase C; ERK: extracellular signal-regulated protein kinase; cPLA$_2$: cytosolic phospholipase A$_2$; sPLA$_2$: secretory phospholipase A$_2$; FA: fatty acid; X: phosphocholine or phosphoinositol.

chemoattractants, which together with the other chemoattractants, including bacterial products and IL8, cause more neutrophils to infiltrate into the inflammatory sites. Once at the sites of inflammation, neutrophils are prevented from leaving by 20:4n-6. As the number of infiltrating cells increases, the levels of fatty acids and metabolites increase. These lipids exert direct effects on the neutrophils and also amplify the responses of the neutrophils to other inflammatory agents such as cytokines.

14. Acknowledgements

We are indebted to all our colleagues who have contributed towards our work and this has been appropriately referenced. Special thanks to our Laboratory Manager, Geoff Harvey, for providing an excellent working environment during the course of our studies and to Lynne Bullen for skilful secretarial assistance.

Our work received funding support from the National Health and Medical Research Council of Australia and the UNDP/World Bank/WHO Special Programme for Research and Training in Tropical Diseases and Channel 7 Children's Research Foundation.

15. References

1. Simopoulos A.P., *Am. J. Clin. Nutr.* **54** (1991), 438–463.
2. Greenfield S.M., *et al.*, *Aliment. Pharmacol. Ther.* **7** (1993), 159–166.
3. Campan P., Planchand P.O. and Duran D., *Bull. Group Int. Rech. Sci. Stomatol. Odontol.* **39** (1996), 25–31.
4. Leslie C.A., *et al.*, *J. Exp. Med.* **162** (1985), 1336–1349.
5. Kremer J.M., *et al.*, *Arthritis Rheum.* **38** (1995), 1107–1114.
6. Sperling R.I., *Rheum. Dis. Clin. North Am.* **17** (1991), 373–389.
7. Zurier R.B., *et al.*, *Arthritis Rheum.* **39** (1996), 1808–1817.
8. Harel Z., Biro F.M., Kottenhahn R.K. and Rosenthal S.L., *Am. J. Obstet. Gynecol.* **174** (1996), 1335–1338.
9. Deutch B., *Eur. J. Clin. Nutr.* **49** (1995), 508–516.
10. Gibson R.A., Neumann M.A. and Makrides M., *Lipids.* **31** (1996), Suppl: S177–S181.

11. Connor W.E, Lowensohn R. and Hatcher L., *Lipids.* **31** (1996), Suppl. S183–S187.

12. Uauy R., *et al., Lipids.* **31 Suppl** (1996), S167–S176.

13. Olsen S.F. and Secher N.J., *Br. J. Nutr.* **64** (1990), 599–609.

14. Bates D., *Ups. J. Med. Sci. Suppl.* **48** (1990), 173–187.

15. Laugharne J.D., Mellor J.E. and Peet M., *Lipids.* **31** (1996), Suppl: S163–S165.

16. Endres S., *N. Engl. J. Med.* **320** (1989), 265–271.

17. Williams W.V., Rosenbaum H. and Zurier R.B., *Pathobiology.* **64** (1996), 27–31.

18. Dennis E.A., *Tibs.* **22** (1997), 1–2.

19. Balsinde J. and Dennis E.A., *J. Biol. Chem.* **271** (1996), 6758–6765.

20. Shikano M., *et al., Biochim. Biophys. Acta.* **1212** (1994), 211–216.

21. Badiani K. and Arthur G., *Biochem. J.* **312** (1995), 805–809

22. Ohkubo S., Nakahata N. and Ohizumi Y.; *Prostaglandins,* **52** (1996), 403–413.

23. Kramer R.M, *et al., J. Biol. Chem.* **271** (1996), 27723–27729.

24. Sipka S., *et al., Ann. Hematol.* **69** (1994), 307–310.

25. Locati M., *et al., J. Biol. Chem.* **271** (1996), 6010–6016.

26. Chang J., Gilman S.C. and Lewis A.J., *J. Immunol.* **136** (1986), 1283–1287.

27. Roshak A.,Sathe G. and Marshall L.A., *J. Biol. Chem.* **269** (1994), 25999–26005.

28. Pearce M.J., *et al., Biochem. Biophys. Res. Commun.* **218** (1996), 500–504.

29. Fleisher-Berkovich S. and Danon A., *Endocrinol.* **136** (1995), 4068–4072.

30. Reddy S.T. and Herschman H.R., *J. Biol. Chem.* **271** (1996), 186–191.

31. Maridonneau-Parini I., Tringale S.M. and Tauber A.I., *J. Immunol.,* **137** (1986), 2925–2929.

32. Gijon M.A., Perez C. Mendez E. and Sanchez-Crespo M., *Biochem. J.* **306**, (1995), 167–175.

33. Bauldry S.A., McCall C.E. Cousart S.L., Bass D.A., *J. Immunol.* **146**, (1991), 1277–1285.

34. Doerfler M.E., Weiss J., Clark J.D. and Elsbach P., *J. Clin. Invest.* **93** (1994), 1583–1591.

35. Madsen L.M., Inada M. and Weiss J., *Infect. Immun.* **64** (1996), 2425–2430.

36. Gilbert J.J. *et al., J. Immunol.* **16** (1996), 2054–2061.

37. Los M., *et al., Embo. J.* **14** (1995), 3731–3740.

38. Cifone M.G., Cironi L., Santoni A. and Testi R., *Eur. J. Immunol.* **25** (1995), 1080–1086.

39. Lam B.K., Yang C.Y. and Wong P.Y., *Adv. Exp. Med. Biol.* **275** (1990), 183–191.

40. Lanni C. and Becker E.L., *Am. J. Pathol.,* **113** (1983), 90–94.

41. Roberts P.J., Williams S.L. and Linch D.C., *Br. J. Haematol.* **92** (1996), 804–814.

42. Wijkander J., O'Flaherty J.T., Nixon A.B. and Wykle R.L., *J. Biol. Chem.* **270** (1995), 26543–26549.

43. McDonald P.P., Pouliot M., Borgeat P. and McColl S.R., *J. Immunol.* **151** (1993), 6399–6409.

44. Schatz-Munding M. and Ullrich V., *Eur. J. Biochem.* **204**, (1992), 705–712.

45. McGarry J.E., in *The textbook of biochemistry with clinical correlations. 3rd edition,* ed. Devlin T.M. (Wiley-Liss, New York, 1993), 387–422.

46. Zhou S.L., *et al., Mol. Cell. Biochem.* **98** (1990), 183–189.

47. Vyska K., *Circ. Res.* **69** (1991), 857–870.

48. Tanaka T. and Kawamura K., *J. Mol. Cell. Cardiol.* **27** (1995), 1613–1622.

49. Sorrentino D., *et al., J. Clin. Invest.* **82** (1988), 928–935.

50. Van-Nieuwenhoven, F.A, *et al., Biochem. Biophys. Res. Commun.* **207** (1995), 747–752.

51. Greenwalt D.E., Scheck S.H. and Rhinehart-Jones T., *J. Clin. Invest.* **96** (1995), 1382–1388.

52. Cooper R.B., Noy N. and Zakim D., *J. Lipid Res.* **30**, (1989) 1719–1726.

53. Rose H., Hennecke T. and Kemmermeier H., *Mol. Cell. Biochem.* **88** (1989), 31–36.

54. Rose H., Hennecke T. and Kammermeier H., *J. Mol. Cell. Cardiol.* **22** (1990), 883–892.

55. Spector A.A., *in Polyunsaturated fatty acids in human nutrition,* ed Bracco U. and Deckelbaum R.J. (Nestle Nutrition workshop series Vol 28, Raven, New York, 1992). 1–12.

56. Poirier H., *et al., Eur. J. Biochem.* **238** (1996), 368–373.

57. Steinbeck M.J., Robinson J.M. and Karnovski M.J., *J. Leukoc. Biol.* **49** (1991), 360–368.

58. Anel A., Richieri G. V. and Kleinfeld A.M., *Bioichemistry.* **32** (1993), 530–535.

59. Bormann B.J., *et al., Proc. Natl. Acad. Sci. USA.*, **81** (1984), 767–770.

60. Traynor J.R. and Authi K.S., *Biochim. Biophys. Acta.* **665** (1981) 571–577.

61. Stewart A.G. and Harris T., *Lipids.* **26** (1991), 1044–1049.

62. Bauldry S.A., Wooten R.E. and Bass D.A., *Biochim. Biophys. Acta.* **1303** (1996), 63–73.

63. Nigam S., Fiore S., Luscinskas F.W. and Serhan C.N., *J. Cell. Physiol.* **143** (1990), 512–523.

64. Krump E., *et al., Biochem. J.* **310** (1995), 681–688.

65. Waterman W.H., *et al., Biochem. J.* **319** (1996), 17–20.

66. Robinson B.S., Johnson D.W., Ferrante A. and Poulos A., *Biochim. Biophys. Acta.* **1213** (1994), 325–334
67. O'Flaherty J.T., *J. Biol. Chem.* **271** (1996), 17821–17828.
68. Nahas N., Waterman W.H. and Sha'afi R.I., *Biochem. J.,* **313** (1996), 503–508.
69. Winkler J.D.,Sung C.M., Hubbard W.C. and Chilton F.H., *Biochem. J.* **291** (1993), 825–831.
70. Glew R.H., in *The textbook of biochemistry with clinical correlations. 3rd edition.* ed: Devlin T.M. (Wiley-Liss, New York., 1993). p423–473.
71. Lewis R.A. and Austen K.F., in *Inflammation: basic principles and clinical correlates,* ed. Gallin J.I. and Snyderman R. (Raven Press. Ltd., New York, 1988), 121–128.
72. Marcus A.J., in *Inflammation: basic principles and clinical correlates.,* ed. Gallin J.I. and Snyderman R., (Raven Press. Ltd., New York, 1988), 129–137.
73. Lokesh B.R., Black J.M., German J.B. and Kinsella J.E., *Lipids.* **23** (1988), 968–972.
74. Ziboh V.A., *Lipids.* **Suppl** (1996). S249–S53.
75. Fischer S., *et al., Biochem. Biophys. Res. Commun.* **120** (1984), 907–918.
76. Careaga-Houck M. and Sprecher H., *Biochim. Biophys. Acta.* **1047** (1990), 29–34.
77. Gadd M.A. and Hansbrough J.F., *J. Surg. Res.* **48** (1990), 84–90.
78. Watanabe S., Onozaki K., Yamamoto S. and Okuyama H., *J. Leukoc. Biol.* **53** (1993), 151–156
79. Taylor S.M., *et al., J. Leukoc. Biol.* **42** (1987), 253–262.
80. Lefkowith J.B., Morrison A., Lee V. and Rogers M., *J. Immunol.* **145** (1990), 1523–1529.
81. Kinsella J.E., Lokesh B. and Stone R.A., *Am. J. Clin Nutr.* **52** (1990), 1–28.
82. Broughton K.S., Whelan J., Hardardottir I. and Kinsella J.E., *J. Nutr.* **121** (1991), 155–164.
83. Surette M.E., *et al., Biochim. Biophys. Acta.* **1255** (1995), 185–191.
84. Laegreid W.W., *et al., Inflammation.* **12** (1988), 503–514.
85. Gibney J. and Hunter B., *Eur. J. Clin. Nutr.* **47** (1993), 255–259
86. Chilton F.H. *et al., J. Clin. Invest.* **91** (1993), 115–122.
87. Nichols R.C. and Vanderhoek J.Y., *J. Exp. Med.* **171** (1990), 367–375
88. Borgeat P., *Can. J. Physio. Pharmacol.* **67** (1989), 936–942.
89. Abbate R., *et al., Prostaglandins Leukot. Essent. Fatty Acids.* **41** (1990), 89–93.
90. Lee T.H., *et al., J. Clin. Invest.* **74** (1984), 1922–1933
91. Tou J.S. and Healey S., *Lipids,* **26** (1991), 327–330.

92. Swendsen C.L., *et al., Biochim. Biophys. Acta.* **919** (1987), 79–89.

93. Venable M.E., Olson S.C., Neito M.L. and Wykle R.L., *J. Biol. Chem.* **268** (1993), 7965–7975.

94. Arai M.,Imai H., Metori A.and Nakagawa Y., *Eur. J. Biochem.* **244** (1997), 513–519.

95. Steinson W.F. and Parker C.W., *Prostaglandins.* **18** (1997), 285–292.

96. Chilton-Lopez., *J. Immunol.* **156** (1996), 2941–2947.

97. Stuning M., Raulf M. and Konig W., *Biochem. Pharmacol.* **34** (1985), 3943–3950.

98. Iversen L., Fogh K., Bojesen G. and Kragballe K., *Agents. Actions.* **33** (1991) 286–291.

99. Vanderhoek J.Y., Bryant R.W. and Bailey J.M., *Biochem. Pharmacol.* **31** (1982), 3463–3467.

100. Ziboh V.A., Fletcher M.P., *Am. J. Clin. Nutr.* **55** (1992), 39–45.

101. von-Schacky C., *et al., Biochim. Biophys. Acta.* **1166** (1993), 20–24

102. McColl S.R., *et al., Br. J. Pharmacol.* **97** (1989), 1265–1273.

103. Vanderhoek J.Y. and Bailey J.M., *J. Biol. Chem.* **259** (1984), 6752–6756.

104. Powell W.S., Gravelle F., Gravel S. and Hashefi M., *J. Lipid.Mediat.* **6** (1993a), 361–368.

105. Zhang Y., Styhler A. and Powell W.S., *J. Leukoc. Biol.* **59** (1996), 847– 854.

106. Powell W.S., *et al., J. Immunol.* **156** (1996), 336–342.

107. Powell W.S., Gravelle F. and Gravel S., *J. Biol. Chem.* **269**, (1994a), 25373–25380.

108. Powell W.S., Zhang Y. and Gravel S., *Biochemistry.* **33** (1994b), 3927–3933.

109. Powell W.S., Gravel S. and Gravelle F., *J. Lipid Res.* **36** (1995), 2590–2598.

110. Ward P.A., Sulavik M.C. and Johnson K.J., *Am. J. Pathol.* **120** (1985), 112–120.

111. Walstra P., *et al., Biochim. Biophys. Acta.* **921** (1987), 312–319.

112. Rosolowsky M., Falck J.R. and Campbell W.B., *Biochim. Biophys. Acta.* **1300** (1996), 143–150.

113. Goetzl E.J. and Sun F.F., *J. Exp. Med.* **150** (1979), 406– 411.

114. Docherty J.C. and Wilson T.W., *Biochem. Biophys. Res. Commun.* **148** (1987), 534–538.

115. Vanderhoek J.Y., Wilhelmi L.L., Ekborg S.L. and Karmin M.T., *Eicosanoids.* **3** (1990), 181–185.

116. Fogh K., Herlin T. and Kragballe K., *Arch. Dermatol. Res.* **280** (1988), 430– 436.

117. Dvorak A.M., *et al., J. Histochem. Cytochem.* **40** (1992), 759–769.

118. Herrmann F., Lindemann A., Gauss J. and Mertelsmann R., *Eur. J. Immunol.* **20** (1990), 2513–2516.

119. Conti P., *Scand. J. Rheumatol.*, **75** (1988), Suppl. 318–324.

120. Mallery S.R., Zeligs B.J., Ramwell P.W. and Bellanti J.A., *J. Leukoc. Biol.* **40** (1986), 133–146.

121. Maxwell W.J., *et al.*, *Gut.* **30** (1989), 1270–1274.

122. Shak S. and Goldstein I.M., *J. Biol. Chem.* **259** (1984), 10181–10187.

123. Serhan C.N. and Reardon E., *Free-Radic. Res. Commun.* **7** (1989), 341–345.

124. Marcus A.J., *et al.*, *J. Biol. Chem.* **263** (1988), 2223–2229.

125. Marcus A.J., *et al.*, *Proc. Natl. Acad. Sci. USA.* **81** (1984), 903–907.

126. Ferrante A., *et al.*, *J. Clin. Invest.* **93** (1994), 1063–1070.

127. Rossi F., Bellavite P. and Papini E., *Ciba. Found. Symp.* **118** (1986) 172–195.

128. Babior B.M., *Adv. Enzymol. Relat. Areas. Mol. Biol.* **65** (1992) 49–95.

129. Segal A.W., *Mol. Med. Today.* **2** (1996), 192–135.

130. Badwey J.A., *et al.*, *J. Biol. Chem.* **259** (1984), 7870–7877.

131. Poulos A., *et al.*, *Immunology.* **73** (1991), 102–108.

132. Nishizuka Y., *FASEB. J.* **9** (1995), 484–496.

133. Curnutte J.T., *J. Clin. Invest.* **75** (1985), 1740–1743.

134. Huang, Z.H., *et al.*, *Biochem. J.* **325** (1997a), 553–557.

135. Bates E.J., *et al.*, *Atherosclerosis.* **116** (1995), 247–259.

136. Ferrante A., *et al.*, *Biology of the Neonate.* **69** (1996), 368–375.

137. Jacobson P.B. and Schrier D.J., *J. Immunol.* **151**, (1993), 5639–5652.

138. Blackwood R.A, *et al.*, *J. Leukoc. Biol.*, **59** (1996), 663–670.

139. Bates E.J., *et al.*, *J Leukoc. Biol.* **53** (1993a), 420–426.

140. Bates E.J. *et al.*, *J. Leuk. Biol.* **54** (1993b), 590–598.

141. Ford-Hutchinson A.W., *Nature.* **286** (1980), 264–265.

142. Bray M.A., *Br. Med. Bull.* **39** (1983), 249–253.

143. Krauss A.H., Nieves A.L., Spada C.S. and Woodward D.F., *J. Leukocyte. Biol.* **55** (1994), 201–208.

144. Feinmark S.J., *FEBS. Lett.* **136** (1981), 141–144.

145. Serhan C.N., *et al.*, *Biochem. Biophys. Res. Commun.* **107** (1982) 1006–1012.

146. Gyllenhammer H., *Scand. J. Clin. Lab. Invest.* **49** (1989), 317–322.

147. Schultz R.M., *et al.*, *Prostaglandins. Leukot. Essent. Fatty Acid.* **43** (1991), 267–271.

148. Goetzl E.J., Brindley L.L. and Goldman D.W., *Immunology.* **50** (1983), 35–41.

149. Goetzl E.J. and Pickett W.C., *J. Immunol.* **125** (1980), 1789–1791.

150. Dowd P.M., *et al.*, *J. Inves.t.Dermatol.* **84** (1985), 537–541.

151. Powell W.S., Gravelle F. and Gravel S., *J. Bio.l Chem.* **267** (1992), 19233–19241.

152. Powell W.S., *et al.*, *J. Biol. Chem.* **268** (1993b), 9280–9286.

153. O'Flaherty J.T., Cordes J., Redman J. and Thomas M.J., *Biochem. Biophys. Res. Commun.* **192** (1993), 129–134.

154. Powell W.S., *et al.*, *J. Immunol.* **159** (1997) 2952–2959.

155. Serhan C.N.,Hamberg M. and Samuelsson B., *Proc. Natl. Acad. Sci. USA.* **81** (1984), 5335–5339.

156. Samuelsson B., *et al.*, *Science.* **237** (1987), 1171–1176.

157. Palmblad J., Gyllenhammer H. and Ringertz B., *Adv. Exp. Med. Biol.* **229** (1988), 137–145.

158. Lerner R., Heimburger M. and Palmblad J., *Blood.* **82** (1993), 948–953.

159. Fogh K., Sogaard H., Herlin T. and Kraballe K., *J. Am. Acad. Dermatol.* **18** (1988), 279–285.

160. Takata S., *et al.*, *J. Clin. Invest.* **93** (1994), 499–508.

161. Ferrante J.V., *et al.*, *J. Clin. Invest.* **99** (1997), 1445–1452.

162. Serhan C.N. and Drazen J. M., Editorial. *J. Clin. Invest.* **99** (1997), 1147–1148.

163. Serhan C.N., *et al.*, *Biochemistry* **34** (1995), 14609–14615.

164. Wise H., *J. Leukoc Biol.* **60** (1996), 480–488.

165. Armstrong R.A., *Br. J. Pharmacol.* **116** (1995), 2903–2908.

166. Mikawa K., *et al.*, *Prostaglandins Leukot. Essent. Fatty Acids.* **51** (1994), 287–291.

167. Boxer L.A., *et al.*, *J. Lab. Clin. Med.* **95** (1980), 672–678.

168. Zurier R.B., *et al.*, *J. Clin. Invest.* **5** (1974), 297–309.

169. Fantone J.C., Marasco W.A., Elgas L.J. and Ward P.A., *J. Immunol.* **130** (1983), 1495–1497.

170. Goldstein I.M., Malmsten C.L., Samuelsson B. and Weissmann G., *Inflammation.* **2** (1977), 309–317.

171. Spagnuolo P.J., Ellner J.J., Hassid A. and Dunn M.J., *J. Clin. Invest.* **66** (1980), 406–14.

172. Mancuso P., *et al.*, *Crit. Care. Med.* **25** (1977), 1198–1206.

173. Matsumoto K., *et al.*, *J. Appl. Physiol.* **81** (1996), 2338–2364.

174. Wiles M.E., *et al.*, *Inflammation* **15** (1991), 181–99

175. Li Y., Ferrante A., Poulos A. and Harvey D.P., *J. Clin. Invest.* **97** (1996), 1605–1609.

176. Hardy S.J., *et al.*, *J. Immunol.* **153** (1994a), 1754–1760.

177. Hardy S.J., *et al.*, *Eur. J. Biochem.* **198** (1991), 801–806.

178. Robinson B.S., Hii C.S., Poulos A. and Ferrante A., *J. Lipid Res.* **37** (1996), 1234–1245.

179. Zhang J.H., Ferrante A., Arrigo A.P. and Dayer J.M., *J. Immunol.* **148** (1992), 177–192.

180. Ferrante A., *Immunology Series Vol. 5 R. G. Cofey, editor.* (Marcel Dekker, New York 1992) 417–436.

181. Ferrante A., Hii C.S.T. and Rathjen D.A., *Today's Life Science.* **7** (1995), 40–47.

182. Kumaratilake L.M., *et al., Infect. Immun.* **65** (1997) 5342–5345.

183. Tan A-M., *et al., Pediatric. Research.* **37** (1995), 155–159.

184. Kumaratilake L.M., *et al., J. Clin. Invest.* **89** (1992), 961–967

185. Ginsburg I. and Kohen R., *Inflammation.* **19** (1995), 101–118.

186. Pryzwansky K.B., Wyatt T., Reed W. and Ross G.D., *Eur. J. Cell. Biol.* **54** (1991), 61–75.

187. Sengelov H., *J. Clin. Invest.* **92** (1993), 1467–1476.

188. Graves V., *Blood.* **80** (1992), 776–787.

189. Tonnesen M.G., *et al., J. Clin. Invest.* **83** (1989) 637–846.

190. Lee T.H., *et al., Clin. Sci.* **74** (1988), 467–475.

191. Nagy L., *et al., Clin. Exp. Immunol.* **47** (1982), 541–547.

192. Hii C.S.T., *et al., Carcinogenesis.* **16** (1995a), 1505–1511.

193. Hardy S.J., *et al., Biochem. J.* **311** (1995), 689–697.

194. Berridge M.J., *Nature.* **365** (1993) 338–389.

195. Clapham D.E., *Cell.* **80** (1995), 259–268.

196. Rakovic S., *et al., Curr. Biol.* **6** (1996), 989–996.

197. Huang J.M., Xian H. and Bacaner M., *Proc. Natl. Acad. Sci. USA.* **89** (1992), 6452–6456.

198. Chow S.C. and Jondal M., *J. Biol. Chem.* **265** (1990), 902–907.

199. Naccache P.H., Molski T.F., Borgeat P. and Sha'afi R.I., *J. Cell. Physio.* **122** (1985), 273–280

200. Reynaud D. and Pace-Asciak C.R., *Prostaglandins Leukot. Essent. Fatty Acids* **56** (1997) 9–12.

201. Abramson S.B. and Leszczynska-Piziak J. and Weissmann G., *J. Immunol.* **147** (1991), 231–236.

202. Curnutte J.T., Erickson R.W., Ding J. and Badwey J.A., *J. Biol. Chem.* **269** (1994), 10813–10819.

203. Bennett P.A., Finan P.M., Dixon R.J. and Kellie S., *Immunology.* **85** (1995), 304–310.

204. Verhoeven A.J. *et al., J. Biol. Chem.* **268** (1993), 18593–18598.

205. Kessels G.C., Krause K.H. and Verhoeven A.J., *Biochem. J.* **292** (1993), 781–785.
206. Murakami K. and Routtenberg A., *FEBS. Lett.* **192** (1985), 189–193.
207. Sekiguchi K., *et al., Biochem. Biophys. Res. Commun.* **145** (1987), 797–802.
208. Shinomura T., *et al., Proc. Natl. Acad. Sci. USA.* **88** (1991), 5149–5153.
209. Hardy S.J., *et al., J. Neurochem.* **62** (1994b), 1546–1551.
210. Hii C.S.T., *et al, J. Biol. Chem.* **270** (1995b), 4201–4204.
211. Marshall L.A. and Roshak A., *Biochem. Cell. Biol.* **71** (1993), 331–339.
212. Bauldry S.A., *et al., Biochim. Biophys. Acta.* **1299**, (1996), 223–234.
213. Smith D.M. and Waite M., *J. Leukoc. Biol.* **52** (1992), 670–678.
214. Mizukami Y., Yoshioka K., Morimoto S. and Yoshida K.I., *J. Biol. Chem.* **272** (1997), 16657–16662.
215. Kim J.S. and Kahn C.R., *Biochem. J.* **323** (1997), 621–627.
216. Cavigelli M., Dolfi F., Claret F. X. and Karin M., *Embo. J.* **14** (1995), 5957–5964
217. Raingeaud J., *et al., J. Biol. Chem.* **270** (1995), 7420–7426.
218. Cui X.L. and Douglas J.G., *Proc. Natl. Acad. Sci. USA.* **94** (1997), 3771–3776.
219. Rizzo M.T. and Carlo-Stella C., *Blood.* **88** (1996), 3792–3800.
220. Hannun Y.A. and Obeid L.M., *Trends Biochem. Sci.* **20** (1995), 73–77.
221. Schutze S., Wiegmann K., Machleidt T. and Kronke M., *Immunobiology.* **193** (1995), 193–203.
222. Robinson B.S., Hii C.S., Poulos A. and Ferrante A., *Immunology.* **91** (1997), 274–280
223. Smirnov S.V. and Aaronson P.I., *Circ. Res.* **79** (1996), 20–31.
224. Wieland S.J., *et al., J. Biol. Chem.* **271** (1996), 19037–19041.
225. Henderson L.M., Banting G. and Chappell J.B., *J. Biol.Chem.* **270** (1995), 5909–1916.
226. De Coursey T.E. and Cherny V.V., *Biophys. J.* **65** (1993), 1590–1598.
227. Tsai M.H., Yu C.L., Wei F.S. and Stacey D.W., *Science.* **243** (1989), 522–526.
228. Chuang T.H., Bohl B.P. and Bokoch G.M., *J. Biol. Chem.* **268** (1993), 26206–26211.
229. Majumdar S., *et al., Biochim. Biophys. Acta.* **1176** (1993), 276–286.
230. El Benna J., Faust L.P. and Babior B.M., *J. Biol. Chem.* **269** (1994), 23431–23436.
231. El Benna J., Faust L.P., Johnson J.L. and Babior B.M., *J. Biol. Chem.* **271** (1996a), 6374–6378.
232. El Benna J., *et al., Arch. Biochem. Biophys.* **334** (1996b), 395–400.

233. Toullec D., *et al.*, *J. Biol. Chem.* **266** (1991), 15771–15781.
234. Alessi D.R., *et al.*, *J. Biol. Chem.* **270** (1995), 27489–27494.
235. Lee J.C., *et al.*, *Nature.* **372** (1994), 739–746.
236. Ogino T., *et al.*, *J. Biol. Chem.* **272** (1997), 26247–26252.
237. McPhail L.C., Shirley P.S., Clayton C.C. and Snyderman R., *J. Clin. Invest.* **75** (1985), 1735–1739.
238. Corey S.J. and Rosoff P.M., *J. Lab. Clin. Med.* **118** (1991), 343–351.
239. Wolf B.A.,Turk J., Sherman W.R. and McDaniel M.L., *J. Biol. Chem.* **261** (1986), 3501–3511.
240. Essien E.U., *Med. Sci. Res.* **21** (1993), 405–406.
241. Curnutte J.T., *et al.*, *J. Biol. Chem.* **259** (1984), 11851–11857.
242. Lin L.L., *et al.*, *Cell.* **72** (1993), 269–278.
243. Yasuda H., Kishiro K., Izumi N. and Nakanishi M., *J. Neurochem.* **45** (1985), 168–172.
244. Duyster J., Schulze-Specking A., Fitzke E. and Dieter P., *J. Cell. Biochem.* **48** (1992), 288–295.
245. Huang, Z.H., et al., *Circ. Res.* **80** (1997b), 149–158.
246. Pitt M., *et al.*, Chem. Phys. Lipids. **92** (1998), 63–69.
247. Pitt M., *et al.*, Synthesis. (1977) 1250–1242.

CHAPTER 5

PRODUCTION OF CYTOKINES BY POLYMORPHONUCLEAR NEUTROPHILS

Marco A. Cassatella[1]

1. Introduction

Neutrophil polymorphonuclear granulocytes (PMN) are the predominant infiltrating cell type present in the cellular phase of the acute inflammatory response, therefore acting as the first line of defence against invading bacteria and other microorganisms. Mature PMN are terminally differentiated cells, and although have been generally considered to be lacking RNA/protein synthesis capacity, numerous recent studies have made it clear that neutrophils are also able of *de novo* protein synthesis. These cells indeed synthesise numerous proteins involved in their effector functions (1), and can also produce a variety of cytokines (1,2). Since the latter molecules exert a broad spectrum of biological activities, it can be reasonably speculated that in addition to playing an important role in eliciting and sustaining inflammation, PMN may significantly contribute to the regulation of immune reactions and other processes. Thus, in some circumstances, the contribution of PMN-derived cytokines can be of foremost importance.

It is my purpose to summarize in this chapter the current knowledge on the production of cytokines by PMN and other biological aspects, concentrating

[1]Correspondence: Marco A. Cassatella, MD, Ph.D., Istituto di Patologia Generale, Strada Le Grazie 4, 37134 Verona, ITALY, tel ++ 39 045 8098130; fax ++ 39 045 8098127

more on the most recent findings. For a more comprehensive report, the reader may turn to my last review (3), which covers all the literature up to mid 1995.

2. General Characteristics of Cytokine Production by Human Neutrophils *in vitro*

Table 5.1 lists all the cytokines which, to date, have been shown to be released by PMN, *in vitro* or *in vivo*, either constitutively or following appropriate stimulation. Most of the studies addressing cytokine synthesis by neutrophils have been conducted principally through the use of sensitive and specific approaches such as molecular biology techniques, *in situ* hybridization (ISH), immunohistochemistry (IH) and immunoassays. Nevertheless, numerous *in vivo* observations have confirmed the validity of the *in vitro* findings, and now remains little doubt that the release of cytokines constitutes an important aspect of neutrophil biology. Convincing evidence that human PMN can express Interleukin-1α (IL-1α) and IL-1β, IL-1 receptor antagonist (IL-1ra), IL-8, IL-12, Tumor Necrosis Factor-α (TNFα), Transforming Growth Factor-β_1 (TGFβ_1), Macrophage Inflammatory Protein-1α (MIP-1α) and MIP-1β, Interferon-α (IFNα), Growth-related gene product-α (GROα) and CD30 ligand (CD30L), has been generated by several groups (reviewed in ref. 3). In contrast, mRNA expression or release of granulocyte colony-stimulating factor (G-CSF), macrophage CSF (M-CSF), IL-3, GROβ, Interferon-γ inducible protein-10 (IP-10), stem cell factor (SCF) and TGFα by neutrophils have been reported in single instances, and therefore, await further confirmation (3). Finally, conflicting data exist in the literature concerning the issue of whether IL-6, Granulocyte-Macrophage CSF (GM-CSF), and Monocyte Chemotactic Protein-1 (MCP-1) expression can be induced in human neutrophils (2,3). Whichever the case maybe, the fact that neutrophils can synthesize, store and release a wide array of cytokines should bring about a redefinition of the role of neutrophils in physiopathology.

It is however important to mention that, at least *in vitro*, the extent of cytokine production by neutrophils is relatively low, especially when compared to peripheral mononuclear cells (MNC) (2). It follows that if one wants to

Table 5.1 Cytokine expressed by neutrophils

in vitro	*in vivo*
IL-1α/-1β	IL-1α
IL-1ra	IL-1β
IL-8	IL-1ra
IL-12	IL-6
TNFα	IL-8
IFNα	IL-10
CD30L	IL-12
GROα, GROβ*	MIP-2
CINC-1,2α,3	KC/GROα
IP-10	CINC
MIG**	MIP-1α
MIP-1α/-1β	MIP-1β
TGFα, TGFβ_1	MCP-1
IL-3, G-CSF, M-CSF	TNFα
GM-CSF (?), IL-6 (?), MCP-1 (?), SCF* (?)	TGFβ_1

*: mRNA only
**: our unpublished observations

investigate whether neutrophils produce a given cytokine (or in any case a protein), it is absolutely mandatory to work with highly purified PMN populations (>99.5%). It is also highly recommended to exclude the possibility of prestimulation of PMN during their isolation procedures (4), which may be driven, for instance, by contamination of reagents, solutions or labware with trace levels of endotoxin, or by the use of ammonium chloride for erythrocyte lysis. In our experiments, >98 % of freshly purified PMN are usually positive for CD62L, indicating that our isolation procedures with Ficoll, dextran sedimentation and hypotonic lysis do not have any stimulatory effects on neutrophils.

A wide range of stimuli able to induce cytokine synthesis in PMN have been identified (2,3). In addition to classical agonists such as lipopolysaccharide (LPS) and cytokines themselves, also phagocytic particles and microorganisms (such as bacteria, fungi and viruses), chemotactic factors [such as formyl-methionyl-leucyl-phenylalanine (fMLP), leukotriene B_4 (LTB$_4$), platelet-activating factor (PAF), the complement component C5a], and neuroimmunomodulatory substances can induce the release of cytokines by PMN (3). In general, not only the magnitude and kinetics of cytokine release vary substantially depending upon the stimulus used, but the pattern of production is also influenced to a great extent by the stimulus used. We have a for long time focused most of our investigations on the effects of LPS, fMLP, and *S.cerevisiae* opsonized with IgG (Y-IgG). For instance, Y-IgG appears to potently trigger the release of only some pro-inflammatory cytokines (TNFα, IL-8 and GROα), whereas LPS induces anti-inflammatory (for example IL-1ra) as well as pro-inflammatory cytokines, including IL-12 and IP-10 (if LPS is used in combination with IFNγ) (3). In contrast, in the case of fMLP, or of the other chemotactic factors, they seem to trigger only a transient release of IL-8 and GROα, but, apparently, not that of any other cytokine (2,3). The fact that chemotactic factors can induce the production of chemoattractants (i.e. IL-8, GROα) could represent a feedback mechanism whereby greater numbers of PMN are attracted to an inflammatory site, ensuring a persistent influx of PMN that perpetuate the inflammatory reaction. IL-8 is likely the main cause of the sustained local accumulation of neutrophils, due to its long-lasting effect (5). By contrast, the other chemoattractancts act more transiently because they are eventually inactivated by oxidation, hydrolysis or enzymatic cleavage (5). A condensed description on the experimental conditions observed to induce the production of the various cytokines by neutrophils *in vitro* follows below.

3. Production of Specific Cytokines by Neutrophils *in vitro*

3.1 *Chemokines*

Chemokines represent a group of chemotactic cytokines whose importance in inflammatory processes is best illustrated by their ability to specifically recruit discrete leukocyte populations (6). However, we now know that chemokines and their receptors are expressed by a wide variety of non-hematopoietic cells, and that chemokine function extend well beyond leukocyte physiology. For instance, the connections among chemokines, their receptors and human immunodeficiency virus infection broaden the previously narrow focus on chemokines as mere chemoattractants (7). Chemokines are usually small, with molecular weights in the range of 8 to 12 kD, but there are exceptions (5,6). Two major groups of chemokines exist, based upon the positions of the first two cysteine residues in their primary sequences: the "C-X-C", and the "C-C" subfamilies. The C-X-C subfamily includes IL-8, the prototype, MIP-2, IP-10, Monokine induced by IFNγ(MIG), GROα, -β,-γ, epithelial cell derived and neutrophil-activating properties, 78 amino acids (ENA-78), cytokine-induced neutrophil chemoattractant (CINC), and others, and predominantly exerts stimulatory and chemotactic activities towards neutrophils (5,6). The C-C subfamily includes monocyte chemotactic proteins (MCP), RANTES and MIP-1α, -1β, -1γ, and predominantly has monocyte-, eosinophil-, basophil- and T lymphocyte-chemotactic properties (5,6). Recently, two different chemokines, which are likely members of novel groups of chemokines, the C and CX$_3$C subfamilies, have been identified (6). To the former belongs lymphotactin, a potent attractant for lymphocytes, whereas to the latter belongs fractalkine or neurotactin, which is an integral membrane protein with a chemokine domain at its N-terminus (6). It is now well established that neutrophils can secrete both C-X-C, as well as "C-C" chemokines.

3.2 *Interleukin-8*

It is worth recalling that IL-8 is one of the potentially most important (and most extensively) studied cytokine produced by neutrophils. The latter cells are the primary targets for IL-8, responding to this mediator by chemotaxis, release of granule enzymes, respiratory burst, up-regulation of CR1 and CD11/CD18 expression on the surface, and increased adherence to unstimulated endothelial cells (5). In addition, IL-8 has chemotactic activities for T lymphocytes and basophils, though much less effectively than for neutrophils, and is also an angiogenic factor (5).

Early studies showed that PMN express significant steady-state levels of IL-8 mRNA and release substantial amounts of IL-8 into the culture supernatants after LPS stimulation (8,9). However, it soon emerged that phagocytosis of Y-IgG represented a much more potent stimulus for the extracellular production of biologically active IL-8 (9). Subsequently, we were able to demonstrate that fMLP (10 nM), as well as other neutrophil chemotactic factors such as C5a and PAF, also induced PMN to release substantial amounts of IL-8 (10). Our results were later substantially confirmed not only for fMLP (11–13) and C5a (14), but even extended to another classic PMN chemotactic factor, LTB$_4$ (15). Secretion of IL-8 in response to fMLP was transient, since maximal production was observed at 2–3 h and then returned to basal levels, contrary to the sustained release of IL-8 induced by Y-IgG or LPS (9,10). Nevertheless, Strieter et al. (16) reported that if neutrophils were exposed to chemotactic agonists in the presence of LPS, the production of IL-8 was synergistically elevated.

In relation to the LPS-induced IL-8 production by neutrophils, this has been recently shown to be inhibited by the protease inhibitor, FUT-175 (17), and by the combined nitric oxide-superoxide donor (3-morpholinosydnonimine, SIN-1)(18), but to be enhanced by the nitric oxide donor (1,2,3,4-oxatriazolium 5-amino chloride, GEA-3162) (18). The latter results may have important implications for the patients with acute lung injury who are commonly treated with inhaled nitric oxide. LPS-induced IL-8 production by neutrophils is also potentiated by PMN binding to solid phase fibrinogen (19), or to plastic surfaces precoated either with fibronectin (Fn), a ligand of the integrin receptor $\alpha5\beta1$, or with laminin (Ln), a ligand of the integrin receptor $\alpha_6\beta_1$ (20). Hypoxia exerted an overall down-regulating effect on LPS-induced IL-8 (TNFα and IL-1β) release, but subsequent reoxygenation restored cytokine production, increasing IL-8 levels even above the normoxic levels (20). However, not only spontaneous IL-8 release was significantly enhanced by PMN binding to Fn or Ln, but reoxygenation itself significantly amplified the responses mediated by Fn and Ln (20).

The range of stimuli shown to induce the production of IL-8 has steadily increased during the past years (Table 5.2). For example, PMN stimulated with TNFα produce IL-8 mRNA in a time- and dose-dependent manner (16,21). In

Table 5.2   Agents able to trigger the production of IL-8 by human neutrophils

LPS from *E.Coli*	cycloheximide*
fMLP	Staurosporine
C5a	
	S.cerevisiae
Leukotriene B$_4$	
	IgG-opsonized *S.cerevisiae*
PAF	zymosan
TNFα	*P. aeruginosa*
IL-1β	*C. albicans* and its derivative products
GM-CSF	*Borrelia burgdorferi* outer surface protein A
PMA	capsular polysaccharide complex (CPC)
	from *Bacteroides fragilis*
A23187	LPS from *A.actinomycetemcomitans*
anti-CD11/CD18 antibodies	LPS from *Fusobacterium nucleatum*
anti-CD30L antibodies	LPS from *Porphyromonas gingivalis*
Substance P	LPS from *Capnocytophaga ochracea*
interaction with Fibronectin or	*Mycobacterium.tubercolosis*
Laminin	
Lactoferrin	Lipoarabinomannan (LAM)
Lactoferricin	*Cryptococcus neoformans*
Protamine	Glucuronoxylomannan
calcium pyrophosphate dihydrate	*Plasmodium falciparum-infected*
(CPPD) microcrystals	erythrocytes
monosodium urate (MSU)	Panton-Valentine leukocidin from
microcrystals	*S.aureus*
Sulfatides*	Erythrogenic toxin A from *Streptococcus*
	pyogenes
Thrombopoietin	Alveolysin from *Bacillus alvei*
IL-2, IL-13, TGFβ	Respiratory Syncitial Virus

*: mRNA only

another study (22), it was found that IL-1β induced a lower level of mRNA expression and a smaller amount of IL-8 than LPS and TNFα after 24 h of incubation. We have also found that IL-1β, over a wide concentration range, is a very weak stimulus for the extracellular production of IL-8 (23). However, we also observed that IL-1β dramatically synergises with TNFα, if used at the same concentrations produced by neutrophils in response to LPS (23). Other studies have identified staurosporine (a non specific inhibitor protein kinase C and of other kinases) (24), the calcium ionophore A23187 (11,13,25), phorbol esters (PMA) (11,22,24), as well as GM-CSF (26-28), as very potent inducers of IL-8 by human PMN. In the case of neutrophils treated with GM-CSF, the immunosuppressive drugs cyclosporin A (CsA), and rapamycin enhanced the release of IL-8, even after a further stimulation with fMLP, whereas FK506 had no effect (29). Also the effect of A23187 on IL-8 production was partially inhibited by a selective PAF antagonist (25), in line with the established capacity of A23187 to stimulate the synthesis of PAF in neutrophils. That PAF receptor antagonists can inhibit IL-8 (and LTB$_4$) release from neutrophils have been also confirmed in a more recent study (30), in which (+)-cis-3,5-dimethyl-2-(3-pyridyl)thiazolidin-4-one hydrochloride (SM-12502) was used prior to stimulation with either A23187, fMLP, or with NaF in the presence of Al^{3+} (an activator of heterotrimetric G-proteins).

The inflammatory microcrystals monosodium urate (MSU) and calcium pyrophosphate dihydrate (CPPD), the major mediators of gout and pseudogout, respectively, were both shown to increase the secretion of IL-8 by neutrophils, but to have no effect on that of MIP-1α (31). Interestingly, the presence of MSU and CPPD synergistically enhanced the production of IL-8 induced by TNFα and GM-CSF, but completely inhibited MIP-1α secretion induced by TNFα (31). Adding new stimuli to the list of the IL-8 inducers, we identified substance P, one of the main mediator of neurogenic inflammation, not only as able to directly stimulate the release of IL-8 from human neutrophils, but also to enhance the effect of TNFα and fMLP (32). Sulfatides (33), which are established ligands for L-selectin, human or bovine lactoferrin (LF), and lactoferricin (LFcin), a peptide derived from the N-terminal region of LF (34), all have been shown to stimulate the release IL-8 from human neutrophils. Interestingly, a basic peptide, protamine, exerted the same effect as that of LF and LFcin, suggesting the importance of the basic nature of LF and LFcin in acting as an inducer of IL-8 release from PMN (34). Thrombopoietin (TPO), which regulates early and late stages of platelet formation as well as platelet activation, is another molecule able to stimulate an early but sustained release of IL-8 from human neutrophils (35). Thus, in addition to sustaining megakaryocytopoiesis, TPO may have an important role in regulating PMN activation. More recently, Wiley and colleagues showed that cross-linked CD30L can transduce a signal to the ligand-bearing cell (36). CD30L, in fact, induced the production of IL-8 by freshly isolated neutrophils when activated by cross-linking with specific monoclonal antibodies (mAbs) or by CD30-Fc fusion protein (36). Indirect effects through CD30 were clearly ruled out, since only CD30L, but not CD30, is expressed on neutrophils (36).

Coincubation of neutrophils with heat-killed *C.albicans* (28), or with zymosan (a yeast cell wall extracts) (25), also resulted in the appearance of immunoreactive IL-8 into the PMN supernatants. In agreement with our previous observations made with unopsonized yeast particles (37), both Au et al. (25), and subsequently Altstaedt et al. (4), showed that opsonization is not a prerequisite for IL-8 stimulation. Evidence that IL-8 release from neutrophils stimulated by zymosan was dependent on a CD11b/CD18 signaling pathway was also provided (25). PMN produce IL-8 (and other pro-inflammatory cytokines such as TNFα, and IL-1β) in response to stimulation with *Cryptococcus neoformans* yeast cells, or to glucuronoxylomannan (GXM), the major *C.neoformans* capsular polysaccharide, being the magnitude of the cytokine response related to the yeast capsule size (38). IL-8 mRNA and protein production is observed also in response to *Plasmodium falciparum*-infected erythrocytes (39), and to various bacterial products or toxins (40). Recently, *Borrelia burgdorferi* outer surface protein A (OspA), but not the unlipidated recombinant OspA, has been shown to induce human PMN to produce IL-8, at levels comparable to those induced by 25 nM LPS (12). Furthermore, purified capsular polysaccharide complex (CPC) from *Bacteroides fragilis* yielded high levels of IL-8 production by PMN, with a response more robust than, and time-dependently different from, that observed in autologous MNC (41). Not only LPS from *Escherichia Coli*, but also LPS from the periodontopathic bacteria *Actinobacillus actinomycetemcomitans, Fusobacterium nucleatum,* and, to lesser extent, *Porphyromonas gingivalis* and *Capnocytophaga ochracea,* have been shown to stimulate PMN to release great amounts of IL-8 (other than TNFα, IL-1α/β and IL-1rα) (42). PMN stimulated with *Mycobacterium tubercolosis*, or with a major mycobacterial cell wall component, lipoarabinomannan (LAM), release both IL-8 and GROα (43). Release of IL-8 critically depended on the PMN: *M.tubercolosis* ratio, being the 1:1 ratio the optimal one. Moreover, treatment of PMN with an inhibitor of LTB$_4$ formation (MK-866), blocked LAM capacity to induce IL-8 (43). Clinical *Pseudomonas aeruginosa* isolates, the mucoid *P.aeruginosa* strain (CF3M) and its nonmucoid revertant (CF3), purified *P.aeruginosa* mucoid exopolysaccharide (alginate), as well as a very low molecular weight (1 kD) product of *P.aeruginosa*, were all shown to produce a significant increase in IL-8 release from human PMN (44,45). Interestingly, simulation of neutrophils with formalin-killed strain *P.aeruginosa* 5276 induced levels of IL-8 production which were more than ten times higher than those induced by LPS or IL-1β, under the same time of incubation (24 h) (46). A moderate inhibitory effect of erythromycin on IL-8 production in formalin-killed *Pseudomonas*-stimulated neutrophils, but not in alveolar macrophages (AM), was demonstrated *in vitro* (46). Erythromycin did not however suppress IL-1β-induced neutrophil and AM-derived IL-8 production. It is important to mention that treatment with erythromycin of patients with chronic airway disease (CAD) and persistent *P.aeruginosa* infection causes significant reductions of the inflammatory parameters in bronchoalveolar lavage fluids (BAL) from these patients (46), an observation having significant implications in the context of cystic fibrosis (CF).

The respiratory syncytial virus (RSV) also provokes an enhancement of IL-8 mRNA steady-state levels, accompanied by the secretion of IL-8 in a time- and dose-dependent manner (11). Konig and colleagues demonstrated that synthesis of IL-8 from PMN depended on the adherence of viral particles and on a phagocytic event, and not on the infection process. The latter was demonstrated by the fact that stimulation of human PMN with viable, heat-inactivated, or UV-inactivated RSV induced IL-8 production (protein + mRNA) to a similar degree (11,47). If the RSV particles were opsonized with mAbs directed to the RSV-fusion protein (F protein), IL-8 release from PMN increased in comparison with RSV alone, and this increase occurred without a concomitant enhancement of IL-8 mRNA levels (11,47). Involvement of the Fcγ-receptors might thus play a role in enhancing the synthesis and/or secretion rate of the *de novo*-synthesized cytoplasmic IL-8 pool, as we also observed in another model (37). Stimulation of human PMN with purified RSV G-protein, a major capsid protein, resulted in an increased IL-8 release from human PMN, but to a significantly lesser degree compared with the intact RSV (47). The knowledge that inactivated RSV, similarly to viable RSV, may induce cytokine release from human PMN may be helpful in developing new strategies to prevent RSV disease.

On a final note, it is also correct to mention here that TGFβ (48), IL-2 (28) and IL-13 (49), were all reported to induce IL-8 mRNA expression and secretion by PMN. However, we (for IL-2 and IL-13, unpublished observations) and others (for TGFβ, ref. 50), could not reproduce such observations. Finally, the presence of IL-8 mRNA in most samples of freshly isolated neutrophils has been recurrently observed (10,11,16,24,28,45). Usually, these constitutive IL-8 transcripts decrease almost completely within a few hours of cell culture in the absence of stimulation (10). Despite the presence of specific mRNA, secretion of IL-8 by unstimulated cultured human neutrophils is always very low (below 100 pg/ml), unless cells have been inadvertently preactivated by the isolation procedures. We do not know whether the constitutive IL-8 mRNA results from mechanical stress during cell preparation, or represents a constitutive RNA pool that may facilitate the appearance of the mature protein when the PMN are stimulated. Cell-associated IL-8 increases several-fold during incubation at 37°C *in vitro*, and much more (200-fold) after treatment with stimuli (13,51). Since cychloheximide (CHX), but not actinomycin D (Act D), inhibits the accumulation of cell-associated IL-8 after culture at 37°C, accumulation of IL-8 in these conditions seems to be under translational rather than transcriptional control (13).

3.3 *Growth related gene product-α and GROβ*

IL-8 is not the only C-X-C chemokine with neutrophil activating properties secreted by PMN. Our studies revealed in fact that activated PMN release GROα (52). A previous work by Haskill and coworkers showed that PMN which have been adhered for 45 min to fibronectin-coated plastic expressed selectively GROα mRNA, whereas monocytes from the same individuals expressed all three GRO isoforms (GROα, GROβ and GROγ) (53). However, these authors utilized only RT-PCR analysis for their studies. In our hands, the release of GROα by stimulated PMN was preceded by an accumulation of GROα mRNA, whose kinetics varied depending on the agonist. Y-IgG-phagocytosis was approximately two- to three-fold more potent than LPS, and much more than TNFα (52). By contrast, LPS was more potent than Y-IgG and TNFα in inducing the production of GROα by monocytes, indicating that the regulation of GROα production is governed by distinct mechanisms depending on the cell type (52). Surprisingly, very small quantities of GROα protein were detected in the cell-free supernatants of PMN stimulated with 10 nM fMLP, in spite of a very high accumulation of GROα mRNA transcripts (comparable to that induced by LPS) (52). Similarly, Y-IgG only caused a moderate GROα mRNA accumulation compared to LPS, TNFα, or fMLP (52), suggesting that GROα production in PMN is controlled at the translational or post-translational level, as was in the case of Y-IgG-stimulated IL-8 release (51).

Other works have recognized neutrophils as cells potentially able to produce GROα. In one of them, Koch et al (54), examined whether PMN obtained from peripheral blood (PB) or from reumathoid arthritis synovial fluids (RA SF) generated GROα. They found that after a 24-h culture, both RA SF PMN and PB PMN constitutively produced very high levels of GROα, and that this production was further increased upon stimulation with LPS (54). In another study, Hachicha et al. (31) assessed the levels of GROα after stimulation of neutrophils for up to 12 h with TNFα, GM-CSF, MSU and CPPD, used either individually or in combination. Low levels of GROα were detected in both control and stimulated cell supernatants, regardless of the triggering conditions (31). Although the number of PMN used in these experiments were not specified, the quantitative results shown with TNFα were essentially in agreement with ours (52). More recently, evidence that PMN activated with *M.tubercolosis* or LAM release GROα has been also provided (43). LAM produced an up to 4-fold increase of GROα release, whereas *M.tubercolosis* stimulated a 15-fold increase. Finally, mRNA expression of KC, which is the murine analogue of GROα, was recently found within exudate neutrophils obtained after intraperitoneal injection of thioglycollate in rats (55).

The ability of PMN to produce GROα is relevant for several reasons. Similar to IL-8, GROα acts as a mediator of inflammation, as it has powerful chemotactic and activatory properties on PMN, including degranulation, increased expression of adhesion molecules and *in vivo* recruitment of neutrophils to sites of injection (5,6). Therefore, generation of GROα by neutrophils may contribute to stimulate the recruitment to, and activation of further neutrophils at sites of inflammation, in addition to IL-8. A recent study by Villard et al. (56), for instance, has shown that the concentrations of GROα and IL-8 were markedly elevated in BAL of three acute pathologic states: bacterial pneumonia (BPN); adult respiratory distress syndrome (ARDS); and *Pneumocystis carinii* pneumonia (PCP). The levels of these two chemokines were higher in the ARDS and BPN groups than in PCP group, and that the levels of GROα were consistently higher than those of IL-8, whereas BAL levels of both IL-8 and GROα were basically undetectable in 16 subjects of control group (56). A biological assay showed that BAL GROα was active, in that specific blocking antibodies against the chemokine significantly reduced (by 51%) neutrophil chemotactic activity *in vitro*. GROα or IL-8 both correlate with the absolute neutrophil number/ml when all groups were studied, again suggesting that GROα maybe as important as IL-8 in acute lung inflammatory process (56). The study did not establish the precise source of GROα and IL-8 in the alveoli, but the results emphasize that other neutrophil chemokines in addition to IL-8 can be produced at higher concentrations and are likely to act in concert with IL-8 in the lung. Moreover, the fact that among its various biological activities, GROα possess mitogenic effects on normal and transformed human melanocyte cell lines (5), raises the possibility that neutrophil-derived GROα might play a role in melanocyte transformation.

It has also been reported that PMN constitutively express GROβ mRNA at very low levels (57). A five-ten fold induction of these GROβ transcripts were however observed upon stimulation with LPS for 24 h, whereas in monocytes the same treatment resulted in a more than 100-fold GROβ mRNA increase (57). Likely because of the lack of available assays to measure the chemokine, nothing is known on the protein secretion.

Finally, rat peritoneal neutrophils incubated with staurosporine and PMA accumulated, in a time dependent manner, high levels of CINC-3 mRNA and released siginificant levels of CINC-3, CINC-1 and CINC-2α, but not of CINC-2β (58). Production of staurosporine- and PMA-induced neutrophil chemotactic factors were inhibited by the protein kinase C inhibitors, H-7, calphostin C and Ro 31-8425, and by the tyrosine kinase inhibitor, genistein (58).

3.4 *Interferon-γ inducible protein-10*

Another member of the C-X-C chemokine family, IP-10, is produced and released by human neutrophils (59). Despite its structural homology to IL-8, IP-10 is predominantly chemotactic for lymphocytes and NK cells, as opposed to neutrophils (60). A possible explanation is that unlike other C-X-C members, IP-10 is devoided of the -E-L-R- motif (an amino acid sequence preceding the first two cysteine residues), whose conservation seems to be essential to confer neutrophil chemoattractant properties to the C-X-C chemokines (5,6). IP-10 is specifically produced in response to IFNγ by monocytes, lymphocytes, keratinocytes and endothelial cells (5,6). Surprisingly, in neutrophils, IFNγ alone had only a modest effect on IP-10 mRNA accumulation (59). However, stimulation of PMN with IFNγ in combination with either TNFα or LPS (but not with Y-IgG or fMLP) resulted in a considerable induction of IP-10 mRNA transcripts, as well as in the extracellular release of the protein. In the latter conditions, accumulation of IP-10 protein in culture supernatants was evident not before 6 h and was dependent on the concentration of LPS or TNFα. By contrast, under the same conditions, IFNγ proved to be the most potent stimulus for IP-10 production by PBMC, suggesting that, depending on the target cell, IP-10 production is controlled in different ways. Another striking difference between PBMC and PMN was that costimulation of IFNγ-treated PBMC with either LPS or TNFα led to a diminished production of IP-10 respective to PBMC treated with IFNγ alone. IL-10, as well as neutralizing antibodies to TNFα, moderately suppressed extracellular production of IP-10 in neutrophils stimulated with IFNγ plus LPS (59). The generation of IP-10 by PMN may significantly contribute to recruit NK cells, monocytes and activated T lymphocytes to sites of inflammation (5). Although it is still too early to speculate on an eventual *in vivo* role of neutrophil-derived IP-10, it is noteworthy that our preliminary experiments indicate that PMN can produce also MIG, another chemokine homologous to IP-10 and with similar biological properties.

3.5 *Macrophage inflammatory protein-1α and MIP-1α*

The ability of stimulated neutrophils to secrete MIP-1α and MIP-1β was documented by Kunkel's group (61,62). MIP-1α and MIP-1β act as potent chemotactic/activating factors for monocytes and subpopulations of T lymphocytes, and also activate several effector functions of macrophages and neutrophils (5,6). Kasama et al. (61) initially observed that cell-free supernatants from human PMN stimulated with increasing concentrations of LPS possessed a chemotactic activity for human monocytes, which was significantly attenuated (by approximately 60%) in the presence of neutralizing anti-human MIP-1α antibodies. By using Northern blot analysis, ELISA and IH, they were able to demonstrate that LPS induced a mRNA expression and extracellular production of MIP-1α (61), and of MIP-1β as well (62). Stimulation of PMN in the presence of both LPS and GM-CSF resulted in a synergistic expression of both MIP-1α mRNA and protein, compared with LPS alone (61). McColl's group extended to other stimuli the ability of inducing neutrophils to secrete MIP-1α (31). Among MSU, CPPD, GM-CSF and TNFα, only the latter exerted a significant effect on MIP-1α mRNA expression and secretion (31). In our unpublished experiments we could confirm that neutrophils express MIP-1α and MIP-1β mRNAs, not only in response to LPS or TNFα, but also to Y-IgG. Importantly, the major finding of a potentially biological significance in McColl's paper (31) was that while secretion of MIP-1α induced by TNFα was completely inhibited in the presence of either MSU or CPPD, the production of IL-8 in the same conditions was synergistically enhanced. These results imply that the failure of inflammatory microcrystals to directly induce MIP-1α production (while inducing that of IL-8), as well as to inhibit the relese of MIP-1α in response to TNFα, can prevent the generation of neutrophil-derived chemotactic signals that could attract MNC to the synovial environment.

The ability of PMN to secrete MIP-1α and MIP-1β is of considerable importance. The fact that neutrophils produce MIP-1α and MIP-1β, other than IL-8, GROα and IP-10 suggests that PMN, once arrived at the inflammatory site, can promote not only the further recruitment of neutrophils, but also the subsequent accumulation and activation of monocytes/macrophages, eosinophils and lymphocytes. It is reasonable to speculate that PMN, through the production of IL-8, GROα, CINCs, MIP-1α, MIP-1β, IP-10 and MIG, could play a pivotal role in regulating the switch of the type of leukocyte infiltration typically observed during the evolution of the inflammatory response from acute to chronic stages.

3.6 *Monocyte chemotactic proteins*

Initial attempts to define whether MCP-1 mRNA expression occurs in adherent or LPS-stimulated neutrophils, failed (8). Furthermore, Van Damme et al. (63) developed sensitive radioimmunoassays for MCP-1 and MCP-2. In agreement with the previous study (8), they could not detect any extracellular release of either MCP-1 or MCP-2 by granulocytes, even though the cells were stimulated for up to 48 h with optimal doses of many agonists, including IL-1β, IFNβ, IFNγ, GM-CSF, PMA, and LPS (63). In contrast, Burn et al. (64) reported that MCP-1 transcripts and antigenic protein were clearly detectable in neutrophils incubated for 20 h in tissue culture medium, as measured by Northern analysis or RT-PCR and by IH, respectively, but were absent in freshly-isolated neutrophils (64). Under similar experimental conditions, we were not able to detect any MCP-1 transcripts by Northern blot (M.P.Russo, unpublished observations). Similarly, Hachicha et al. (31) reported that mRNAs for MCP-1, MCP-2, MCP-3, RANTES or I-309 were undetectable in unstimulated PMN, or in PMN stimulated for 3 h with TNFα, GM-CSF, MSU and CPPD, either alone or in combination. Therefore, further studies are necessary to clarify whether or not, or under which conditions, human neutrophils express MCP-1 mRNA and protein.

3.7 *Tumor necrosis factor-α*

Molecular evidence of the ability of PMN to either express TNFα mRNA or secrete the related protein *in vitro* was shown to occur in response to LPS (65,66) or to the opportunistic fungus, *C.albicans* (66). Proof of TNFα gene expression in PMN was previously provided by Lindemann and colleagues (67), who observed that neutrophils stimulated with GM-CSF for up to 24 h accumulated TNFα mRNA transcripts without releasing the protein. Furthermore, indirect evidence for the involvement of released TNFα in the granulocyte-mediated killing of two extremely TNFα-sensitive cell lines, namely WEHI sarcoma 164, and L929 cells, was published almost in the same period by Mandi et al. (68). This same group subsequently reported that human neutrophils could indeed be stimulated by *Candida albicans*, *E.coli*, *Stapylococcus aureus, Klebsiella pneumonia*, PMA and LPS, to produce TNFα, being heat-killed *S.aureus* the most potent condition (69). We also showed that phagocytosis of Y-IgG induces an extracellular release of TNFα at levels much higher than those detected after treatment with endotoxin (70). Interestingly, maximal yields of TNFα in neutrophil supernatants in response to Y-IgG (70), as well as to LPS (65,66,70–72), were detected after 5–6 h of stimulation and then declined over time. Thus, if TNFα measurement is carried after 24 h of PMN stimulation, it is possible to find no TNFα in cell-free supernatants (4). It is not clear yet why the yield of TNFα decays with time, but phagocytosis carried out in the presence of protease inhibitors such as α1-antitrypsin increased the recovery of TNFα (37), suggesting that the stability of TNFα in the culture medium is influenced by proteolytic enzymes. Elastase and cathepsin G are known to specifically degrade TNFα (73,74). Furthermore, very high doses of LPS determine a more sustained TNFα release over time (38).

Table 5.3 lists the stimuli that induce TNFα expression in human neutrophils. The latter include sulfatides (33), MP-F2, a β1-2 oligomannoside *Candida* constitutent (75), *Listeria monocytogenes* and *Yersinia enterocolitica* (76), *C.neoformans* and its derivatives (38), LPS from various periodontopatic bacteria (42), and *P.falciparum*-infected erythrocytes (39).

Table 5.3   **Agents able to trigger the production of TNFα by human neutrophils**

LPS	
	C. albicans and its derivative products
fMLP	*Staphilococcus aureus*
TNFα	*Escherichia Coli*
IL-1β	LPS from *A.actinomycetemcomitans*
IL-2	LPS from *Fusobacterium nucleatum*
GM-CSF	LPS from *Porphyromonas gingivalis*
PMA	LPS from *Capnocytophaga ochracea*
Sulfatides*	*Listeria Monocytogenes*
Concanavalin A	*Klebsiella Pneumoniae*
Interaction with Fibronectin or Laminin	*Yersinia Enterocolitica*
	Cryptococcus neoformans
S.Cerevisiae	
IgG-opsonized *S.Cerevisiae*	Glucuronoxylomannan
	Plasmodium falciparum-infected
zymosan	erythrocytes

*: mRNA only

Boxer's group have recently reported that activation with fMLP (100 nM) of PMN plated onto fibrinogen stimulated detectable release of TNFα within 45 min of incubation, with maximal production by 90 min (77). PMN preparations, which were stated to be greater than 95%, with a monocyte contamination of less than 1% (77), released both H_2O_2 and lactoferrin with parallel kinetics to those of TNFα. Since it was well known that TNFα is a potent agonist of adherent PMN (78), the authors investigated the effect of anti-TNFα antibodies. Neutralizing rabbit anti-TNFα antibodies inhibited both H_2O_2 and lactoferrin release stimulated by fMLP, whereas rabbit IgG, anti-HLA-A,B,C, anti-CD14, and anti-interleukin-8 antibodies were without effect. Furthermore, treatment of PMN with either Act D or CHX resulted in a partial (33%) inhibition of H_2O_2 and lactoferrin release, suggesting that protein synthesis was required for this fMLP-mediated activation of adherent PMN. The addition of TNFα to either CHX or of Act D-treated PMN overcame the inhibition, indicating that the effect was specific for TNFα. Finally, the addition of a combination of both antibodies against the 55- and 75-kD TNFα receptors resulted in a significant inhibition of fMLP-mediated activation of H_2O_2 and lactoferrin release. Taken together, these findings supported the hypothesis that TNFα release and ligation of TNFα receptors are central for fMLP stimulated oxidant release from PMN adherent to fibrinogen. Regarding the ability of fMLP to trigger TNFα expression, others (79), and we (2,3), have never been able to demonstrate such effect. However, in our experimental conditions, neutrophils are usually suspended in medium plus 10% FBS, treated with fMLP (usually at 10 nM), and then plated into tissue culture plates or flasks for up to 24 h (3,51). Derevianko and colleagues too (20), were unable to measure any TNFα release from PMN adhered to plastic surfaces, or to surfaces precoated either with Fn or Ln and stimulated with 100 nM fMLP for up to 24 h. Importantly, under these same experimental conditions, fMLP induced the release of IL-8 (20). If true, it thus appears that production of TNFα by PMN stimulated with fMLP occurs under specific conditions (77).

Another agonist demonstrated able to induce TNFα gene expression and secretion in PMN is IL-2 (80). Again, we could not reproduce these findings even though we used three different commercial preparations of IL-2 (at doses ranging from 1 to 10000 U/ml) (our unpublished observations). Nevertheless, the recent observations by Girard et al. (81) provide a clue, insofar as they found that IL-2 alone did not modify the level of *de novo* RNA and protein synthesis in neutrophils, similarly to what we observed. However, when the PMN were stimulated with IL-2 in combination with a fixed concentration of GM-CSF, but not of TNFα or fMLP, a dose-dependent effect of IL-2 in potentiating the induction of both RNA and protein synthesis by GM-CSF was observed (81). Although a great donor-to-donor variability existed, the data suggested that IL-2 may actually function in neutrophils, but only if they are specifically "primed" by GM-CSF.

Some controversies exist also concerning the ability of LPS to induce TNFα production in neutrophils. Takeichi et al. (82) for example, reported that, despite TNFα mRNA induction, neither LPS, nor Concanavalin A (Con A), nor zymosan were effective stimuli for TNFα release by neutrophils. Similar findings were reported by Altstaedt et al. (4), and by Terashima et al. (83). Takeichi et al. (82) attributed these conflicting results to the fact that their

TNFα assay was not sensitive enough. Moreover, in a more recent study (84), the same group reported that highly purified PMNs (>99.5%) isolated from periapical exudates (PE) expressed significant levels of mRNA for TNFα (and IL-1α/β), but antigenic TNFα was not detected in PE. They invoked again a low sensitivity of the ELISA with respect to RT-PCR, or that TNFα produced by PMN was adsorbed by active TNF-receptors expressing cells (84). In spite of the latter negative reports, there is enough compelling evidence that PMN release TNFα in response to LPS, based on more data generated by several other laboratories, including our own (50,51,85). What is more, Haziot et al. were able to confer to surface CD14 an important role in mediating the secretion of TNFα by LPS-treated neutrophils, as anti-CD14 mAbs severely inhibited this response (86).

TNFα is a potent stimulus of PMN themselves, promoting adherence to endothelial cells and to particles, and leading to increased phagocytosis, respiratory burst activity and degranulation (87). The ability of PMN to release TNFα in response to so many different stimuli, suggest that granulocytes may exert host defense functions that go beyond the killing of invading microorganisms in septic infections, and may therefore represent a manner whereby neutrophils can activate themselves in an autocrine/paracrine fashion.

3.8 *CD30 Ligand*

CD30, a member of the NGF/TNF receptor superfamily, is preferentially expressed by Th2-type CD4+ T cell clones as well as by CD8+ T cell clones showing a Th2 profile of cytokine secretion (88). The natural ligand for CD30, CD30L, has been shown to be a type II transmembrane glycoprotein of the TNF ligand superfamily (88). CD30L has been found to be expressed by B lymphocytes, as well as by a subset of activated macrophages and T cells (88). CD30 triggering induces nuclear factor-kB activation in human T cells, and may provide a critical costimulatory signal for the development of Th2 responses and HIV replication (88).

By Northern blot analysis, Gruss et al. (89) observed that PMN constitutively express CD30L mRNA, but not CD30 mRNA, and that after 24-h treatment with LPS, IFNγ, or GM-CSF, the steady-state levels of CD30L mRNA were slightly increased. They also found that in reactive lymph nodes and tonsils, CD30L was expressed by a small subset of lymphoid cells, histiocytes, and also granulocytes, as detected by immunostaining and flow cytometry (90). Higher levels of CD30L expression were noted in Hodgkin disease (HD) lesions among bystander cells, which included T cells and granulocytes (90). Remarkably, native CD30L displayed at the cell surface was functionally active, as shown by the ability of fixed granulocytes to interact with CD30 positive cell lines and induce their proliferation (90). Our unpublished experiments confirm that PMN express high levels of CD30L mRNA, especially after stimulation with LPS or fMLP. In addition, by immunofluorescence analysis, we found a variable CD30L protein expression in neutrophils, depending on the donor. The biological implication of CD30L expression in neutrophils requires to be furtherly investigated. For instance, it is known that the interaction between CD30L and CD30 triggers the replication of HIV (91). In addition, Ho et al. (92) showed that human neutrophils can potentiate HIV replication in infected mononuclear leukocytes, but did not identify the mechanisms or the molecules implicated in these effects. In the light of the potential ability of neutrophils to express CD30L, one obvious candidate for this interesting effect could be just CD30L.

3.9 *Interleukin-1*

For a long time a considerable dispute has existed regarding the ability of PMN to synthesize and secrete IL-1 (93–96), but nowadays there is little doubt that neutrophils can be induced to produce small amounts (hundreds of picograms as a maximum) of IL-1. That human PMN produce an IL-1-like activity after stimulation with particulate and soluble agents, such as zymosan and PMA, respectively, was clearly documented by Tiku et al. (97). This IL-1-like activity was detected in the supernatants of PMN only if stimulated for at least 4.5 h, and was also induced by A23187 plus cytochalasin B, as well as by LPS, albeit at much lower levels (97). Subsequently, neutrophils stimulated with GM-CSF were observed to express the mRNA and release both IL-1α and IL-1β (98,99). Partial elucidation of the mechanisms whereby GM-CSF regulates IL-1β gene expression in PMN has been recently reported by Fernandez et al. (100), who demonstrated actions at both the transcriptional and post-transcriptional levels. In another study (101), human PMN produced both forms of IL-1 in response to LPS over a 72-h culture period, being IL-1β produced and released before IL-1α. Similar patterns of IL-1α and IL-1β production in response to zymosan, LPS or Con A, were also described by Takeichi et al. (82). Lord et al. (102) not only provided evidence that PMN transcribe and translate the IL-1α and IL-1β genes after stimulation with LPS or IL-1α, but also established that IL-1α and IL-1β synthesis attributed to PMN could not be accounted for by the low level of contaminating PBMC. IL-1β mRNA accumulation is induced in a dose-dependent manner also by IL-1β and/or TNFα (103). While the relative levels of the cell-associated antigenic IL-1β induced by TNFα and/or IL-1β strongly correlated with the induction of IL-1β mRNA, no IL-1β antigen was detected in the supernatants of PMN incubated with or without cytokines for less than 4 h (103). In agreement with these observations, we also found that neutrophils produce and release IL-1β not before 5–6 h following stimulation with TNFα (51). Increase of IL-1β mRNA expression induced by TNFα is not affected by difluoromethylornithine (DFMO), a selective inhibitor of ornithine decarboxylase (104). Interestingly, neonatal PMN can express antigenic IL-1β when stimulated by TNFα and LPS, and this expression seems consistently higher than that of adult PMN (79). Also fMLP (100 nM) induced release of detectable amounts of IL-1β by PMN over a 24-h period, and precoating of tissue culture plates with the matrix proteins Fn and Ln enhanced both spontaneous and fMLP- and LPS-stimulated IL-1β release (20). We (2,3), and others (79), have never been able to measure any extracellular IL-1β in response to fMLP (10–100 nM). Therefore, as discussed in the case of TNFα, elaboration of cytokines in response to fMLP, if true, seems to be modulated at multiple levels by integrin-extracellular matrix interactions.

Included in the list (Table 5.4) of stimuli able to trigger the production of IL-1β from PMN, are: phagocytosis of yeast particles (37,72), *Listeria monocytogenes* and *Yersinia enterocolitica* (76), *C.neoformans* (38), *C.albicans* or MP-F2, its capsular material (75), a streptococcal preparation termed

Table 5.4   Agents able to trigger the production of IL-1 by human neutrophils

LPS	*C. albicans* and its derivative products
fMLP	
	S.cerevisiae
TNFα	
	IgG-opsonized *S.cerevisiae*
IL-1α	zymosan
IL-1β	LPS from *F.mortiferum*
GM-CSF	LPS from *A.actinomycetemcomitans*
PMA, A23187	LPS from *Fusobacterium nucleatum*
Anti cytoplasmic (ANCA) antibodies	LPS from *Porphyromonas gingivalis*
anti-CD32 (FcγRII) antibodies	LPS from *Capnocytophaga ochracea*
Concanavalin A	*Yersinia Enterocolitica*
MSU, CPPD	*Listeria Monocytogenes*
Interaction with Fibronectin or	*C.neoformans*
Laminin	
Streptococcal OK-432	Glucuronoxylomannan
Staphilococcus aureus	Epstein Barr Virus

*: mRNA only

OK-432 (105), the non-oral organism *F.mortiferum* (106), and LPS from *F.nucleatum and A.actinomycetemcomitans* and, and to lesser extent, LPS from *P.gingivalis* and *C.ochracea* (42). A very recent study (107) has demonstrated that neutrophils can be stimulated to express mRNA and protein for IL-1β by anti-neutrophil cytoplasmic antibodies (ANCA), which are present in patients with systemic vasculitis. Both human ANCA and mAbs to a variety of autoantigens recognized by ANCA, including proteinase 3, myeloperoxidase (MPO), bactericidal/permeability increasing protein and elastase, were effective (107). This response could be inhibited by Act D and CHX, but not by FK506 or cyclosporin A (107). Besides, human anti-MPO IgG F(ab)$_2$ were completely without effect on IL-1β production (and on superoxide production), suggesting the requirement for Fc receptors involvement. Indeed, the mAbs Fab IV.3 (anti FcγRII) induced IL-1β production from neutrophils treated with normal serum

(107). Since neutrophils accumulate in the acute blood vessel lesions of patients with autoimmune systemic vasculitis, the data suggest that, in these individuals, ANCA may stimulate PMN to release IL-1β, other than activating neutrophils to produce reactive oxygen radicals and to degranulate (108). The possibility that neutrophil-derived IL-1β may contribute to augment the local inflammatory response by the activation of vascular endothelial cells and infiltrating leucocytes must thus be considered for therapeutical intervention. In other studies, McColl and colleagues tested the capacity of neutrophils to synthesize and release IL-1α/β species after phagocytosis of MSU and CPPD, alone, or in combination with TNFα and GM-CSF (109,110). Acute gout and pseudogout are associated with phagocytosis of MSU and CPPD crystals by joint neutrophils. The latter are the major, if not the only cell type within the SF in the initial phase of such crystal-induced attacks. Initially, it was shown that MSU crystals were more potent inducers of both IL-1α and IL-1β generation than CPPD or unopsonized zymosan (109). With all the three stimuli, the syntesis of IL-1β was 5 to 14 fold greater than that of IL-1α, and up to 10 times more IL-1β than IL-1α was usually secreted (109). Colchicine, a clinical specific and effective drug in the treatment of acute gout, partly inhibited the secretion of IL-1 by neutrophils during phagocytosis of solid particles (109). These results suggested that neutrophil-derived IL-1 contribute to the pathogenesis of crystal-induced arthritis. Then (110), they observed that treatment of PMN with GM-CSF and TNFα before incubation with suboptimal concentrations of the crystals enhanced the total synthesis of IL-1 induced by microcrystals by five- to nine-fold, over a 12-h incubation period. Under the same conditions, the levels of total IL-1ra produced by neutrophils were approximately 35 to 43% lower than the expected amounts produced by cytokine-treated cells (110). As a result of this shift in IL-1 and IL-1ra production by GM-CSF- and TNFα-activated neutrophils, the net biologic activity of IL-1 secreted in response to the microcrystals was enhanced. Treatment of neutrophils with colchicine prior to incubation with GM-CSF or TNFα inhibited the crystal-induced IL-1 production by 50 to 55%, but failed to affect that of IL-1ra. In this situation therefore, the IL-1ra to IL-1 ratio increased significantly by 185–220% (110). Altogether, these results not only demonstrated that IL-1 and IL-1ra production by human neutrophils were differentially regulated, but that the combined presence of GM-CSF or TNFα and microcrystals favor the production of biologically active IL-1 over that of IL-1ra, thereby potentially amplifying the inflammatory response associated with crystal-induced diseases. In addition, because colchicine selectively inhibited IL-1 without affecting IL-1ra production, they uncovered another putative site of action of the drug.

IL-1α and IL-1β production by neutrophils can have profound effects during inflammation and, as a consequence, pathophysiological implications. The latter might be: recruitment and regulation leukocye function, priming of neutrophils for oxidative activity, phagocytosis, degranulation and stimulation of the production of arachidonic acid metabolites, regulation of fibroblast, osteoclasts and synovial cells activation, induction of fever, and so forth (111).

3.11 *Interleukin-1 receptor antagonist*

Release of IL-1 in concert with TNFα fulfils immunomodulatory functions that may be beneficial for the host, but, if not controlled, may contribute to the pathogenesis of the diseases in which IL-1 is involved (111). In this regard, the biologic effects of IL-1 can be regulated by natural inhibitors such as for instance the IL-1 receptor antagonist (IL-1ra) (112). IL-1ra is usually made by the same cell types that secrete IL-1, and specifically inhibits the pro-inflammatory actions of IL-1 by binding to its cognate receptors located on target cell and without initiating any signal transduction (113). As IL-1ra blocks the activities of IL-1 both *in vitro* and *in vivo*, the production of relatively large amounts of IL-1ra by neutrophils could be of major biological significance since it could inhibit an established inflammatory response mediated by IL-1 (112).

The first report suggesting that neutrophils might secrete products featuring IL-1-inhibitory activity were those by Tiku et (97,114), but the molecular demonstration that this IL-1 inhibitory activity corresponded to IL-1ra was provided six years later by McColl's group (115). The latter authors not only were able to confirm the data that neutrophils constitutively produce IL-1ra (114,116), but also that following activation with TNFα and GM-CSF, PMN express the mRNA and secrete increased amounts of IL-1ra protein over a 24-h period (approximately 0.5 ng/ ml/10^6 cells)(115). The same authors concluded that IL-1ra constitutes one of the major *de novo*-synthesized product of activated neutrophils. They also calculated that IL-1ra is produced in excess of IL-1 by a factor of at least 100; such a ratio fits perfectly with the reported amounts of IL-1ra needed to inhibit the pro-inflammatory effects of IL-1 (111,113). Ulich et al. (117) concomitantly found that PMN were able to express increased levels of IL-1ra mRNA and protein after incubation with LPS. Interestingly, extent of IL-1ra mRNA expression found in PMN was in magnitude similar to, or even greater than that found in PBMC (117). LPS proved to be a very efficient stimulus for the production of IL-1ra in PMN also in our hands, being much more potent than Y-IgG (118). Consistent with a poor ability of Y-IgG to induce IL-1ra in neutrophils, Malyak et al. (116) also reported that adherent IgG did not trigger the production of IL-1ra from PMN. It is noteworthy that the stimulation of human monocytes with LPS or IgG, these latter either in a soluble form (119), or attached to plastic surfaces (120), led instead to approximately the same amount of IL-1ra production. Whether this difference between monocytes and neutrophils is due to a greater ability of the monocyte Fcγ-receptors to generate intracellular signals for expression, translation and secretion of IL-1ra, remains to be investigated. In this respect, data by Chang et al. (121) indicate that adherent anti-FcγRIII (CD16) mAbs, but not anti-FcγRI or anti-FcgRII mAbs, induce the production of IL-1ra from PMN. However, in a recent publication by Ohlsson et al. (72), it has been shown that pre-opsonized yeast particles were more efficient than LPS in inducing *de novo* synthesis and release of IL-1ra in neutrophils and MNC. The discrepancy with our data might be related to the fact that Ohlsson et al. (72) stimulated cells with 25 particles per cells of pre-opsonized yeasts while we used a particle cell ratio of 2 to 1 (118). In any case, if one examines the IL-1ra/IL-1 ratio under those stimulatory conditions, in each of the two studies an anti-inflammatory balance was found, being IL-1ra secreted in a greater excess than IL-1 (72,118).

Elegant studies performed by Colotta and collaborators showed that in addition to LPS and GM-CSF (122), IL-4 (122), IL-13 (123) and TGFβ_1 (124) are efficient inducers of IL-1ra mRNA expression and secretion in PMN. That IL-4 and TGFβ significantly enhance the spontaneous production of IL-1ra by human PMN has been recently confirmed in other studies (116,125). In the latter's paper, while LPS and TNFα had an additive effect on the production of IL-1ra, there was no significant enhancement following further addition of IL-4 or IL-10 (125). Interestingly, the studies by Colotta's group (123,124) also revealed that in PMN, either IL-13 or TGFβ_1 induce the mRNA expression of the intracellular form of IL-1ra (icIL-1ra), whose biological function remains obscure. The observation that TGFβ1 is able to trigger the production of IL-1ra, might explain one of the mechanism(s) whereby IL-1ra is constitutively produced by PMN (114–116,118). TGFβ_1 is in fact constitutively expressed by PMN (126), and could therefore stimulate the same cells to produce IL-1ra through an autocrine loop. Very recently, Muzio et al. (127) cloned and characterized a new intracellular isoform of IL-1ra expressed in PMN and other cells, which was termed icIL-1ra type II (icIL-1raII). icIL-1raII was found to be potentially biologically active, and to differ from the previously known icIL-1ra (icIL-1raI) only by an additional stretch of 21 amino acids located within the NH$_2$-terminal portion of the molecule (127).

Table 5.5 summarizes the list of the agents able to induce IL-1ra production in PMN. These include A23187, zymosan (114), MSU, CPPD (110), and *P.falciparum*-infected erythrocytes of the Malayan Camp strain *in vitro* (39),

Table 5.5   Agents able to trigger the production of IL-1ra by human neutrophils

LPS	zymosan
anti-CD16 (FcγRIII) antibodies	
	IgG-opsonized yeast particles
TNFα	*C. albicans*
IL-1β	LPS from *A.actinomycetemcomitans*
IL-4	LPS from *Fusobacterium nucleatum*
IL-13	LPS from *Porphyromonas gingivalis*
GM-CSF	LPS from *Capnocytophaga ochracea*
TGFβ_1	*Bacteroides forsythus*
PMA	*F.mortiferum*
A23187	*Plasmodium falciparum*-infected erythrocytes
MSU, CPPD	Epstein Barr Virus

*: mRNA only

but it is worth spending a few more words on other situations in which IL-1ra is expressed in neutrophils. For instance, functional studies have shown that stimulation of PMN with a number of periodontopathic bacteria results in the production of an IL-1 inhibitor.

Yamazaki et al. (106) have shown in 1989 that PMN stimulated with the periodontopathic bacteria *Bacteroides gingivalis, Bacteroides forsythus, A.actinomycetemcomitans F.nucleatum and F.mortiferum*, produce an IL-1 inhibitor, likely IL-1ra. More recently, Yoshimura et al. (42) confirmed these data, showing that substantially great amounts of IL-1ra were released from PMN stimulated with each LPS from the periodontopathic bacteria, *P.gingivalis, A.actinomycetemcomitans, C.ochracea* and *F.nucleatum,* other than non-oral bacterium *E.coli.* The inhibitory effects of IL-1ra on the biological activity of IL-1 in the supernatants of PMN were examined by the thymocyte comitogen proliferation assay. The supernatants of PMN stimulated with each LPS showed less biological IL-1 activity as compared with the same doses of recombinant human IL-1β detected by enzyme-linked immunosorbent assay. Furthermore, no activity was detected in the supernatants of PMN stimulated with *P.gingivalis* or *C.ochracea* (42). These findings demonstrated that LPS from periodontopathic bacteria are capable of stimulating PMN to release not only pro-inflammatory cytokines but also their inhibitors, such as IL-1ra. Different secretion levels of these cytokines and their biological activities induced by the various LPS might be important in the onset and progression of periodontal diseases.

In another series of papers, Gosselin's group analyzed in detail the effect of Epstein-Barr virus (EBV) on gene expression and protein synthesis of IL-1 and IL-1ra in human peripheral blood neutrophils (128,129). EBV was found to induce a rapid accumulation of IL-1 and IL-1ra mRNA in neutrophils, associated with a later appearance of considerable amounts of IL-1α, IL-1β and IL-1ra proteins. Approximately 3200 and 610 times more IL-1ra than IL-1α or IL-1β, respectively, was secreted by neutrophils in response to EBV. Heat-inactivated virus was unable to stimulate cytokine synthesis, whereas UV-irradiated virus retained the full IL-1- and IL-1ra-inducing potential of the native particle (129). Pretreatment of cells with CHX or phosphonoacetic acid (the latter, known to inhibit viral DNA polymerase activity), did not abrogate the effect of EBV, suggesting that EBV does not penetrate the cell, but that a virion's structural molecule is required to induce such an effect. In this respect, neutralization of the viral particles with the mAb 72A1, which is known to react with glycoprotein gp350 of the viral envelope, inhibited the production of IL-1 and IL-1ra, suggesting that gp350 could be involved in this process. Therefore, EBV may directly activate certain cellular genes when it binds to the cells. Furthermore, the effect induced by EBV did not reflect an overall metabolic activity of neutrophils: EBV failed to induce GM-CSF synthesis, while MSU crystals, in the same experiments, were potent activators (129). The elevated levels of IL-1ra produced by EBV-stimulated PMN might be part of mechanisms used by the virus to avoid rejection at the early stage of its infectious process, and thus to evade the immune system.

3.12 *Interleukin-6*

Whether or not human PMN express and release IL-6 is still a matter of discussion. The controversy started with the paper published by Cicco et al. (130), who reported that stimulation of PMN with GM-CSF, and to a lesser extent with TNFα, leads to a rapid accumulation of IL-6 mRNA, and subsequent secretion of the related protein. LPS, PMA and CHX were also reported to induce IL-6 transcripts in PMN (130). Previously, Kato and colleagues (131), had shown that in a whole blood culture system, the IL-6-expressing cells after stimulation with LPS or Con A, were exclusively monocytes. In agreement with the latter data, we provided clear molecular evidence for a complete lack of IL-6 gene expression in PMN cultured for up to 18 h in the presence of LPS or Y-IgG (70). Since then, we consider the presence of IL-6 mRNA as a marker for monocyte contamination, and we screen for IL-6 transcripts every Northern blot made with RNA isolated from PMN. Actually, even by RT-PCR we do not find IL-6 mRNA transcripts in any of our neutrophil preparation, either in resting conditions or after treatment with LPS, GM-CSF and CHX (M.P.Russo et al., unpublished observations). Incidentally, other studies have emphasized that if production of IL-6 is detected in the cultures of human PMN, this is accounted for by contaminating monocytes. In one of them, Wang and colleagues (50) demonstrated that if neutrophils are prepared with extreme caution, so that monocyte contamination is kept below 0.7%, IL-6 release from PMN is undetectable. What is more, they also show, as we did (70), that after LPS stimulation only monocytes express IL-6 mRNA. In another study, Takeichi et al. (82) characterized cytokine secretion by peripheral blood PMN, monocytes and lymphocytes stimulated with zymosan, Con A and LPS. Both monocytes and lymphocytes produced high levels of IL-6, while PMN did not. In addition, as revealed by a very sensitive radioactive RT-PCR analysis, PMN stimulated with zymosan showed stronger expression of IL-1α, IL-1β, and TNFα mRNA than cells stimulated with LPS or Con A, but IL-6 mRNA was never detected under any condition. In contrast, stimulated monocytes or lymphocytes expressed all cytokine transcripts at very high levels (82). Identical results were even observed if PMN were isolated from the gingival crevicular fluid from patients affected by periodontitis (82), or, from alveolar bone-derived PMN (84). Finally, in a study in which the ability of *P.falciparum*-infected erythrocytes to induce cytokine production from blood cells was investigated, granulocytes did not release IL-6, while autologous PBMC (mainly monocytes) secreted large amounts of the cytokine (39).

There are however several published articles showing that PMN express IL-6. Palma et al. (71) for example, reported a time-dependent extracellular production of IL-6 in response to LPS, with maximal release after 24 h (400 pg/ml/10^6 cells). This secretion was preceded, in Northern blot analysis, by an augmentation of IL-6 mRNA by LPS. Surprisingly, PMN displayed a substantial expression of IL-6 transcripts under resting conditions (71). Melani et al. (132) also found a constitutive IL-6 mRNA expression in circulating human granulocytes immediately purified from fresh blood (98% neutrophils, 1.2% eosinophils, 0.8% mononucleated cells). For this investigation they used either RT-PCR or ISH. Interestingly, this constitutive IL-6 expression was very weak if neutrophils were isolated from buffy coats instead of fresh heparinized peripheral blood. Furthermore, IL-6 expression disappeared if PMN were left on ice or at 37°C in Dulbecco's modified Eagle's medium for 1 h, but it was still inducible by the additon of GM-CSF (50 ng/ml) for another hour (132). Altstaedt and coll. (4) could not detect any IL-6 signals by RT-PCR in freshly isolated neutrophils, but these were detectable after stimulation with LPS or zymosan for 1 or 3 h. However, no IL-6 protein was found in supernatants of these stimulated neutrophils (4). Induction of IL-6 mRNA levels after *in vitro* treatment of blood neutrophils (>97% pure) with GM-CSF were also reported by Quayle et al. (133). A more recent study (purity of PMN only >96%) has reported a detailed analysis on the ability of LPS and dexamethasone to modulate IL-6 mRNA expression (by RT-PCR) and production in PMN (134). Curiously, neither GM-CSF, nor PMA had an effect on IL-6 mRNA abundance (134), in contrast with the data of Cicco et al. (130). Arnold and colleagues reported not only a constitutive IL-6 mRNA expression, but also that after phagocytosis of *L.monocytogenes*, *Y.enterocolitica* and *E.coli*, PMN secrete large amounts of IL-6, IL-1β and TNFα (76). In a different paper, they also showed that after exposure to RSV particles, PMN secrete IL-6 in a dose- and time-dependent manner (11). But the same authors precised that their neutrophil preparations were less than 98% pure (11,76). Results by Retini et al. (38) demonstrated that in response to *C.neoformans* yeast cells, PMN (purity greater than 98%) from normal subjects produce IL-6 to levels comparable to those induced, in their hands, by LPS. Even culture of PMN (and PBMC) with OK-432, a streptococcal preparation, resulted in a concentration-dependent increase in the production of IL-6 (and IL-1β) (105). However, while PMN shared a purity of over 97%, surprisingly (2), the relative amount of cytokine release by PMN and PBMC, on a per cell basis, were very similar (105). Finally, in a series of papers in which PMN from subjects at different stages of HIV infection were assayed, Cassone et al. (135) initially reported that neutrophils produced significant amounts of IL-6 after stimulation with MP-F2, with no differences between HIV-negative (HIV⁻) and HIV-positive (HIV⁺) PMN. However, in a subsequent study (75), the same group reported that production of IL-6 was much more elevated in PMN from HIV⁺patients at all stages of infection, both under basal conditions and after stimulation with LPS or MP-F2. In the last work (136), they substantially confirm that production of IL-6 from HIV⁺ subjects was three-six times higher than that of HIV⁻ individuals, but they also state (and show) that PMN from normal donors produce little IL-6 mRNA and protein even after stimulation, in accordance with the recognized low or no production of IL-6 in PMN from other studies (50,70).

In summary, although it cannot be definitively and formally ruled out that certain stimuli, or some pathological conditions might specifically induce IL-6 from human PMN, the compelling evidence accumulated by now emphasizes the need to exclude any possible monocyte contamination, as we (70) and others (50,82,131) did. In contrast to the human system, Romani and colleagues (137) reported that neutrophils purified from the peritoneal cavity of mice, and cultured *in vitro* with IFNγ plus LPS, or with different strains of *C.albicans* cells, express IL-6 messages (as revealed by RT-PCR), and produce substantial amounts of immunogenic IL-6, as measured by ELISA.

3.13 *Interleukin-12*

IL-12 is a heterodimeric factor of 70 kD (p70), formed by two covalently-linked glycosylated chains of approximately 40 kD (p40) and 35 kD (p35), whose co-expression is necessary for biologic activity. IL-12 is produced mainly by mononuclear phagocytic cells, B cells, neutrophils and other types of antigen presenting cells (APC). IL-12 triggers several biologic activities of NK cells and T lymphocytes, on which it induces the production of lymphokines, particularly IFNγ, enhancement of cell-mediated cytotoxicicity, and mitogenic effects. In addition, IL-12 is required for optimal differentiation of cytotoxic T lymphocytes and appears to have an obligatory role as inducer of differentiation of Th1 and to suppress IgE synthesis. The first demonstration that mature human neutrophils produce and release both the IL-12p40 free chain and the IL-12p70 heterodimer was produced in my laboratory (138). Our experiments showed that among a wide range of stimuli tested, including TNFα, fMLP, PMA and Y-IgG, only LPS in combination with IFNγ efficiently induced a significant production of biologically active IL-12. This was because on the one hand, LPS induced a 100-fold increase in IL-12p40 mRNA without having an effect on IL-12p35 mRNA accumulation, on the other, IFNγ directly induced a several-fold increase in the accumulation of IL-12p35 mRNA and enhanced the LPS-induced accumulation of IL-12p40 mRNA. Therefore, the combined effect of LPS and IFNγ induced sufficient expression of both IL-12p40 and IL-12p35 mRNAs to attain production of the biologically active

IL-12p70 heterodimer at physiologically relevant concentrations (138). Interestingly, the kinetics of LPS plus IFNγ-induced IL-12p40 and IL-12p70 production by PMN were relatively delayed (peaking at 48 h) compared to those of TNFα, IL-1β, IL-8 or IL-1ra. Furthermore, IL-10 suppressed the LPS-induced IL-12p40 mRNA and protein secretion in PMN (138), as previously observed in monocytes (139). Our results have been recently confirmed and extended by Cassone and colleagues (136). Neither LPS, nor MP-F2 were found able to induce biologically active IL-12 production by PMN, whereas the two microbial imunomodulators alone were capable of inducing appreciable IL-12 release by monocytes. However, after addition of IFNγ, both MP-F2 and LPS were capable of inducing PMN to produce IL-12 (136).

IL-12 expression has been observed also in murine neutrophils stimulated *in vitro*. Thioglycollate-elicited neutrophils were cultured in the presence of either IFNγ plus LPS or *C.albicans* cells for 24 h (137). The *C.albicans* cells utilized were the agerminative live vaccine strain PCA-2, which provoke healing infections, and the highly virulent CA-6 strain, which induces nonhealing infections. Low levels of bioactive IL-12 and IL-10 were found in PMN cultures stimulated with IFNγ plus LPS. IL-12, but not IL-10 was produced in response to the agerminative strain PCA-2, while the opposite pattern occurred in response to CA-6 (137). A similar profile of cytokine production was observed in stimulated neutrophils from peripheral blood. As revealed by RT-PCR, IL-10 and IL-12p40 messages, together with those of TNFα and IL-6 were present in elicited neutrophils cultured with LPS plus IFNγ for 2 h. In contrast, in peritoneal macrophages were present IL-6 and TNFα messages, but not IL-10 and IL-12p40 mRNA. Finally, the presence of IL-10 and IL-12 in neutrophils was also documented by an immunophenotype and fluorescence microscopic analyses (140). In another work, Kanangat et al. (141) investigated whether IL-12 induction occurs in response to herpes simplex virus (HSV) infection of the mouse eye. The authors could show an early induction and continued maintenance of IL-12p40 mRNA in the cornea and draining lymph node upon ocular infection with HSV (141). IL-12p40 protein also was detected in the cornea upon ocular HSV infection (141). However, due to the difficulties of isolating individual cell types from the cornea and to assess their IL-12p40 responsiveness, different purified cell populations, including neutrophils, were studied for their responsiveness *in vitro* to exposure to infectious or inactivated HSV. Cultured corneal cells failed to generate IL-12p40 upon exposure to HSV. However, unfractionated splenocytes and enriched populations of dendritic cells, macrophages, and neutrophils (80% pure) isolated from the peritoneal cavity after thioglycollate administration), all responded to UV-inactivated or live HSV, as well as to LPS, by up-regulating the expression of IL-12p40 mRNA (141). Curiously, by far the most prominent cell in the HSV-infected cornea soon after the infection is exactly the neutrophils. The data indicated that inflammatory cells that infiltrate the cornea in response to HSV-1 infection might be the main source of IL-12. IL-12 possesses important immunoregulatory functions, in particular the induction of IFNγ production and facilitation of Th1 type responses. Therefore, the ability of neutrophils to produce IL-12 suggests that they may play an active role in the regulatory interactions between innate resistance and adaptive immunity, and, at the same time, favor a Th1-type immune response. The ability of neutrophils to produce IL-12 *in vivo*, and the meaning and importance of such function in the context of mounting Th1/Th2 responses, is described below.

3.14 *Interferon-α*

Molecular demonstration of the ability of neutrophils to express and release the IFNα protein was reported by Shirafuji et al. (142). By Northern blot analysis, they were able to demonstrate that G-CSF induced the mRNA for IFNα type 1 in neutrophils, but not in MNC (142). In addition, by a specific radioimmunoassay they revealed that the levels of IFNα in the culture media of these G-CSF-treated neutrophils rose in a time-dependent manner (142). Under the same experimental conditions, neither LPS, nor fMLP effectively stimulated the expression of IFNα in PMN (142). In a subsequent work, and using the RT-PCR, Brandt et al. (143) were able to show that PMN accumulate IFNα mRNA in a constitutive manner or upon infection with the Sendai virus, being IFNα-1, IFNα-2, and IFNα-4 the species predominantly expressed (143). A biological assay revealed that the antiviral activity of supernatants recovered from PMN stimulated with Sendai virus was very similar to that detected in MNC, but much more abundant than those measured from purified T and B cells (143). The fact that neutrophils can be significant sources of IFNα, also in the bovine system (144), emphasize the potentially important role of PMN in host defense against viral infection, or in other biological processes in which interferons are implicated.

3.15 *Transforming growth-factor-β*

Grotendorst and colleagues (126) reported that cultured human neutrophils constitutively express TGFβ_1 mRNA and secrete high levels of the protein in a fully active form. Interestingly, after activation of neutrophils with LPS, fMLP or immune complexes for 24 h, no difference in the levels of TGFβ_1 protein were detected, relative to untreated cells (approximately 50 ng/ml/10^6 cells). However, as opposed to neutrophils, stimulation with LPS, fMLP or immune complexes resulted in a strong increase of TGFβ secretion by monocytes (126). Remarkably, unstimulated PMN secreted approximately five times more TGFβ than an equal number of unstimulated monocytes, over a 24 h-period in culture (126). That PMN may represent an important potential source of TGFβ in inflammatory infiltrates was confirmed by the studies of Fava et al. (145), who reported that a pre-existing TGFβ-bioactivity could be released from freshly isolated peripheral PMN, if incubated with PMA at 37° for 30 min. The identity of this activity as TGFβ_1 was immunologically confirmed. However, in contrast with the findings of Grotendorst et al. (126), Fava et al. (145) found a little detectable TGFβ_1 activity released from unstimulated PMN, but this might be explained by the fact that neutrophils were only cultured for 30 min, as opposed to 24 h (126). Our unpublished observations confirm that neutrophils constitutively express high levels of TGFβ_1 mRNA, and that these levels are unaffected in LPS- or fMLP-activated cells. The ability of neutrophils to produce TGFβ may play an important role in situations such as wound repair, chronic immuno-driven inflammations and immune responses, or in the pathogenesis of fibrotic disease.

3.16 *Other cytokines*

Isolated observations would indicate that neutrophils can express or produce other cytokines. For example, Lindemann et al. (67) reported that stimulation of PMN with GM-CSF induces the mRNA expression and release of G-CSF and M-CSF. Ramenghi et al. (146), evaluated by RT-PCR the cell types in peripheral blood that express the mRNA for stem cell factor (SCF), the ligand of the c-kit proto-oncogene. Only granulocytes, and not isolated lymphocytes, monocytes, or the total cell population obtained by Ficoll purification, appeared to express transcripts encoding both the soluble and transmembrane forms of SCF (146). In similar experiments, we could demonstrate neither constitutive or induced SCF mRNA, nor secretion of the related protein (our unpublished observations). Clearly, further experiments are mandatory before making any speculation on the possible biological significance of SCF expression by PMN. Kita and coworkers (147), on the basis of indirect effects, assumed that neutrophils stimulated with PMA in combination with ionomycin (a calcium ionophore), produce IL-3 and GM-CSF. They were, however, unable to directly measure by specific immunological techniques IL-3 and GM-CSF in neutrophil culture supernatants (147). Similarly, Contrino et al. (79) failed to detect the GM-CSF protein in cell lysates and supernatants from PMN stimulated (for 3 and 24 h) with TNFa, LPS, fMLP, or IL-1β. In contrast, Roberge and colleagues (129), more recently, identified MSU crystals, but not EBV, as able to induce the syntesis of GM-CSF.

Very recently, Calafat and colleagues (148), using immunoelectron microscopy, have clearly demonstrated that monocytes and neutrophils store TGFα in cytoplasmic vescicles. TGFα is a polypeptide belonging to the family of EGF-related protein and exerts several effects on target cells, such as mitogenic signaling and promotion of neovascularization. It has also been suggested that TGFα is involved in wound healing and in tumor development. No colocalization of TGFα with components of azurophilic or specific granules or secretory vesicles was observed in neutrophils, suggesting that TGFα-containing granules differ from the three main kinds of granules or from the rapidly mobilizable pool of secretory vesicles. This implies that TGFα is stored in a novel, not previously described compartment. Monocytes and neutrophils were also pelleted and lysed to quantify TGFα using ELISA. Monocytes were found to contain approximately 257 pg of TGFα/10^6 cells, but neutrophils much less: 2.5 pg of TGFα/10^6 cells. Other findings indicated that the TGFα gene was expressed early in myeloid development, and the protein is stored in granules. Interestingly enough, a previous report (149) also showed that granulocytes stimulated with fMLP plus cytochalasin B were able to release immunoreactive TGFα, but, even though neutrophils were not excluded as possible source, it was demonstrated that eosinophils were the major manufacturers. The findings that neutrophils contain TGFα might help to explain complications caused by chronic inflammation, such as fibrosis and neoplastic transformation.

Finally, as observed for RANTES, MCP-2, MCP-3, and I-309 (31), human neutrophils neither seem to produce any IL-2 activity (101), nor IL-10 or IL-13 (M.A. Gougerot-Pocidalo, personal communication). In contrast, and as already mentioned above, Romani and coworkers (137) reported that, *in vitro*, purified murine neutrophils can produce IL-10, but not IL-4, in response to either IFNγ plus LPS, or to *C.albicans*.

4. Modulation of Cytokine Production in Human Neutrophils

An increasing number of studies have documented that, at least *in vitro*, agonist-induced cytokine release by neutrophils can be influenced (either positively, or negatively) by immunomodulating agents, such as IFNγ, IL-4, and IL-10 (2,3 for reviews). These molecules, usually (but not always), do not directly trigger by themselves any functional responses of neutrophils. The effects of IL-10 and IFNγ can be briefly summarised as follows. IL-10 inhibits the LPS-induced extracellular release of TNFα (23,50), IL-1α/β (23,50) IL-8 (23,50,62), GROα (52), IP-10 (59), MIP-1α/β (62) and IL-12 (138), while it potentiates that of IL-1ra (118). By contrast, the effects of IFNγ are usually opposite to those of IL-10, except in the case of IL-1ra (P.P.McDonald et al., unpublished observations). The fact that the release of cytokines is modulated by IL-10 and IFNγ raises the intriguing possibility that both Th1 and Th2 lymphocytes might play a role also in influencing the production of cytokines by PMN.

Studies performed *in vitro* with IL-10 and IFNγ, both in our laboratory and in others, have revealed the existence of a PMN-centered cytokine network regulating IL-8 release by LPS-stimulated PMN (depicted in Figure 1 of reference 2). Briefly, the extracellular production of IL-8 in neutrophils stimulated with LPS starts after 30–60 min, slowly increases up to 5–6 h, and, after this period, dramatically increases up to 18–20 h (23). The mechanisms underlying these kinetics resulted to be a direct effect of LPS, accounting for the initial release of IL-8 (up to 5–6 h), and an endogenous production of TNFα and IL-1β, which synergize in an autocrine/paracrine manner with LPS in inducing the late phase of IL-8 production (2,23). Supporting this network were the fundamental observations made with the use of IL-10 and IFNγ. In the presence of IL-10, the initial production of IL-8 by PMN stimulated with LPS does not change, but the late IL-8 release is completely suppressed (23). This reflects the fact that IL-10 significantly inhibits the release of TNFα and IL-1β (23). Indeed, the late production of IL-8 in PMN stimulated with LPS in the presence of neutralizing antibodies against TNFα and IL-1β is inhibited at levels comparable (but not identical) to those obtained when the cells are co-stimulated with IL-10 and LPS (23). Furthermore, IL-10 potentiates the release of IL-1ra induced by LPS (118), and this inhibitor of IL-1 action (10 μg/ml), in turn, might reduce the LPS-stimulated IL-8 production *in vitro* (150). In the presence of IFNγ, the LPS-induced production of TNFα and IL-1β are strongly potentiated, and this results in a massive production of IL-8 at later times: again, such release can be completely blocked by anti-TNFα and anti-IL-1β neutralizing antibodies (51). Remarkably, based on the results of Kasama and coworkers, a similar *in vitro* network probably also exists for MIP-1α and MIP-1β release in LPS-stimulated neutrophils. These authors reported that production of MIP-1α and MIP-1β features similar kinetics, is equally affected by the action of neutralizing anti-TNFα antibodies, and is influenced by IL-10 and IFNγ in a very similar manner to those of IL-8 (62,85). Even the time course of GROα release in LPS-treated PMN, and the effects of IL-10 and IFNγ thereupon were very similar to those observed in the case of IL-8 (52). It is therefore tempting to speculate that GROα production is regulated in a manner similar to that of IL-8. Moreover, the profile of TNFα, IL-1β and IL-8 secretion by PMN in response to *C.neoformans* was recently reported to have many analogies with the above described network (38). However, other findings suggest that the observations made *in vitro* do not always reflect the various molecular interactions occurring *in vivo*. For instance, Pang et al. (151) reported that neutrophils isolated from sputum of subjects with chronic bronchial sepsis constitutively secreted large amounts of IL-8, IL-1β, and TNFα, with little increase in the presence of LPS. In addition, IL-10 inhibition of IL-8 production by sputum neutrophils was significantly less than that noted with LPS-stimulated blood neutrophils. Moreover, antibody to IL-1β, but not to TNFα, inhibited IL-8 secretion by sputum neutrophils, contrasting with results found using blood neutrophils (151), and suggesting that in purulent sputum an autocrine loop involving IL-1α maintains IL-8 secretion by PMN within the bronchus lumen. Obviously, it is possible that additional factors *in vivo*, such as time and exposure to other cell types and growth factors condition the development of a particular neutrophil phenotype in term of cytokine release.

5. Molecular Regulation of Cytokine Production in Neutrophils

Studies addressing cytokine release by neutrophils at the molecular level have revealed that the induction of a cytokine production in PMN is usually preceded by an increased accumulation of the related mRNA transcripts. Molecular approaches and other related techniques have also yielded important insights into the molecular mechanisms regulating cytokine gene expression in PMN. As in other cell types, cytokine expression in neutrophils can be regulated at transcriptional, post-transcriptional, translational and post-translational levels (3). For instance, nuclear run-on assays (a technique which allows a direct evaluation of the transcriptional activity of a given gene) demonstrated that neutrophils cultured for 4 h actively transcribe the IL-1β, IL-8 and MIP-1α genes only if LPS was present in the medium, but not constitutively (152,153). As opposed to transcriptional regulation, cytokines regulated at the level of mRNA stability are IL-1β, IL-8, MIP-1α/β and IL-1ra, whereas a translational or secretional control have been clearly shown, respectively, for IL-1 and MIP-1α, and for IL-1ra and IL-8 (see reference 3 for a detailed review). Important information on the mechanisms involved in gene regulation has also derived from the effects of metabolic inhibitors, such as Act D, a blocker of RNA synthesis, or CHX, puromycin, and emetine, which are inibitors of protein synthesis. In particular, the use of CHX have made it clear that the influence of *de novo* protein synthesis towards the steady state level of a given cytokine mRNA can considerably vary depending upon the triggering stimulus.

The mechanisms underlying some of the modulatory actions of IL-10 and IFNγ towards cytokine mRNA accumulation in LPS-treated neutrophil have also been extensively analyzed. For instance, our nuclear run-on analyses revealed that LPS-mediated transcriptional activation of the IL-8 gene was markedly inhibited by IFNγ or IL-10 (152). Other investigators reported that the inhibitory effect of IL-10 towards LPS-induced IL-8 mRNA accumulation correlated with an enhancement of IL-8 mRNA degradation (50,62). MIP-1α represents another gene whose modulation by IL-10 and IFNγ in PMN is regulated at the level of both mRNA stability and transcription (62,153). Yet, another cytokine mRNA that was found to be mainly regulated at the post-transcriptional level in neutrophils is that encoding IL-1ra. For instance, the augmented expression of IL-1ra mRNA in PMN treated with IL-13 (123) and TGFβ$_1$ (124) was shown to depend on a marked increase of IL-1ra transcripts stability. Furthermore, the half-life of IL-1ra mRNA was prolonged in PMN stimulated in the presence of IL-10 and LPS, as compared with cells stimulated with LPS alone, whereas the half-life of IL-1β mRNA was unchanged (118). Finally, clear direct evidence that IL-8 production can be modulated by IFNγ at the level of secretion was also provided (51).

6. Production of Cytokines by Neutrophils Isolated from Individuals Affected by Different Human Pathologies

Studies that have examined the capacity of neutrophils to produce cytokines in human pathological conditions are not as many as those regarding MNC, but the number of such studies is rapidly growing. A concise description of what has been reported so far is presented below.

6.1 *Production of IL-8*

Some investigators have examined the IL-8 producing capacity of PMN in the context of various diseases. For example, Kuhns et al. (154) observed that during the evolution of the inflammatory response associated with skin lesions raised by suction, IL-8 reached levels up to 175 ng/ml in the media bathing the lesions. Accumulation of IL-8 strictly correlated with the accumulation of the exudative neutrophils at this inflammatory site (13). Furthermore, these neutrophils exhibited 100-fold greater levels of cell-associated IL-8, and spontaneously released up to 50-fold more IL-8 than freshly isolated peripheral blood neutrophils from the same donor (13). These data indicated that neutrophils that have migrated to a inflammatory focus, have upregulated their production of IL-8, and suggested that, by releasing IL-8, PMN play a role in the autocrine regulation of the inflammatory response. Other observations indicated that neutrophils isolated from sputum of subjects with bronchiectasiasis are a significant source of IL-8, IL-1β, and to lesser extent, TNFα, and that an autocrine loop involving IL-1β was responsible of the maintainance of IL-8 production within the bronchus lumen (151). Even neutrophils isolated from the sputa of patients with CF were found to release elevated amounts of IL-8 and nitrite, being PMN from sputa of subjects with disease exacerbations more active than corresponding cells from stable subjects (155). Accordingly, significant levels of IL-8 and nitrite were present in the soluble phase of sputa of CF subjects, again at much higher levels in patients with disease exacerbations (155). IL-8 and nitric oxide produced by neutrophils and other cells could thus become novel therapeutic targets to block lung damage in CF. In this context, low dose and long-term erythromycin treatment of patients affected by chronic airway disease (CAD) has proved to be effective (46). Interestingly, one of the possible mechanisms whereby erythromycin exerts these effects was shown to be a moderate *in vitro* inhibitory effect on IL-8 production in *Pseudomonas*-stimulated neutrophils but not in AM (46). Thus, the clinical efficacy of erythromycin therapy for CAD patients might be partly mediated through a reduced IL-8 production, which in turn diminishes neutrophil accumulation and subsequent damage.

The role of IL-8 in inducing neutrophil accumulation in the nasal discharge of patients with chronic sinusitis was examined by Suzuki and colleagues (156). Chronic sinusitis is a common inflammatory paranasal sinus disease, which is clinically characterized by edematous hypertrophy of the paranasal mucosa and persistent purulent nasal discharge and paranasal sinus effusion with selective and vigorous recruitment of neutrophils. By IH and ISH, Suzuki and colleagues examined the nasal discharge and mucosal specimens obtained from two groups of patients, those with chronic sinusitis and those with allergic rhinitis. The IL-8 levels in nasal discharge were significantly higher in the chronic sinusitis group than in the allergic rhinitis group (156). Immunoreactivity to IL-8 was observed in emigrated PMN of nasal smear, in nasal gland duct cells, and in epithelial cells of the chronic sinusitis group, whereas those of the allergic rhinitis group mostly showed little or no reaction. Similar patterns of localization were shown by ISH for IL-8 mRNA. That neutrophils from neither asthmatic or atopic dermatitis patients express significantly more IL-8 than control neutrophils was also confirmed by Simon et al. (157). The results of Suzuki et al. (156) suggest that chemotactic factors in sinus effusion, including IL-8 derived from nasal gland duct cells and epithelial cells, firstly attract neutrophils out of mucosa, and then, neutrophils that have emigrated into the sinus effusion secrete IL-8. This might induce a further neutrophil accumulation in the sinus of chronic sinusitis patients. Involvement of PMN as mediators of lung injury in the pathogenesis of pulmonary complications associated with cocaine abuse has been supported by Baldwin et al. (158). As a matter of fact, they investigated whether controlled *in vivo* administration of cocaine (inhaled or intravenously) alters the function of neutrophils in a manner capable of contributing to acute lung injury. While exposure to cocaine *in vivo* enhanced the antibacterial and antitumor activities of PMN, it also potentiated their ability to release IL-8 (measured, however, in response to IL-2) (158).

Lin and Huang, in another work, evaluated IL-8 gene expression and release by PMN and peritoneal macrophages (PM) during peritonitis caused by *S.aureus,* in uremic patients on continuous ambulatory peritoneal dialysis (CAPD) (159). Their previous study indicated that IL-8 was detectable in drain dialysate of these patients during the early acute stage of peritonitis, at variable levels depending on the microorganism type (160). These authors revealed that both the IL-8 levels and the amount of IL-8 mRNA expression were highly correlated with the PMN count found in the drain dialysate, since both were high at the onset of peritonitis and then decreased together progressively (159). However, PM expressed more IL-8 mRNA than PMN. These data suggest that through the release of IL-8, also PMN may be considered potential contributors to the pathogenesis of peritoneal injury.

Finally, several investigators (161,162) examined the expression of neutrophil-specific chemoattractants in psoriatic lesions. Dense focal accumulation of neutrophils in the upper epidermis is in fact a hallmark of psoriasis, but the signals for neutrophil diapedesis and migration *in vivo* are not fully understood. The studies presented evidence for differential expression of neutrophil-attracting chemokines such as IL-8, GROα, and ENA-78, in psoriatic lesions. ISH and IH of serial sections were employed to identify and localize the cells producing these chemokines. A series of observations were made. Along with keratinocytes, a major portion of lesional IL-8 messages were produced by neutrophils themselves residing in microabscesses in the stratum corneum (161). As opposed to IL-8, GROα was highly expressed by single cells in the papillary dermis (vessel-associated cells and infiltrating cells) (161,162). GROα mRNA expression was highly variable and, in the upper epidermidis, GROα as well as IL-8 messages were tipically coexpressed by clusters of keratinocytes (161,162). Focal expression of GROβ and IL-8 in the epidermis was associated with a focal infiltration of neutrophils (161,162). mRNA expression of the highly homologous chemokine ENA-78 was absent (162). GROα hybridization pattern did not correspond to the distribution pattern of neutrophils, indicating that neutrophils were not a major source for GROα (161,162). Taken together, the data indicate GROα is an important chemoattractant for neutrophil diapedesis *in vivo*, whereas further migration of neutrophils and formation of micro-pustules appear to be influenced by the cooperative action of both GROα and interleukin-8.

6.2 *Inflammatory bowel disease*

Since neutrophils are important cellular mediators in some inflammatory bowel diseases (IBD), and IL-8 is found in increased quantities in inflamed mucosa,

Grimm et al. (163) studied IL-8 gene expression in uninflamed intestinal tissue resected for colon carcinoma and in inflamed colonic tissue resected from IBD. IL-8 mRNA was detected by ISH in macrophages and neutrophils adjacent to ulceration in inflamed bowel, as well as in many neutrophils in lamina propria, ulcer slough and crypt abscesses, but was not detected in uninflamed mucosa displaying intact epithelium or from carcinoma resections (163). IL-8 protein, as detected by IH, was present in the same distribution as IL-8 mRNA. Recently recruited CD14+ macrophages were also responsible for some of this IL-8 expression, but epithelial cells in normal and inflamed tissue showed neither IL-8 mRNA nor IL-8 protein. These results show that neutrophils and recently recruited macrophages are responsible for production of IL-8 in IBD, suggesting a mechanism for a continuing cycle of neutrophil attraction and activation.

TNFα is another cytokine implicated in the pathophysiology of IBD (164). Beil and colleagues (165) used an ultrastructural immunogold morphologic and morphometric analysis to identify the cellular and subcellular sites of TNFα in colonic biopsies obtained from patients with Crohn's disease (CD). In contrast to ulcerative colitis, which is another type of inflammatory bowel disease, neutrophils are not a frequent infiltrating cell type in bowel tissues of CD (164). Interestingly, Beil's study identified TNFα as expressed in tissue neutrophils, in addition to eosinophils, macrophages, mast cells, fibroblasts, epithelial and Paneth cells. In neutrophils, TNFα was not present in cytoplasmic granules, but rather, it was associated with the membranes of Golgi structures and cytoplasmic vesicles, or in lipid bodies (165). Thus, while numbers of neutrophils are small in colonic CD samples, when present they contain TNFα.

6.3 *Neutrophil-derived cytokines in rheumatoid arthritis and systemic lupus erythematosus*

Rheumatoid arthritis (RA) is a systemic autoimmune disease characterized by chronic inflammation of the synovium, which often leads to the destruction of articular cartilage and juxta-articular bone. Although the etiology of RA is unknown, considerable evidence suggests that cytokines play a critical role in its pathogenesis (166). In view of the fact that SF from patients with active RA are heavily infiltrated with neutrophils (167), several groups have investigated whether these cells can be a potential source of cytokines. Malyak et al. (168), for example, found a very strong correlation between SF IL-1ra levels and the number of neutrophils present in these fluids, in contrast to the number of MNC. Isolated SF PMN contained preexisting IL-1β and IL-1ra protein in the absence of detectable mRNA, and both LPS and GM-CSF induced modest increases in IL-1β and IL-1ra mRNA and protein by cultured SF PMN, as well as by normal cultured PMN. So, with regard to the IL-1β and IL-1ra proteins, PMN isolated from inflammatory SF were found to be qualitatively similar to PMN from normal peripheral blood, and, not to be activated *in vivo*. Interestingly, SF samples from patients with non-inflammatory arthropathies contained undetectable levels of IL-1ra, and therefore it can be inferred that normal SF does not contain IL-1ra (168). Malyak et al. (168) concluded that neutrophils might significantly contribute to the total IL-1ra levels in SF in patients with active RA. The ability of RA blood- and SF-derived PMN to produce IL-1α and IL-1β, in the absence or presence of LPS, was also assessed by Dularay et al. (99). In contrast with Malyak et al. (168), no production of IL-1β (or IL-1α) by SF-PMN was found, whereas blood PMN from 3/8 RA patients produced IL-1 (99). Conflicting results were also reported by Edwards and colleagues (133,169). This group, initially reported that in RA patients, SF-PMN, but not blood PMN, contained levels of IL-1β mRNA ranging from 0.5 to 3% of the maximal levels that could be induced by GM-CSF treatment of blood neutrophils (133). Subsequently, they detected IL-1β mRNA transcripts in blood PMN of patients with RA, at much greater levels than those detected in paired SF-PMN (169). In two patients with seronegative arthritis and two patients with ankylosing spondylitis, the hybridization signals for IL-1β mRNA in the blood neutrophils were undetectable. The results of this second study (169) implied that activation of IL-1β expression by PMN in RA occurs in the circulation before the cells enter into diseased joints. As a consequence, only a small sub-population of SF PMN expressing IL-1β can be found at any moment, namely those one which have most recently been attracted into the inflamed joint. Of note, it was that both RA- and blood-PMN expressed high levels of TGFβ mRNA, but no TNFα mRNA (133). To complicate these various discrepancies, Beaulieu and McColl (170) found RA SF-PMN to be significantly less efficient in producing IL-1ra, compared with matched blood PMN. The spontaneous, GM-CSF- or TNFα-induced production of IL-1ra by SF-neutrophils was significantly decreased when compared with blood neutrophils isolated from the same individuals. Under the same experimental conditions, production of both IL-1β and IL-8 was up-regulated, suggesting that there was no a general down-regulation of cell function in SF PMN. These results were also paralleled by a comparable modulation at the level of cytokine mRNA expression (170). Beaulieu and McColl therefore concluded that neutrophils are likely to be an important source of IL-8 and IL-1β in the RA joint, and that SF-neutrophils appear incapable of mounting a response as high as that of blood neutrophils in terms of IL-1ra production (170). Koch et al. (54) found significantly greater levels of antigenic GROα in SF from patients with RA as compared with osteoarthritis (OA) or other noninflammatory arthritides. Remarkably, this GROα accounted for 28% of the chemotactic activity for PMN found in RA SF (54), suggesting that also GROβα plays an important role in the migration of PMN into the inflamed RA joints. Both RA SF PMN, and normal blood PMN, produced significant amounts of GROα, either constitutively or after stimulation with LPS (54). Therefore, production of IL-8 (170), GROα (54) and other chemokines by neutrophils and other cells may lead to the recruitment of more leukocytes to the joint, and therefore perpetuate RA. Neutrophils possess the greatest capacity to directly induce cartilage degradation and therefore to act as mediators in the pathogenesis of tissue damage observed in RA (recently reviewed in ref. 167).

PMN from patients with systemic lupus erythematosus (SLE) are known to exhibit several functional abnormalities (171), leading, as a consequence, to an increased susceptibility to infections, which is actually one of the hallmark of SLE (172). Hsieh et al. (173) found that the spontaneous and LPS-stimulated production of IL-8 by the peripheral blood PMN of active SLE patients were impaired as compared to inactive SLE or healthy individuals. This impaired IL-8 production by SLE-PMN was not linked to the administration of steroids, because incubation of normal PMN or inactive SLE-PMN with prednisolone for 24 h did not significantly affect IL-8 production (173). However, the possibility that a long-term immunosuppressive treatment may lead to a defective IL-8 production in active SLE patients could not be excluded. The same group also reported that the spontaneous and LPS-stimulated production of IL-1ra by PMN, but not by PBMC, of active SLE were significantly lower than that of inactive SLE or normal groups (174). This impaired IL-1ra production by SLE-PMN seemed, again, not to be due to the administration of corticosteroids, because prednisolone did not affect the IL-1ra production of normal neutrophils *in vitro*, either spontaneously or after LPS-stimulation (174). Moreover, the IL-1ra production by active SLE-PMN increased concomitantly with clinical and laboratory improvement after effective treatment, but failed to recover in the patients without response to the treatment (174). The results of Yu's group (173,174) suggest that decreased IL-8 and IL-1ra productions constitute specific functional defects of PMN in patients with active SLE, that not only might predispose to infections, but that may also be regarded as novel indicators of disease activity in patients with active SLE.

6.4 *Neutrophil-derived cytokines in patients with sepsis*

McCall et al. (175) reported that circulating PMN of patients with the sepsis syndrome (sepsis-PMN) were, *in vitro*, tolerant to endotoxin-induced expression of the IL-1β gene. This tolerance consisted in a combined reduction in LPS-stimulated levels of IL-1β mRNA and a decreased synthesis of the immunoreactive IL-1β protein. It was excluded that the mechanisms responsible for the tolerance of sepsis-PMN were due to the loss of the CD14 surface protein, the receptor required for endotoxin-mediated gene induction in PMN (86), or that they were the result of a global reduction in the functional responses of PMN (175). The down-regulation of IL-1β gene in sepsis-PMN occurred concomitantly with an upregulation of the constitutive expression of the type II IL-1 receptor (IL-1RII) (176), and did not persist in PMN of patients recovering from the sepsis syndrome. Tolerance involved specific signal transduction pathways triggered by LPS, since sepsis-PMN normally synthesized IL-1β in response to *S.aureus,* and secreted elastase (2). Interestingly, tolerance was not limited to infection by Gram-negative bacteria, but was also observed when the sepsis syndrome was induced by Gram-positive bacteria, Rickettsia, Candida, and staphylococcal exotoxins. In a more recent report, Cavaillon's group demonstrated that, in addition to the circulating form of IL-8, high levels of cell-associated IL-8 could be detected in blood samples from patients with sepsis syndrome (177). Other than erythrocytes, already known as "sink" for IL-8, PMN and PBMC contributed to the detection of cell-associated IL-8. On a per cell basis, the amount of IL-8 associated with PMN was twice that found with PBMC, and 2 to 7 times that found in erythrocytes (177). Taking into account the relative number of circulating cells, 78.5% to 92% of the detectable cell-associated IL-8 in blood were linked to PMN. Previously, others (13) and we (51) had also shown that cell-associated IL-8 is measurable in neutrophils *in vitro* (51) and *in vivo* (13). This analysis of cell-associated cytokines was extended to another component of the inflammatory response, IL-1ra, which also can exist as an intracellular form. Cell-associated IL-1ra was indeed detected in septic patients (177). What is more, IL-8, as well IL-1ra mRNA were detected in PBMC and PMN from some septic patients and from some healthy controls, thus illustrating that circulating cells can contribute to the production of both IL-8 and IL-1ra (177). The authors concluded that measurement of cell-associated pro-inflammatory and anti-inflammatory cytokines in sepsis patients is not only a more reliable reflection of their production than is the simple measurement in plasma, but may provide useful indications to further understand the inflammatory process.

6.5 *Neutrophil-derived cytokines in patients with bacterial infections*

To determine, at the single-cell level, the cytokine-producing cells during the early and late stages of shigellosis, Raqib et al. (178) examined by IH, cryopreserved tissues from *Shigella*-infected patients. *Shigella* infection is usually accompanied by an intestinal activation of epithelial cells, T cells, and macrophages within the inflamed colonic mucosa. Histopathologically, *Shigella* infection is characterized by the presence of chronic inflammatory cells with or without neutrophils and microulcers in the lamina propria, crypt distortion, and, less frequently, crypt abscess. Raqib and coworkers found that *Shigella*-infected patients had significantly higher numbers of cytokine producing cells for all the cytokines studied (IL-1α/β, IL-1ra, IL-4, IL-6, IL-8, IL-10, IFNγ,

TNFα, Lymphotoxin-α, TGFβ_1, -β_2, and -β_3), than the healthy controls. However, production of the various cytokines in the rectal biopsies during acute and convalescent periods was not significantly different between the two periods, with the exceptions of TGFβ and IL-1ra (178). In the acute *Shigella* infection, the PMN present in the crypt abscess were clearly seen to contain IL-1β (178). This observation is revelant in view of current evidence that IL-1 is a key player in the cascade mediating invasion and inflammation of the intestinal mucosa.

Meningitis is an acute inflammatory disease of the pia and arachnoid and the fluid in the subarachnoid space. Meningitis is accompanied by a differential immigration of leukocytes into the subarachnoid space, but the mechanisms regulating leukocyte invasion during meningitis are still incompletely understood. Findings by Sprenger et al. (179) suggested that the local production of the CXC-chemokines, IL-8 and GROα and of the CC-chemokines, MCP-1 represents the major chemoattractant stimuli for the differential recruitment of leukocytes into the subarachnoid space during meningitis. In 48 paired CSF and serum samples from patients hospitalized for meningitic symptoms, high levels of IL-8, GROα, and MCP-1 were in fact detected in the cerebrospinal fluid (CSF) during bacterial and abacterial meningitis, whereas MIP-1α or RANTES were below detection limits. Elevated chemokine levels were not found in the blood serum samples taken in parallel (179). IL-8 and GROα levels significantly correlated with the number of immigrated granulocytes in the CSF of patients with bacterial meningitis. A similar correlation was found when MCP-1 levels and the mononuclear cell count were analyzed in abacterial meningitis (179). In another work (180), the protein concentrations and mRNA expression of TNFα and TGFβ_1 in CSF in 23 patients with bacterial or viral meningitis were instead investigated. High amounts of both cytokines at protein and mRNA level (especially of TNFα) were detected in bacterial as well viral infections (180). While a preponderance of TNFα compared to TGFβ_1 mRNA was visible in CSF cells of patients with bacterial meningitis, a balance of TNFα and TGFβ_1 mRNAs or a higher expression of TGFβ_1 mRNA was detected in viral meningitis. Remarkably, in the acute phase of the disease in bacterial meningitis, but even in viral infections, neutrophils expressed more TNFα and TGFβ_1 mRNA than lymphocytes and monocytes/macrophages, which instead were dominating the cytokine synthesis during the healing phase. In addition, TNFα and TGFβ_1 were expressed by neutrophils at the time of significant clinical worsening (180). Considering that TGFβ_1 has suppressive effects, PMN-derived TGFβ_1 might be involved in the down-regulation of the inflammatory activity and may act as a factor that could contribute to positive outcomes.

Takeichi and colleagues focused on adult periodontitis, a chronic infectious disease associated with active tissue damage. PMN usually constitute the great majority (>95%) of cells in gingival crevicular fluid (GCF) obtained from gingival inflammation. Furthermore, in GCF, it was possible to reveal, with considerable frequency, significant levels of both IL-1 and TNFα (181). Takeichi et al. (82) found significant levels of biologically active IL-1α and IL-1β, but not TNFα or IL-6, in GCF. Very elegantly, by using RT-PCR associated with a slot blot analysis, they provided a clear evidence that highly purified PMN (>99.5%) collected from GCF express IL-1α, IL-1β and TNFα mRNA, but not IL-6 transcripts. Also Takahashi et al. (182) examined the IL-1β mRNA-expressing cells in GCF obtained from patients with periodontitis and healthy controls. GCF was done at 15 diseased sites from five patients with adult periodontitis and eight clinically periodontal healthy sites from three volunteers. ISH showed IL-1β transcripts in both PMN and MNC, but not in epithelial cells, in all GCF samples from diseased and healthy sites. The latter case was not surprising, because a small inflammatory reaction to bacterial plaque is constantly present even in clinically healthy sites. PMN were the predominant leucocytes in diseased and healthy sites, and the percentages of IL-1β mRNA-positive PMN in GCF samples from diseased and healthy sites were 92.3 and 80.9%, respectively. Besides, the mean amounts of IL-1β mRNA expression in PMN were higher than that of MNC in all samples and there was heterogeneity within the populations of PMN and MNC in their ability to express the IL-1β gene (182). The findings of Takahashi et al. (182) indicate that IL-1β is predominantly produced by PMN in the gingival crevice of patients with adult periodontitis and healthy controls. In line with these observations, Hendley et al. (183) showed that freshly obtained oral PMN accumulated IL-1β mRNA and released the soluble cytokine after 3 h of culture, but failed to respond to further stimulation with GM-CSF. In contrast, peripheral PMN cultured in the absence of stimulus did not express or produce this cytokine. Furthermore, the amount of IL-1β produced by oral PMN was strikingly greater than that produced by circulating PMN *in vitro* (183). This finding implies that PMN enter the oral cavity from the peripheral circulation and then are maximally activated *in situ* in the gingival tissues and oral cavity, presumably in response to the oral flora. IL-1β might thus play a central role in oral immunity and inflammatory disease states.

In a different study, Tonetti et al. (184) performed ISH of IL-8 and MCP-1 genes in frozen tissue sections from patients affected by periodontal infections. Maximal IL-8 expression was found in the junctional epithelium adjacent to the infecting microorganisms, where PMN infiltration was more prominent, whereas MCP-1 was expressed in the chronic inflammatory infiltrate and along the basal layer of the oral epithelium where only cells of the monocyte/ macrophage lineage were present (184). These topographically specific tissue locations of chemokine mRNA expression was consistent with an hypothetical establishment of a discrete chemotactic source for an effective local host defenses. In a more recent work, Takeichi's group (84) characterized alveolar bone-derived PMN for their ability to produce pro-inflammatory cytokines *in vivo*. IL-1α, IL-1β, and TNFα are known to induce osteoblastic bone resorption, inhibit bone formation *in vitro*, and decrease bone collagen synthesis. Periapical exudates (PE) were collected from periapical lesions with chronic periapical periodontitis through root canals. Chronic apical periodontitis is an infectious disease, characterized by granuloma formation and progressive bone resorption around the apex of the tooth. The authors detected high concentrations of IL-1α, IL-1β and IL-6 in PE, but not of TNFα. Since PE contains predominantly PMN with a few percent of lymphocytes and/or macrophages, the latter were purified and analyzed for cytokine mRNA expression using a cytokine-specific RT-PCR. Highly purified PMN (>99.5%) isolated from PE expressed significant levels of mRNA for IL-1α, IL-1β, and TNFα. IL-6 mRNA was not detected, despite a high concentration of IL-6 detected in supernatants of PE (84), likely deriving from macrophages, T lymphocytes, osteoblasts, or fibroblasts around periapical lesions. These data strongly suggest that human PMN derived from alveolar bone can spontaneously produce IL-1α, IL-1β, and TNFα at sites of inflammation, and probably initiate inflammation and regulate augmentation of bone resorption *in vivo*. PMN could also regulate bone formation and resorption with osteoblasts synergistically.

6.7 *Neutrophil derived cytokines in patients with viral infections*

Bortolami and colleagues assessed the effect of different doses of IFNα on TNFα production by resting and LPS-activated human neutrophils from normal and hepatitis C virus (HCV)-infected patients (185). Their results revealed that none of the IFNα concentrations (25–5000 U/ml) alone induced TNFα from PMN, and that TNFα production by PMN after LPS stimulation was similar in normal and HCV-infected patients. However, various doses of IFNα associated with LPS induced a marked increase in TNFα secretion by PMN from HCV-infected patients, but had minimal effects on healthy control PMN (185). The data uncovered a new biological property of IFNα, which may be taken into account during therapy for HCV-related chronic hepatitis. Cassone et al. (135) reported that neutrophils from HIV-infected patients (HIV[+]) were able to synthesize amounts of IL-1β and IL-6 comparable to those made by neutrophils of healthy subjects, suggesting that cells from HIV[+]patients were good responders to activating signals (135). More recently, their analysis of neutrophil ability of AIDS patients to produce cytokines has been extended (75,136). IL-1β, IL-6, IL-8 and TNFα production by PMN from 21 HIV[+], including 11 full-blown AIDS, and 20 HIV-uninfected (HIV[−]) subjects (matched for age and sex to HIV[+]ones) was studied by RT-PCR and ELISA. In all subjects, cytokine gene expression was strongly stimulated by MP-F2 or LPS, and inhibited by IL-10. In contrast with their previous findings (135), they reported that PMN from HIV[+] subjects showed increased IL-6 and TNFα gene expression and produced more IL-6 and TNFα than PMN from HIV[−] controls. Quantitatively similar expression of beta-actin and IL-1β transcripts, and production of IL-1β and IL-8 proteins were observed in cells from HIV[+] and HIV[−] subjects (75,136). We also investigated the ability of neutrophils isolated from HIV[+] patients to produce pro-inflammatory cytokines (our unpublished observations). We determined the *in vitro* responsiveness of PMN and PBMC to LPS, used in the presence or absence of IFNγ, in 47 HIV[+] patients with advanced stages of virus infection. Release of TNFα and IL-8 from HIV[+.] PMN has been found to be higher than that of normal PMN. Conversely, release of IL-1β and IL-1ra in response to LPS, or to LPS plus IFNγ, was found to be lower in PMN from HIV[+] patients than from controls. The release of IL-12 induced by LPS, or by LPS plus IFNγ, did not significantly differ between PMN from HIV[+] patients and healthy donors. Importantly, the capacity of IFNγ to modulate the production of the various cytokines seemed not to be modified in HIV[+] patients. However, the production of TNFα and IL-12 in response to LPS, or to LPS plus IFNγ, were found to be significantly higher in PBMC isolated from HIV[+] patients, whereas the release of IL-1β was significantly lower. In the case of IL-8, no statistically significative difference was found between PBMC isolated from HIV[+] patients and healthy donors. Collectively, ours and Cassone's data suggest that in HIV[+] patients with advanced stages of disease, the ability of PMN (and PBMC) to produce specific cytokines in response to LPS is significantly altered, and this might play a role into the evolution of HIV disease.

7. Cytokine Production by Neutrophils *in vivo*

A growing number of *in vivo* studies have confirmed the possibility that PMN are a significant source of cytokines. Remarkably, in specific experimental animal models, the production of cytokines by neutrophils appears to be fundamental for the evolution and/or resolution of the induced pathological process.

7.1 *Effects of LPS administration in vivo on neutrophil-derived cytokines*

To study neutrophil cytokine expression *in vivo*, the most widely used experimental system is an LPS-induced acute inflammation in animals. One such example is the intratracheal injection (IT) of endotoxin, which in rats causes a dramatic influx of PMN into the bronchoalvolar space. When the kinetics of cytokine mRNA expression in the lung were investigated by

Northern analysis, it was found that IL-1α mRNA peaked at 2 to 6 h, whereas IL-1β/IL-1ra mRNAs peaked at 6 h, concurrent with the maximum influx of neutrophils. Fractionation of AM-enriched and PMN-enriched subpopulations from the BAL cells revealed that neutrophils were the predominant source for both IL-1α/β and IL-1ra mRNAs (117). Production of IL-1 by PMN may play a role in the activation of lymphocytes during the transition between acute neutrophilic and chronic mononuclear inflammation, whereas the synthesis of IL-1ra might function as a negative feedback mechanism by which neutrophils downregulate their own influx into inflammatory sites. Using a similar rat model, Xing et al. (186) provided *in vivo* evidence that PMN can represent a significant source of TNFα at sites of acute inflammation. By Northern blot analysis, they found that PMN displayed several times more TNFα mRNA than AM at 6 and 12 h after IT instillation of LPS. By ISH, most of the cells positive for TNFα mRNA were PMN localized within the inflamed tissue near bronchioles or vessels. By IH, TNFα protein was localized mainly to AM at early times after LPS challenge (1 to 3 h), whereas thereafter (6–12 h), PMN were the predominant source of TNFα protein (186). In another more extensive study (187), the same group demonstrated that LPS triggers in lung PMN and AM, a distinct cytokine response, by selectively increasing mRNA transcripts encoding TNFα, IL-1β, IL-6, and MIP-2 (which is functionally equivalent to IL-8), but not RANTES or TGFβ_1. At a time (1 h) when only a minimal PMN infiltration was present, AM appeared to be the predominant source of all cytokines examined, whereas at later times (6 and 12 h) when PMN infiltration became maximal (88% PMN), PMN were the prominent source of these cytokines. A low, basal, noninducible signal for TGFβ_1 (but not for RANTES) mRNA was detected in both AM and PMN. Interestingly, ISH of the lung tissue, revealed that amongst the cells which stained for MIP-2 mRNA in response to LPS, were, particularly, the PMN located in the vicinity of bronchioles and vasculature, but not within the vasculature itself (187). Under similar experimental conditions (IT instillation of LPS), recruited PMN could rapidly (30 min) and persistently (up to 16 h) be induced to express MIP-2 and KC (the latter being the murine analogue of GROα/MGSA) (55). Although Northern analyses were performed on pooled BAL cell RNA, these BAL cell population changed from predominantly (>95%) macrophages to mostly PMN (60% within 2 h, 91% after 16 h) after LPS instillation (55). Furthermore, expression of MIP-2 and KC mRNA was also observed within exudative neutrophils obtained after intraperitoneal (IP) injection of thioglycollate (55). Collectively, these observations support the notion that in this lung model of LPS-elicited inflammation, infiltrating PMN represent a significant source of pro-inflammatory cytokines. Recently, production of TNFα, IL-1β, IL-8, and IL-1ra was analyzed in a model of local Shwartzman reaction (LSR) prepared in rabbit lung (188). In this model, myeloperoxidase activity, representing neutrophil accumulation, peaked at 1–2 h and was sustained for 48 h after IV challenge with LPS. Kinetics of cytokine production revealed that TNFα was the first to appear, peaking at 0.5 h, whereas IL-1β and IL-8 increased later and peaked at 2 h (188). IL-1ra was present even before the challenge, and its production increased showing a dual peak: at 0.5–2 h, and at 48 h. The authors speculated that endogenous IL-1ra might serve to suppress part of IL-1 activity and function through a negative feedback mechanism. IH showed that the cellular source of these cytokines were AM and infiltrating neutrophils (188), and it was inferred that production of cytokines was not a direct mediator for the initiation of LSR, but likely the consequence of events following leukocyte infiltration.

Circulating PMN can also constitute a prominent source of cytokines. Williams et al. (189) showed that following IV infusion of LPS for 2 h in rats, PMN rather than MNC in the pulmonary vasculature were the major source of IL-1β transcripts. In contrast, no induction of IL-1β expression was observed in airway or circulating leukocytes. A recent study by Cirelli et al. (190) confirmed that an accumulation of intravascular mononuclear phagocytes and neutrophils in the pulmonary circulation is observed during a continuous infusion of endotoxin in sheep. These authors detected an increased cytoplasmic TNFα immunoreactivity in both mononuclear phagocytes and neutrophils sequestered in pulmonary arterioles, capillaries, and venules. Coincidentally, plasma levels of TNFα significantly increased, suggesting that both neutrophils and mononuclear phagocytes contributed to the rise in the circulating levels of TNFα, and the development of acute lung injury (190). Moreover, in a study recently performed to investigate the *in vivo* effects of ethanol on LPS-induced TNFα and iNOS expression in the lung, ethanol intoxication was found not to affect TNFα mRNA expression in AM or recruited neutrophils, but instead to inhibit that of iNOS (191).

Terebuth et al. (192) performed IH to localize cells expressing IL-6 in selected organs of normal and endotoxin-challenged mice. In normal mice, a constitutive cytoplasmic IL-6 immunoreactivity was detected in blood monocytes and their precursors, in bone marrow and splenic stromal macrophages, and in granulocytes as well (192). While significant serum levels of IL-6 were absent, cell-associated IL-6 bioactivity was found in circulating PMN but not in lymphocytes. However, after IP injection of LPS, there was a two- to three-fold increase in PMN cell-associated IL-6 bioactivity from 1 to 3 h, followed by an almost complete depletion at 6 h. Concomitantly, serum levels of IL-6 peaked at 3 h after LPS challenge and dropped significantly by 6 h. Interestingly, constitutive and increased intracellular IL-6 in circulating PMN was detected in the absence of IL-6 mRNA, which was instead present in granulocytic/monocytic progenitors in the bone marrow. In the latter cells, IL-6 transcripts increased with a similar time course after LPS challenge (192). These data suggest a scenario in which circulating granulocytes bear IL-6 as a stored component, likely acquired during bone marrow maturation:, during endotoxemia, they release IL-6 as a result of appropriate signals received, for example, during margination or chemotaxis. More recently, Nill et al. (193) compared the temporal sequence of endotoxin-induced TNFα, IL-1α, and IL-10 gene expression and cellular localization of cytokine proteins in pulmonary tissue of two strains of mice that have a genetically based differential sensitivity to endotoxin. Cytokines were studied by RT-PCR and ISH in lung tissue harvested from endotoxin-sensitive C3H/HeN and endotoxin-resistant C3H/HeJ mice at different times, after IP injection of LPS (193). Although levels of TNFα mRNA and protein in the two mouse strains were similar at 1–2 h, the IL-1α gene and protein expression in pulmonary tissue isolated from endotoxin-resistant mice was lower at any time point examined (193). IL-10 mRNA and protein levels were upregulated and continued to increase over a 12-h time period in C3H/HeN mice, whereas they were basically undetectable in CH3/HeJ endotoxin-resistant mice. In both types of mouse strains, TNFα, IL-1α, and IL-10 immunoreactive proteins were localized primarily to the infiltrating neutrophils, as well as to AM and type II pneumocytes (193). However, quantitation of neutrophil infiltration into pulmonary tissue demonstrated that there was a significantly decreased inflammatory infiltrate in pulmonary tissue isolated from CH3/HeJ mice following LPS-administration, which correlated with decreased levels of immunoreactive cytokine proteins within pulmonary cells (193). These results unequivocally implicate that infiltrating neutrophils are important cellular mediators of pulmonary tissue damage induced by endotoxin in the CH3H/HeN endotoxin-sensitive mice.

7.2 Other in vivo models of acute inflammation involving neutrophils

Mori et al. (194) examined by Northern blot analysis the expression of 12 different genes in peritoneal exudate neutrophils, harvested at 5 and 24 h after IP injection of casein. While IL-1α, TNFα and MCP-1 mRNAs were below the detection levels during the entire inflammatory period of observation, the remaining nine genes were classified into three categories (194). The first group included γ-actin, MRP-8 and MRP-14, the latter two being calcium-binding proteins and components of a complex molecule with inhibitory activity against casein kinase I and II. These messages were constitutively expressed in blood neutrophils and were also rapidly induced after emigration into inflammatory sites. The second group of genes included IL-1β, IL-8, MIP-1β and the fMLP-R, which were induced rapidly after the onset of inflammation (2–5 h), but returned to basal levels of expression by 24 h. The functions of the products of the genes in the second group relate especially to chemotaxis, one of the hallmarks of early inflammation. Expression of IL-1β was in agreement with previous findings reported by the same group using IH studies (195). To the third group of expressed genes, only ferritin-related mRNAs (F and H chains) were ascribed, because they were induced slowly (4–7 h), and increased with the progression of the inflammatory process. This finding suggests in any case that neutrophils retain the potential for biosynthesis at later stages of inflammation. The study of Mori et al. (194) not only underlined that neutrophils contribute to the acute inflammatory reactions by synthesising a variety of proteins for a fairly long period, but also evidenced that such response is regulated and subjected to a programmed sequence.

In a rat model of transient retinal ischemia, a condition which leads to neuronal damage, Hangai et al. (196) studied the levels of IL-1 gene expression by semi-quantitative PCR, and used also ISH and IH. Little expression of IL-1α and IL-1β genes was observed in normal retina, but this was highly up-regulated after ischemia and subsequent reperfusion, in a time-dependent manner (196). Time courses of IL-1α and IL-1β mRNA expression were also different, in that induction of IL-1α mRNA occurred before that of IL-1β mRNA. For IL-1β, three types of cells, including neutrophils, were identified as cellular origin of its mRNA. The authors speculated that neutrophils recruited after ischemia are activated and then synthesize IL-1, which then promotes secretion of products that damage microvasculature and retinal tissue (196).

In another paper aiming to identify the neutrophil chemoattractants generated in a model of myorcadial infarction in the rabbit, Ivey et al. (197) attributed important roles to the complement fragment C5a, and to the chemokine IL-8. Ischemia induces all the typical changes characteristic of an acute inflammatory response, amongst which an early neutrophil accumulation is a prominent feature. A determinant step in neutrophil accumulation is the local generation of chemical signals responsible for leukocyte recruitment. Neutrophil accumulation is markedly accelerated during reperfusion after ischemia, and early studies have implicated PMN in the generation of tissue damage associated to reperfusion (198). In their study, Ivey et al. (197) demonstrated that immunoreactive C5a and IL-8 were present in myorcardial tissue after ischemia and reperfusion, but the time course of their appearance was quite different. C5a was detected already after 5 min of the initiation of reperfusion, while IL-8 concentrations rose slowly and were significantly elevated at 1.5 h and highest at 4.5 h, in close parallel with leukocyte infiltration. Further experiments revealed that neutrophil depletion virtually abolished IL-8 generation in the myocardium, but had no influence on C5a generation. C5a was probably liberated from preformed substrates as early as a few minutes after the initiation of reperfusion and induced a first phase of neutrophil infiltration. Once in the tissue, neutrophils became the source of IL-8 in the myocardium, and this IL-8 generation was responsible for a subsequent wave of neutrophil accumulation (197). Other results have involved locally produced IL-8 as a pivotal mediator of cerebral reperfusion (199). Reperfusion to rabbit brain, after a transient focal ischemia, induced neutrophil infiltration and aggregation, neither of which were observed in rabbit brain rendered ischemic alone for the same time interval (199). Brain tissue levels of IL-8 increased significantly at 6 h after reperfusion, but without a noticeable elevation of plasma IL-8 levels. Moreover, IL-8 protein was detected by IH in the vascular wall and, to a lesser degree, in infiltrated neutrophils, suggesting a local production of IL-8 in reperfused brain tissues. In addition, a neutralizing anti-IL-8 antibody significantly reduced brain edema and infarct size in comparison to rabbits receiving a control antibody (199), suggesting that IL-8 might be considered as a novel target for the intervention of this injury.

In a rat model of lung injury obtained by IT instillation of bleomycin, which subsequently leads to fibrosis, Sakanashi et al (200) investigated the kinetics and the molecular mechanisms underlying macrophage infiltration. Northern blot analysis revealed that the expression of MCP-1 mRNA in the lung was most prominent the first day after instillation and declined thereafter, thus preceding the numerical change of the exudate monocytes. IH disclosed that the main sources of MCP-1 production were alveolar and interstitial macrophages, as well as PMN (200). Based on these results, the authors speculated that MCP-1 produced by PMN and by alveolar and interstitial macrophages induced the infiltration of blood monocytes in the very early phase, and that the subsequent accumulation of macrophages was enhanced by the MCP-1 production by monocyte-derived exudate macrophages (200). In contrast, in rabbit BAL cells exposed to hyperoxia (201), a quantitative ISH showed that both IL-8 and MCP-1 were expressed in AM, whereas only IL-8 was present in recruited PMN. Interestingly, IL-8 mRNA production in PMN was elevated throughout the time that PMN were available for analysis, and although no data on IL-8 protein were produced, the presence of increased levels of IL-8 mRNA in PMN entering the alveolus implies an autocrine role for this cytokine in PMN activation (201).

Using the model of anti-glomerular basement membrane (anti-GBM) nephritis in rats, Wu et al. (202) investigated the mechanisms underlying *in situ* chemokine expression and the *in vivo* function of these molecules during the acute phase of this inflammatory model. Previous studies had in fact established that CXC chemokines are important for the acute influx of PMN in anti-GBM nephritis and the consequent damage to the glomerulus (manifested as proteinuria). Other studies have also implicated CC chemokines in the pathophysiology of glomerulonephritis. Wu et al. (202) were able to observe that during the evolution of anti-GBM nephritis, CXC chemokine expression (MIP-2 and CINC) was monophasic and paralleled neutrophil influx, whereas CC chemokine expression (MIP-1α, MIP-1β and MCP-1) was biphasic with peaks coinciding with the influx of PMN and then macrophages. IL-1β and TNFα mRNA expression exhibited features intermediate between those of CXC and CC chemokines. The initial peak of chemokine expression was attenuated by decomplementation (which selectively attenuates PMN influx), neutropenia (by cell depletion with a specific antiserum), and irradiation-induced leukopenia. The delayed peak was attenuated only by leukopenia, but was augmented in the accelerated form of this disease model, corresponding to an increase in macrophages influx. Differential expression of chemokines by PMN and macrophages was not an intrinsic property of these cells, as these leukocytes expressed similar profiles of chemokines *in vitro*, either after adherence or with endotoxin stimulation (202). In general, macrophage expression of chemokine mRNA was quantitatively more modest than in PMN. IH for MIP-1α in acute nephritis validated that expression during acute nephritis was accompanied by local protein production. Moreover, neutralizing Abs to MIP-1α attenuated the acute phase proteinuria, but not the accompanying influx of PMN or macrophages. In comparison, neutralizing Abs to CINC inhibited both PMN influx and proteinuria. A combination of the two antibodies was not significantly more effective than either antibodies alone (202). The study conclusively established that myeloid cells are necessary for glomerular chemokine expression during nephritis, and that the differential expression of CXC and CC chemokines not only relates specifically to the differential influx of leukocyte subsets, but must involve additional factors. In addition, this study argued against the simplified scheme that CXC chemokines are mediators of acute inflammation, and CC chemokines are mediators of chronic inflammation.

7.3 *Neutrophil-derived cytokines during in vivo infections*

To better clarify the pathogenesis of arthritis, Matsukawa et al. (203) used a model of rabbit arthritis induced by intra-articular injection of LPS. Initially, these authors observed that both leukocyte infiltration and loss of proteoglycan were largely initiated by IL-1β produced by macrophages and neutrophils in the synovial exudate (203). Destruction of cartilage was the consequence of leukocyte-derived cartilage-degrading substances, such as elastase and superoxide anion (203). They also investigated the generation kinetics of IL-1ra, and its significance in the pathogenesis of LPS-arthritis (which subsides within 48 h). Production of IL-1ra (by leukocytes) was delayed compared to IL-1β, was sustained for 1 week and was 180–200-fold molar excess of IL-1β. LPS-induced leucocyte infiltration was inhibited by 70–75% by rabbit IL-1ra, suggesting that endogenous IL-1ra may suppress a part of IL-1 activity at the site, but its amount was too low for suppression of all the biologic effects of IL-1β. Subsequently, the same group injected homologous IL-8 in rabbit knee joints and investigated the inflammatory response (204). In these experiments, IL-8 induced a massive accumulation of neutrophils (but no appreciable numbers of lymphocytes) and provoked the release of neutrophil elastase, which led to cartilage destruction. In addition, injection of IL-8 induced bioactive and immunoreactive IL-1β and IL-1ra, but not TNFα in the joint cavity. As determined by IH, IL-1β- and IL-1ra-positive cells were infiltrating leukocytes (204). Production kinetics of immunoreactive IL-1ra in SF overlapped that of IL-1β, but the peak concentration of IL-1ra exceeded that of IL-1β by a 40–50 fold molar ratio. Strikingly, in neutrophil-depleted rabbits, IL-8 induced no cartilage destruction and far lesser concentrations of IL-1β and IL-1ra as compared with normal rabbits (204), proving that infiltrating neutrophils were the main producers of these cytokines and that they were responsible for cartilage destruction. What is more, IL-8 induced little macrophage/lymphocyte accumulation in neutrophil-depleted rabbits, suggesting that early neutrophil accumulation may affect the later accumulation of macrophages or lymphocytes, likely through the production of specific chemoattractans. The authors thus concluded that IL-8 is a potent neutrophil activator *in vivo* and may have a crucial role in the biology of inflammation and the pathogenesis of inflammatory processes, including septic arthritis (204). In a more recent paper, the same group investigated the network and involvement of inflammatory cytokines in their rabbit model of LPS-induced arthritis (205). The study was based on the assumption that production of TNFα precedes that of IL-1β and IL-1ra and that IL-8 is detectable after the production of IL-1. Surprisingly, maximum levels of TNFα and IL-8 were detected 2 h after LPS-injection, whereas IL-1β and IL-1ra were detected after 6 and 9 h, respectively. By IH, synovial lining cells were positive for TNFα and IL-8, and infiltrating leukocytes were positive for IL-1β and IL-1ra and IL-8. In neutrophil-depleted rabbits, the levels of TNFα and IL-8 were similar to those in normal rabbits. In contrast, no IL-1β was detected in neutrophil-depleted rabbits and the levels of IL-1ra were much lower (205). The effects of inhibitors against TNFα, IL-1β, and IL-8 led to the following observations. TNFα and IL-8 were produced by synovial lining cells, were the first cytokines appearing at the site of inflammation, and induced subsequent production of IL-1β and IL-1ra by neutrophils. IL-1β induced further production of IL-1β. Endogenous IL-1ra down-regulated the production of IL-1β but not that of TNFα or IL-8 (205). Interestingly, the early phase of the leukocyte influx was not inhibited by inhibitors of each cytokine, indicating that this phase was dependent on other chemoattractants, such as for instance C5a, PAF or LTB$_4$ (205). Furthermore, late accumulation of neutrophils was inhibited only by 40 to 60% by anti-TNFa mAbs, recombinant IL-1ra or anti-IL-8 IgG, suggesting that factor(s) other than IL-8 (maybe GROα, MIP-2, or ENA-78) were involved in the late phase of leukocyte influx in LPS-induced arthritis (205).

In a very interesting study, Jordan et al. (206) determined the endogenous mediators involved in the induction of IL-1ra during the oral infection of mice with the enteropathogenic *Y.enterocolitica*. These bacteria initially proliferate in the tissue of the terminal ileum, predominantly in the Peyer's patches (PP), where the immediate antibacterial host defence is characterized by an infiltration of granulocytes and monocytes. By ISH, northern blot and IH, Jordan et al. found expression of IL-1ra mRNA and synthesis of IL-1ra in PP, as well as in non infected organs such as spleen, but not in the liver (206). In contrast, the mRNA for IL-1β in PP was expressed considerably earlier, as sessile macrophages were its primary source. No temporal differences were observed between IL-1α and IL-1ra (206). Circulating and recruited neutrophils, but not PBMC, were identified to be the primary source of IL-1ra in tissues, whereas approximately 20% of the positive IL-1ra-staining cells were accounted for by inflammatory macrophages. In addition, ISH of adjacent sections of PP revealed a distinct hybridization pattern for each cytokine, suggesting that IL-1α,

IL-1β and IL-1ra were produced independently by different cell types, or alternatively by cells of the same phenotype located within different tissue areas. Strikingly, neutralization with an antiserum of IL-6, a cytokine which was also promptly induced by *Y.enterocolitica* infection, caused a suppression of both IL-1ra mRNA in PP, and synthesis of IL-1ra in circulating neutrophils. In support of these *in vivo* findings, IL-6 induced IL-1ra expression in cultures of macrophages and PMN *in vitro*, and anti-IL-6 antiserum blocked these effects of IL-6 (206). In this respect, previous studies in humans, had demonstrated that IL-6 infused into cancer patients rapidly increased the levels of circulating IL-1ra (207). Altogether, the observations of Jordan et al. (206) uncovered important inter-relationships among IL-1, IL-6 and IL-1ra in *Y.enterocolitca* infections. For example, after the production of IL-1 and IL-6 early after *Yersinia* infection, IL-6 in turn induces IL-1ra, which then may inhibit IL-1 activities through a negative feedback loop, thus facilitating the resolution of the inflammatory response locally and presumably at remote sites of infection.

More insights into the mechanisms underlying neutrophil influx in the airways during chronic bacterial infection were uncovered by Inoue et al. (44), who studied the effect of *P.aeruginosa* supernatant delivered in the dog trachea *in vivo* on the expression and localization of IL-8 mRNA in airways. The latter procedures caused IL-8 mRNA expression in epithelial and gland duct cells but also in recruited neutrophils (44). The molecule responsible for this IL-8 induction was a small molecular weight (1 kD) product of *P.aeruginosa* (44). IL-8 expression in recruited neutrophils might provide a potential mechanism for amplifying the inflammatory response and for a positive feedback of a protective antibacterial response, for example by rendering phagocytosis more effective.

In vivo expression of TNFα- and IL-1α-transcripts, but not of IL-6, in *Listeria monocytogenes*-elicited neutrophils was recently demonstrated by Dai et al. (208). Such observations have been made in elicited peritoneal PMN from IFNγ receptor-deficient (IFNγR-/-) mice, which were used as a model to study the innate immune responses during infection with *L.monocytogenes* (208). In agreement with previous reports on the essential role of IFNγ to limit bacterial spread, these mutant mice were unable to limit bacterial growth and died of sepsis even with an infection dose of 70 Listeria. The authors detected large inflammatory foci of infection in the spleen or liver of IFNγR-/- mice, which were populated mainly by PMN that, interestingly, were fully able to kill *Listeria* (208). Nevertheless, despite their obvious contribution in innate immune responses against *Listeria*, IFNγR-/-, neutrophils were unable to rescue mice from fatal listeriosis, arguing for their limited protective role in IFNγR-/- mice. Very recently, Thomas and colleagues investigated the role of neutrophils in herpetic stromal keratitis (HSK) (209). HSK is an immunopathologic response observed in immunocompetent mice after corneal infection with herpes simplex virus-1. The earliest sign of disease is a specific neutrophil infiltration, which lasts for 48 to 72 h and then disappears. This rapid PMN response most likely contributes to curtailing viral replication and to minimize viral dissemination. In search of how PMN exert antiviral effects, the group performed ISH experiments. Preliminary results revealed TNFα and iNOS signals in cells resembling PMN in acute inflamed cornea (209). These molecules might thus play an antiviral activity against HSV. However, a secondary neutrophil infiltration most likely orchestrated by CD4+ T cells, this time more massive, occurred, beginning 8 to 9 days postinfection, a time in which HSK became clinically evident (209). Suppression of PMN during this secondary phase (by antibodies-mediated depletion) considerably diminished the severity of HSK. In summary, the results of Thomas and colleagues (209) suggest that herpes simplex virus infection of the cornea rapidly invokes recruitment of neutrophils that may aid in viral clearance, but that, or indirectly, serve as agonists in perpetuating a CD4+ T cell-mediated inflammatory reaction. In addition, results from the same group showed that enriched PMN from mice peritoneum can produce IL-12 upon exposure to HSV (141).

Romani et al. (137,140) have provided seminal information on the role of neutrophils in the generation of murine T helper responses to *C.albicans*. It is well known that subsets of CD4+ T helper cells can be characterized on the basis of their pattern of cytokine production either in mice (210) or human systems (211). Th1 cells predominantly produce IL-2, IFNγ and lymphotoxin, and are effective inducers of delayed type hypersensitivity (DTH), while Th2 mainly produce IL-4, IL-5 and IL-10, and provide more effective help for B cells. Human Th1-like cells preferentially develop during infections by intracellular bacteria, protozoa, and viruses, whereas Th2-like cells predominate during helmintic infestations and in response to common environmental allergens (211). Strongly polarized human Th1-type and Th2-type responses not only play different roles in protection, but they can also promote different immunopathological reactions (211). For example, *C.albicans* is a commensal microorganism that, especially in immunonocompromised hosts, may represent an important cause of morbidity and mortality. Studies in mice have clearly established that multiple mechanisms may control the outcome of experimental infections. In immunized mice such outcome is greatly conditioned by the type of predominant T helper cell subset activated by the initial exposure to the yeast: Th1 cell activation leads to resistance and onset of durable protection, whereas Th2 cell responses are associated with susceptibility to progressive disease (212,213). Previous studies in Romani's lab had indicated that numerous factors are involved in the preferential induction of murine Th1 or Th2 cell reponses to *Candida* (212,214). Cytokines emerged, obviously, as key regulators in the development of CD4+ subsets from precursor Th cells (210), and for the Th1-responses several evidence indicated production of IL-12 as fundamental (214). Importantly, depletion of granulocytes in resistant mice led to the onset of Th2 rather than Th1 responses, indicating that the latter cells may participate in *Candida* driven Th1-development (212). Interestingly, neutropenia constitutes in humans one of the major factor responsible for fungal dissemination to visceral organs. Using live vaccine strain or virulent challenge in mucosal or systemic infection of mice with *C.albicans*, Romani et al. (137) initially examined the effect of depletion of neutrophils on the course of primary and secondary challenge and on development of CD4+ cell-dependent immunity. They obtained evidence of deleterious effects of neutrophil depletion occurring at the time of infection under all conditions of testing, both in naive and in previously immunized mice (137). Neutrophil depletion concurrent with infection also resulted in the selective appearance of the IL-4 message in purified CD4+ splenocytes, an early indicator of Th2 development. In contrast, neutrophil depletion appeared to benefit the hosts late in the course of an overwhelming systemic infection. In an attempt to correlate neutrophil function with the nature of the T cell response, the authors also tested the ability of neutrophils to produce cytokines associated with functionally distinct CD4+

Th cell responses to *Candida*. They found that neutrophils were endowed with the capacity to secrete IL-12 and IL-10 *in vitro* in response to either different strain of *C.albicans* or to IFNγ plus LPS. In particular, IL-10 and bioactive IL-12, but not IL-4, were found in cultures stimulated with IFNγ plus LPS. IL-12 but not IL-10 was produced in response to the live vaccine strain PCA-2, which causes healing infection, while the opposite pattern was observed in response to the highly virulent CA-6 strain which causes nonhealing infection (137). The authors therefore concluded that neutrophil ablation early in the course of Th1-associated self-limiting infection appeared to change the qualitative development of the T cell response, and rendered mice susceptible to infection (137).

Subsequently, the ability of neutrophils to release IL-12 and IL-10 *in vivo*, during the course of *C.albicans* systemic infection, was investigated by injecting intravenously the live vaccine strain PCA-2, or the CA-6 strain (140). Under those conditions, neutrophils expressed secreted IL-12 and IL-10, correlating with the respective development of self-limiting (Th1-associated) and progressive (Th2-associated) disease (140). Importantly, macrophages were characterized as cells with a poor ability to secrete IL-10 and, even less, IL-12 (140). Neutrophil depletion prevented the development of protective Th1 responses in healer mice, but exogenous IL-12 was effective in protecting neutropenic hosts susceptible to infection, consistent with a role for neutrophil-derived IL-12 in Th1 development (140). Neutrophil depletion however increased resistance later in infection of susceptible host, the latter finding being related to a decreased IL-10 production (140). Another very important observation in the study of Romani and colleagues was that the balance between IL-10 and IL-12 productions by neutrophils was modified by exogenous IL-12, in that PMN-release of IL-10 increased after IL-12 treatment in both uninfected and infected mice (140). Although this IL-12-induced production of IL-10 by neutrophils might have been the result of indirect mediators stimulating PMN, this mechanism could act as a regulatory response to challenge with IL-12. In addition, such effect of IL-12 might account for an observation previously made by the same Romani, of a paradoxical effect of IL-12 in the resistant host. They in fact reported that administration of IL-12 not only fails to promote (enhance) protective anticandidal immunity in nongranulocytopenic mice, but actually promoted Th2 development in a healing infection with detectable levels of circulating IL-10/IL-4 (140). The increased production of IL-10 by neutrophils after IL-12 treatment might be the explanation or could contribute to the failure of IL-12 to exert protective effects in mice with candidiasis (140). In summary, the results of Romani et al. (137,140) are very important because demonstrate that PMN, through the release of IL-12 and IL-10, may significantly contribute to the patterns of susceptibility and resistance in mice with candidiasis. More strikingly, the work of Romani et al. (137,140) reports for the first time that neutrophils, via their ability to release cytokines, play an active role in determining the qualitative development of the T cell response (215). Further evidence for an *in vivo* role of IL-12-producing neutrophils as initiators of a Th-1-cell mediated immunity has been observed in response to *Toxoplasma gondii* or in the IFNγR-/- mice, as mentioned in reference. 216. All the latter concepts likely originated from the work of my group (138)

7.4 *Further experimental situations of in vivo neutrophil-derived cytokines*

Other studies have indicated that the potential production of cytokines by PMN might also significantly affect other processes, such as for instance the immune and the antitumor responses, and so forth. In a series of papers published by Sendo and coworkers (217–220) for example, cell-mediated immune responses and antibody production were analyzed in rats which were depleted of PMN using a specific anti-neutrophil monoclonal antibodies designated RP-3. Those experiments demonstrated that both the priming and the elicitation phases of delayed type hypersensitivity (DTH) to sheep red blood cells (SRBC) (217), and the accompanying MNC recruitment (218), were partially inhibited in PMN-depleted rats, suggesting that neutrophils enhance DTH to SRBC. Of great relevance, the same group previuosly demonstrated that IL-8-induced CD4+ T lymphocyte recruitment into subcutaneous tissues of rats were inhibited by the RP-3 treament (219). Furthermore, by assessing the direct or indirect splenic plaque-forming cell (PFC) response to SRBC in rats depleted of PMN 6–12 h before immunization, they detected an increased number of anti-SRBC antibody-producing cells (220). This phenomenon was observed only when the antigen was administered intraperitoneally and not with IV immunization (220) and suggested that neutrophils could suppress antibody production in certain situations. Of great interest, using a similar experimental animal model, the same group also demonstrated that transplantation immunity against cancer and generation of CD8+ effector T cells to tumor associated antigens were abrogated by selective depletion of neutrophils (221,222). Although the precise mechanisms underlying all these phenomena were not elucidated, it can be envisaged that they could be related to the lack of PMN-derived cytokines, which would affect leukocyte recruitment (IL-8, IP-10, MIP-1α/MIP-1β, and MIP-2), antigen presentation (IL-1), lymphocyte proliferation and activation (IL-1, TNFα) and macrophage activation (TNFα). Moreover, since PMN have been shown to express class II molecules if treated with G-CSF plus either GM-CSF, IL-3 or IFNγ (223), it is possible that they could also function as antigen-presenting cells. Collectively, these findings make it tempting to speculate that PMN, in specific situations, can influence the balance between humoral and cell-mediated immunity in the early stages of the immune response.

The potential ability of PMN to mediate antitumor activity in vivo has been clearly evidentiated by Stopacciaro et al. (224). They took advantage of the murine colon adenocarcinoma C-26 cell line engineered to release G-CSF (C-26/G-CSF), to study the mechanisms responsible for inhibition of tumor take in syngeneic animals, and of regression of an established tumor in sublethally irradiated mice injected with these cells. Using C-26/G-CSF they identified the cell types that infiltrate the tumor and the cytokines expressed *in situ*. It was found that inhibition of tumor take and regression of an established tumor in sublethally irradiated mice occurred through different mechanisms. In the former case, PMN were the main cells responsible for inhibiting the take of C26/G-CSF. In the latter one, PMN, macrophages and T cells, including CD8+ T cells which are required for IFNγ-mediated tumor regression, determined the rejecton of a C26/G-CSF nodule initially grown in sublethally irradiated mice. Both depletion of CD8+T cells, or neutralization of IFNγ- produced by CD8+T cells resulted in a reduction of PMN number and TNFα expression, and therefore in tumor progression (224). Notably, as evidenced by IH and ISH, either newly recruited granulocytes surrounding the injected neoplastic cells, or, in sublethally irradiated mice, the PMN infiltrating the C-26/G-CSF tumor during its initial growing phase, expressed transcripts for IL-1α, IL-1β and TNFα (224). More recently (225), the analysis of the phenotypic changes resulting from the cytokines activities during the rejection of C26/G-CSF, and the inhibition of such changes by anti-cytokine antibodies, indicated that TNFα was instrumental in tumor regression. C-26/G-CSF regressing tumors were characterized by an hemorragic necrosis dependent on the infiltrating leukocytes and the cytotoxic cytokines they produced (225). Complete tumor regression was the result of tumor cell hypoxia following the damage of the tumor microvasculature that was the target of both cytotoxic cytokines (TNFα) and PMN (225). Locally produced IL-1 and TNFα induced VCAM-1 and E-selectin on tumor vessels, and thus indirectly attracted T lymphocytes (225). Treatment with monoclonal antibodies to IFNγ or TNFα blocked tumor regression by inhibiting VCAM-1 and E-selectin expression on tumor-associated endothelial cells, and this resulted in a reduced number of infiltrating leukocytes. Thus, whereas tumor inhibition was mediated mainly by PMN, tumor regression occurred because of the cooperation of PMN and T cells, as well as of a combination of cytokines, for which T-cell derived IFNγ, and PMN-derived TNFα were necessary.

The importance of IL-1β in the pathogenesis of acute pancreatitis has been demonstrated by dramatic attenuation of pancreatic destruction and significant increases in survival when its actions are inhibited. Hypothesizing that infiltrating leukocytes contribute substantially to the intrapancreatic production of IL-1β, Fink and Norman (226) examined the specific role of those cells. Therefore, mice were assigned to one of four groups 48 hr prior to induction of pancreatitis: (a) PMN depletion via anti-murine PMN antiserum. [PMN-d], (b) macrophage (Mo) depletion via anti-macrophage antiserum [Mo-d], (c) PMN and Mphi depletion [PMN+Mo-d], and (d) immunocompetent pancreatitis. Edematous pancreatitis was then induced in all experimental groups by caerulein, and intrapancreatic IL-1β production was determined by IH and RT-PCR (226). The experiments performed by Fink and Norman demonstrated that intrapancreatic IL-1β production was primarily attributable to the leukocytes which infiltrate the gland during the progression of the disease. IH techniques suggested that the macrophage was the major contributor of IL-1 protein. On the other hand, there was greater attenuation of IL-1 mRNA levels in animals that were devoid of neutrophils (226). Elimination of either macrophages or neutrophils (and their inflammatory products, including IL-1β) could thus have beneficial effects and significantly decreases the severity of pancreatic destruction.

To get more insights into the pattern of cytokine expression in wound tissues, and in their regulation during the repair process, Hubner and colleagues (227) have been able to show a strong and early induction of IL-1α, IL-1β and TNFα expression after cutaneous injury in normal mice. The highest levels of these cytokines were seen as early as 12–24 h after wounding, and after completion of the proliferative phase of wound healing, mRNA levels of these cytokines returned to the basal level. Remarkably, during the early phase of wound repair, pro-inflammatory cytokines were predominantly expressed in PMN. At later stages of the repair process, expression of IL-1α, IL-1β and of TNFα was also seen in macrophages. Induction of these cytokines after injury was significantly reduced during wound repair in healing-impaired glucocorticoid-treated mice (227). These findings demonstrate that wound healing defects are associated with impaired IL-1α, IL-1β and TNFα expression and suggests that the early induction of these genes is important for normal repair. More importantly, the data provided evidence for a novel function of PMN as regulators of inflammatory process but also as initiators of proliferative processes, thus appearing to play a pivotal role in the transition between inflammation and wound repair. This hypothesis was supported by the co-localization of cytokine expressing PMN and -for example- KGF-expressing fibroblasts at the wound edge. Thus, the early expression of pro-inflammatory cytokines by PMN that invade the wound seem to be of major significance for induction of growth factor expression and thus for the initiation of wound repair. In another model of local wounding response secondary to the injury to the spinal cord in mouse, Bartholdi et al. (228) investigated the expression pattern of pro-inflammatory and chemoattractant cytokines. They could show by ISH that transcripts for TNFα and IL-1 as well as MIP-1α and MIP-1β were upregulated within the first hours following injury. In this early phase, the expression of the pro-inflammatory cytokines was restricted to cells in the surroundings of the lesion area probably resident CNS cells. While TNFα was expressed in a very early time window, IL-1 could be detected in a subset of PMN which immigrated into the spinal cord around 6 h. Messages for the chemokines MIP-1α/β were expressed in a generalized way in the grey matter of the entire spinal cord around 24 h and got again restricted to the cellular infiltrate at the lesion site at 4 days following injury. The data suggested that resident CNS cells, most probably microglial cells, and not peripheral inflammatory cells, were the main source for cytokine and chemokine mRNAs (228). Lastly, the time course of appearance of the TGFβ and its localization in developing endochondral bone was examined by Carrington and colleagues (229). These authors used the demineralized matrix-induced bone forming system in rats. For the first time, TGFβ was detected in developing endochondral bone in vivo. Intracellular immunohistochemical localization of TGFβ revealed that the cell types in which TGFβ could be detected varied with the time after implantation of the demineralized matrix: first were inflammatory cells, and then cells in late hypertrophying and calcifying cartilage, the osteoblasts and, interestingly, also bone marrow granulocytes (229). Therefore, production of TGFβ by granulocytes may contribute to the regulation of ossification during endochondral bone development.

8. Conclusion

The classical role attributed to neutrophils is still based on the obsolete view that PMN are terminally differentiated, short-lived cells, with minimal, if any, transcriptional or translational activity. However, the studies that were summarized in this chapter clearly demonstrate the ability of neutrophils to synthesize and release various cytokines. Although relatively novel, the research on cytokine production by neutrophils has brought forward new and exciting discoveries. The fact that neutrophils clearly predominate over other cell types under various *in vivo* conditions suggests that, under some circumstances, the contribution of PMN-derived cytokines can be of foremost importance. Nevertheless, with the exception of some particular cases, it is still premature to assess the actual biological significance of cytokine production by neutrophils. The full appreciation of cytokine synthesis by neutrophils as a new dimension of neutrophil biology opens novel perspectives as to the potential role of these cells in the context of inflammmatory and immune responses, and is likely to also provide new insights into therapy of many disorders known to be influenced by PMN.

9. References

1. Loyd A.R. and Oppenheim J.J., *Immunol. Today* **13** (1992), 169–172.
2. Cassatella M.A., *Immunol. Today* **16** (1995), 21–26.
3. Cassatella M.A., *Cytokines produced by polymorphonuclear neutrophils: molecular and biological aspects.* (R.G. Landes Company, Austin, TX, USA, 1996), 1–199.
4. Altstaedt J., Kirchner H. and Rink L., *Immunology* **89** (1996), 563–568.
5. Baggiolini M., Dewald B. and Moser B., *Annu. Rev. Immunol.* **15** (1997), 675–705.
6. Rollins B.J., *Blood* **90** (1997), 909–928.
7. Pantaleo G. and Fauci A.S., *Springer Semin. Immunopathol.* **18** (1997), 253–256.
8. Strieter R.M., *et al.*, *Biochem. Biophys. Res. Commun.* **173** (1990), 725–730.
9. Bazzoni F., *et al.*, *J. Exp. Med.* **173** (1993), 771–774.
10. Cassatella M.A., *et al.*, *J. Immunol.* **148** (1992), 3216–3220.
11. Arnold R., *et al.*, *Immunology* **82** (1994), 184–191.
12. Morrison T.B., Weis J.H. and Weis J.J., *J. Immunol.* **158** (1997), 4838–4845.
13. Kuhns D. and Gallin J.I., *J. Immunol.* **154** (1995), 6556–6562.
14. Ember J.A., *et al.*, *Am. J. Pathol.* **144** (1994), 393–403.
15. McCain R., *et al.*, *Am. J. Respir. Cell. Mol. Biol.* **10** (1994), 651–657.
16. Strieter R.M., *et al.*, *Am. J. Pathol.* **141** (1992), 397–407.
17. Kikuchi M., *et al.*, *Res. Commun. Mol. Pathol. Pharmacol.* **87** (1995), 269–274.
18. Cuthbertson B.H., Galley H.F. and Webster N.R., *Br. J. Anaesth.* **78** (1997), 714–717.
19. Pakianathan D.R., *J. Leuk. Biol.* **57** (1995), 699–702.
20. Derevianko A., D'Amico R. and Simms H., *Clin. Exp. Immunol.* **106** (1996), 560–567.
21. Cassatella M.A., Guasparri I., Ceska M., Bazzoni F. and Rossi, F., *Immunology* **78** (1993), 177–184.

22. Fujishima S., *et al., J. Cell. Physiol.* **154** (1993), 478–485.

23. Cassatella M.A., *et al., J. Exp. Med.* **178** (1993), 2207–2211.

24. Cassatella M.A., *et al., Biochem. Biophys. Res. Commun.* **190** (1993), 660–667 [published erratum in **192** (1993), 324].

25. Au B., Williams T. J. and Collins P. D., *J. Immunol.* **152** (1994), 5411–5419.

26. McCain R.W., Dessypris E.N. and Christman J.W., *Am. J. Respir. Cell. Mol. Biol.* **8** (1993), 28–34.

27. Takahashi G.W., *et al., Blood* **81** (1993), 357–364.

28. Wei S., *et al., J. Immunol.* **152** (1994), 3630–3636.

29. Hilger R.A., Koller M. and Konig W., *Int. Arch. Allergy Immunol.* **107** (1995), 259–260

30. Hilger R.A., Koller M. and Konig W., *Inflammation* **20** (1996), 57–70.

31. Hachicha M., Naccache P.H. and McColl S.R., *J. Exp. Med.* **182** (1995), 2019–2025.

32. Serra M.C., *et al., Immunology* **82** (1994), 63–69.

33. Laudanna C., *et al., J. Biol. Chem.* **269** (1994), 4021–4026.

34. Shinoda I., *et al., Biosci. Biotechnol. Biochem.* **60** (1996), 521–523.

35. Brizzi M.F., *et al., J. Clin. Invest.* **99** (1997), 1576–1584.

36. Wiley S.R., Goodwin R.G. and Smith C.A., *J. Immunol.* **157** (1996), 3635–3639.

37. Cassatella M.A., *et al., Fund. Clin. Immunol.* **1** (1993) 99–106.

38. Retini C., *et al., Infect. Immun.* **64** (1996), 2897–2903.

39. Wahlgren M., *et al., Scand. J. Immunol.* **42** (1995), 626–636.

40. Konig B., *et al., Infect. Immun.* **62** (1994), 4831–4837.

41. Gibson F.C. 3rd, Tzianabos A.O. and Onderdonk A.B., *Infect. Immun.* **64** (1996), 1065–1069.

42. Yoshimura A., Hara Y., Kaneko T. and Kato I., *J. Periodontal. Res.* **32** (1997), 279–286.

43. Riedel D. and Kaufmann., *J. Leuk. Biol.* **51** (1996), a232, 51.

44. Inoue H., *et al., Am. J. Respir. Cell. Mol. Biol.* **11** (1994), 651–663.

45. Konig B., *et al., Int. Arch. Allergy Immunol.* **106** (1995), 357–365.

46. Oishi K., *et al., Infect. Immun.* **62** (1994), 4145–4152.

47. Konig B., Krusat T., Streckert H.J. and Konig W., *J. Leuk. Biol.* **60** (1996), 253–260.

48. Cavaillon J. M., Marie C., Pitton C. and Fitting C., *Proceedings 3rd International Congress on the immune consequences of trauma shock and sepsis*, (Pabst Science Publishers, 1995), 23–25.

49. Girard D., Paquin R., Naccache P.H. and Beaulieu A.D., *J. Leuk. Biol.* **59** (1996), 412–419.

50. Wang P., *et al.*, *Blood* **83** (1994), 2678–2683.

51. Meda L., Gasperini S., Ceska M. and Cassatella M.A., *Cell. Immunol.* **57** (1994), 448–461.

52. Gasperini S., Calzetti F., Russo M.P., De Gironcoli M. and Cassatella M.A., *J. Inflamm.* **45** (1995), 143–151.

53. Haskill S., *et al.*, *Proc. Natl. Acad. Sci. USA* **87** (1990), 7732–7736.

54. Koch A.E., *et al.*, *J. Clin. Invest.* **155** (1995), 3660–3666.

55. Huang S., *et al.*, *Am. J. Pathol.* **41** (1992), 981–988.

56. Villard J., *et al.*, *Am. J. Respir. Crit. Care. Med.* **152** (1995), 1549–1554.

57. Iida N. and Grotendorst G.R., *Mol. Cell. Biol.* **10** (1990), 5596–5599.

58. Edamatsu T., Xiao Y.Q., Tanabe J., Mue S. and Ohuchi K., *Br. J. Pharmacol.* **121** (1997), 1651–1658.

59. Cassatella M.A. *et al.*, *Eur. J. Immunol.* **27** (1997), 111–115.

60. Taub D.D., *et al.*, *J. Exp. Med.* **177** (1993), 1809–1817

61. Kasama T., *et al.*, *J. Exp. Med.* **178** (1993), 63–72.

62. Kasama T., *et al.*, *J. Immunol.* **152** (1994), 3559–3569.

63. Van Damme J., *et al.*, *J. Immunol.* **152** (1994), 5495–5502.

64. Burn T.C. *,et al.*, *Blood* **84** (1994), 2776–2783.

65. Dubravec D.B., Spriggs D.R., Mannick J.A. and Rodrick M.L., *Proc. Natl. Acad. Sci. USA* **87** (1990), 6758–6761.

66. Djeu J.Y., Serbousek D. and Blanchard D.K., *Blood* **76** (1990),1405–1409.

67. Lindemann A., *et al.*, *J. Clin. Invest.* **83** (1989),1308–1312.

68. Mandi Y., Degre M. and Beladi I., *Int. Arch. Allergy Appl. Immunol.* **90** (1989), 411–413.

69. Mandi Y., *et al.*, *Int. Arch. Allergy Appl. Immunol* **96** (1991), 102–106.

70. Bazzoni F., *et al.*, *J. Leuk. Biol.* **50** (1991), 223–228.

71. Palma C., *et al.*, *Infect. Immun.* **60** (1992), 4604–4611.

72. Ohlsson K., Linder C., Lundberg E. and Axelsson L., *Scand. J. Clin. Lab. Invest.* **56** (1996), 461–470.

73. Scuderi P., *et al.*, *Cell. Immunol.* **135** (1991), 299–313.

74. Van Kessel K.P., Van Strip J.A. and Verhoef J., *J. Immunol.* **147** (1991), 3862–3868.

75. Torosantucci A., *et al.*, *Clin. Exp. Immunol.* **107** (1997), 451–457.

76. Arnold R., *et al.*, *Infect. Immun.* **61** (1993), 2545–2552.

77. Balazovich K.J., Suchard S.J., Remick D.G. and Boxer L.A., *Blood* **88** (1996), 690–696.
78. Nathan C.F., *J. Clin. Invest.* **80** (1987), 1550–1560.
79. Contrino J., *et al.*, *Pediatr. Res.* **34** (1993), 249–252.
80. Wei S., *et al.*, *J. Immunol.* **150** (1993), 1979–1987.
81. Girard D., *et al.*, *Blood* **86** (1995), 1170–1176.
82. Takeichi O., *et al.*, *Cell. Immunol.* **156** (1995), 296–309.
83. Terashima T., *et al.*, *Am. J. Respir. Cell. Mol. Biol.* **13** (1995), 69–73.
84. Takeichi O., Saito I., Tsurumachi T., Moro I. and Saito T., *Calcif. Tissue Int.* **58** (1996), 244–248.
85. Kasama T., *et al.*, *J. Invest. Med.* **43** (1995), 58–67.
86. Haziot A., Tsuberi B.Z. and Goyert S.M., *J. Immunol.* **150** (1993), 5556–5565.
87. Fantone J.C. in Cytokines in health and disease, ed. Remick D. and Friedland J. S. (Marcel Dekker, New York, 1997), 373–380.
88. Gruss H.J., Pinto A., Duyster J., Poppema S. and Herrmann F., *Immunol Today* **18** (1997), 156–163.
89. Gruss H.J., *et al.*, *Leukemia* **8** (1994), 2083–2094.
90. Gruss H.J., *et al.*, *Am. J. Pathol.* **149** (1996), 469–481.
91. Biswas P., et al., *Immunity* **2** (1995), 587–596.
92. Ho J.L., *et al.*, *J. Exp. Med.* **181** (1995), 1493–1505.
93. Hanson D.F., Murphy P.A. and Windle B.E., *J. Exp. Med.* **151** (1980), 1360–1371.
94. Windle B.E., Murphy P.A. and Cooperman S., *Infect.I mmun.* **39** (1983), 1142–1146.
95. Jupin C., *et al.*, *Inflammation* **11** (1987), 53–61.
96. Goto F., *et al.*, *Immunology* **53** (1984), 683–692.
97. Tiku K., Tiku M.L. and Skosey J.L., *J. Immunol.* **136** (1986), 3677–3685.
98. Lindemann A., *et al.*, *J. Immunol.* **140** (1988), 837–839.
99. Dularay B., Westacott C.I., and Elson C.J., *Br. J. Rheum.* **31** (1992), 19–24.
100. Fernandez M.C., Walters J. and Marucha P., *J. Leuk. Biol.* **59** (1996), 598–603.
101. Goh K., *et al.*, *Int. Arch. Allergy Appl. Immunol.* **88** (1989), 297–303.
102. Lord P.C.W., *et al.*, *J. Clin. Invest.* **87** (1991), 1312–1321.
103. Marucha P.T., Zeff R.A. and Kreutzer D.L., *J. Immunol.* **145** (1990), 2932–2937.
104. Walters J.D., *et al.*, *J. Leuk. Biol.* **57** (1995), 282–286.
105. Ueta E., Umazume M., Yamamoto T. and Osaki T., *Int. J. Immunopharmacol.* **16** (1994), 7–17.
106. Yamazaki K., *et al.*, *Oral. Microbiol. Immunol.* **4** (1989), 193–198.

107. Brooks C.J.. *et al., Clin. Exp. Immunol.* **106** (1996), 273–279.
108. Falk R.J., Terrel R.S., Charles L.A. and Jennette J.C., *Proc. Natl. Acad. Sci. USA* **87** (1990), 4115–4119.
109. Roberge C.J., *et al., Agents Actions* **34** (1991), 38–41.
110. Roberge C.J., *et al., J. Immunol.* **152** (1994), 5485–5494.
111. Dinarello C.A., *FASEB J.* **8** (1994), 1314–1324.
112. Arend W.P., *Adv. Immunol.* **54** (1993), 167–227.
113. Dripps D.J., Brandhuber B.J., Thompson R.C. and Eisenberg S.P., *J. Biol. Chem.* **266** (1991),10331–10336.
114. Tiku K., *et al., J. Immunol.* **136** (1986), 3686–3692.
115. McColl S.R., *et al., J. Exp. Med.* **176** (1992), 593–598.
116. Malyak M., *et al., J. Clin.I mmunol.* **14** (1994), 20–30.
117. Ulich T.R. *et al., Am. J. Pathol.* **141** (1992), 61–68.
118. Cassatella M.A., Meda L., Gasperini S. and Bonora S., *J. Exp. Med.* **179** (1994), 1695–1699.
119. Poutsiaka D.D., *et al., Blood* **78** (1991)1275–1281.
120. Arend P.W. *et al., J. Immunol.* **147** (1991), 1530–1536.
121. Chang D.M., *Clin. Immunol. Immunopatol.* **74** (1995), 23–30.
122. Re F., *et al., Eur. J. Immunol.* **23** (1993), 570–573.
123. Muzio M., *et al., Blood* **83** (1994), 1738–1743.
124. Muzio M., *et al., Eur. J. Immunol.* **24** (1994), 3194–3198.
125. Marie C., *et al., Cytokine* **8** (1996), 147–151.
126. Grotendorst G.R., Smale G. and Pencev D., *J. Cell. Phys.* **140** (1989), 396–402.
127. Muzio M., *et al., J. Exp. Med.* **182** (1995), 623–628.
128. Beaulieu A.D., Paquin R. and Gosselin J., *Blood* **86** (1995), 2789–2798.
129. Roberge C.J., Poubelle P. E., Beaulieu A.D., Heitz D. and Gosselin J., *J. Immunol.* **156** (1996), 4884–4891.
130. Cicco N.A., *et al., Blood* **75** (1990), 2049–2052.
131. Kato K., *et al., J. Immunol.* **144** (1990), 1317–1322.
132. Melani C., *et al., Blood* **81** (1993), 2744–2749.
133. Quayle J.A., Adams S., Bucknall R.C. and Edwards S.W., *FEMS Immunol. Med. Microbiol.* **8** (1994), 233–239.
134. Mianji S., Hamasaki Y., Yamamoto S. and Miyazaki S., *Int. J. Immunopharmacol.* **18** (1996), 339–346.
135. Cassone A., *et al., J. Clin. Microbiol.* **31** (1993),1354–1357.
136. Cassone A., Chiani P., Quinti I. and Torosantucci A., *J. Leuk. Biol.* **62** (1997), 60–66.

137. Romani L., *et al.*, *J. Immunol.* **158** (1997), 2356–2362.
138. Cassatella M.A., *et al.*, *Eur. J. Immunol.* **25** (1995), 1–5.
139. D'Andrea A., *et al.*, *J. Exp. Med.* **178** (1993), 1041–1048.
140. Romani L., *et al.*, *J. Immunol.* **158** (1997), 5349–5356.
141. Kanangat S., Thomas J., Gangappa S., Babu J.S. and Rouse B.T., *J. Immunol.* **156** (1996), 1110–1116.
142. Shirafuji N., *et al.*, *Blood* **75** (1990), 17–19.
143. Brandt E.R., Linnane A.W. and Devenish R.J., *Br. J. Hematol.* **86** (1994), 717–725.
144. Rouse B.T., Babiuk L. and Henson P., *J. Infect. Dis.* **141** (1980), 223–230.
145. Fava R.A., *et al.*, *J. Exp. Med.* **173** (1993), 1121–1132.
146. Ramenghi U., *et al.*, *Stem Cells* **12** (1994), 521–526.
147. Kita H., *et al.*, *J. Exp. Med.* **174** (1991), 745–748.
148. Calafat J., *et al.*, *Blood* **90** (1997), 1255–1266.
149. Bry K., Hallmann M. and Lappalainen U., *Prostaglandins* **48** (1994), 389–399.
150. DeForge L.E., Tracey D.E., Kenney J.S. and Remick D.G., *Am. J. Pathol.* **140** (1992), 1045–1054.
151. Pang G., Ortega M., Zighang R., Reeves G. and Clancy R., *Am. J. Respir. Crit. Care Med.* **155** (1997), 726–731.
152. Cassatella M.A., Gasperini S., Calzetti F., McDonald P. and Trinchieri G., *Biochem. J.* **310** (1995), 751–755.
153. Cassatella M.A., *Immunol. Letters* **38** (1996), 79–82.
154. Kuhns D., *et al.*, *J. Clin. Invest.* **89** (1992), 1734–1740.
155. Francoeur C. and Denis M., *Inflammation* **19** (1995), 587–598.
156. Suzuki H., *et al.*, *J. Allergy Clin. Immunol.* **98** (1996), 659–670.
157. Simon H.U., *et al.*, *Int. Arch. Allergy Immunol.* **107** (1995), 124–126.
158. Baldwin G.C., Buckley D.M., Roth M.D., Kleerup E.C. and Tashkin D.P., *Chest* **111** (1997), 698–705.
159. Lin C.Y. and Huang T.P., *Nephron* **68** (1994), 37–441.
160. Lin C.Y., Lin C.C. and Huang T.P., *Nephron* **63** (1993), 404–408.
161. Gillitzer R., Ritter U., Spandau U., Goebeler M. and Brocker E.B., *J. Invest. Dermatol.* **107** (1996), 778–782.
162. Kulke R., *et al.*, *J. Invest. Dermatol.* **106** (1996), 526–530.
163. Grimm M.C., Elsbury S.K., Pavli P. and Doe W.F., *Gut* **38** (1996), 90–98.
164. Derkx B., *et al.*, *Lancet* **342** (1994), 173–174.
165. Beil W.J., *et al. J. Leuk. Biol.* **58** (1995), 284–298.
166. Arend W.P. and Dayer J.M., *Arthritis Rheum.* **33** (1990), 305–315.

167. Edwards S.W. and Hallett M.B., *Immunol. Today* **18** (1997), 320–324.
168. Malyak M., Swaney R.E. and Arend W.P., *Arthritis Rheum.* **36** (1993), 781–789.
169. Quayle J.A., *et al.*, *Ann. Rheum. Dis.* **54** (1995), 930–933.
170. Beaulieu A.D. and McColl S., *Arthritis Rheum.* **37** (1994), 855–859.
171. Landry M., *Arch. Dermatol.* **113** (1977), 147–154.
172. Staples P.J., *et al.*, *Arthritis Rheum.* **17** (1974), 1–10.
173. Hsieh S.C., *et al.*, *Clin. Exp. Rheum.* **12** (1994), 627–633.
174. Hsieh S.C., *et al.*, *Br. J. Rheumatol.* **34** (1995), 107–112.
175. McCall C.E., *et al.*, *J. Clin. Invest.* **91** (1993), 853–861.
176. Fasano M.B., *et al.*, *J. Clin. Invest.* **88** (1991), 1452–1459.
177. Marie C., *et al.*, *Infect. Immun.* **65** (1997), 865–871.
178. Raqib R., *et al.*, *Infect. Immun.* **63** (1995), 289–296.
179. Sprenger H., *et al.*, *Clin. Immunol. Immunopathol.* **80** (1996), 155–161.
180. Ossege L.M., Sindern E., Voss B. and Malin J.P., *J. Neurol. Sci.* **144** (1996), 1–13.
181. Kabashima H., *et al.*, *Infect. Immun.* **58** (1990), 2621–2627.
182. Takahashi K., Poole I. and Kinane D.F., *Arch. Oral. Biol.* **40** (1995), 941–947.
183. Hendley T.M., Steed R.B. and Galbraith G.M., *J. Periodontol.* **66** (1995), 761–765.
184. Tonetti M.S., *et al.*, *Infect. Immun.* **62** (1994), 4005–4014.
185. Bortolami M., *et al.*, *Fund. Clin. Immunol.* **3** (1995), 153–156.
186. Xing Z., *et al.*, *Am. J. Pathol.* **143** (1993), 1009–1015.
187. Xing Z., *et al.*, *Am. J. Respir. Cell. Mol. Biol.* **10** (1994), 148–153: erratum *Am. J. Respir. Cell. Mol. Biol.* **10** (1994), following 346.
188. Imamura S., Matsukawa A., Ohkawara S., Kagayama M. and Yoshinaga M., *Pathol. Int.* **47** (1997), 16–24.
189. Williams J.H., *et al.*, *Am. J. Respir. Cell. Mol. Biol.* **8** (1993), 134–144.
190. Cirelli R.A., *et al.*, *J. Leuk. Biol.* **57** (1995), 820–826.
191. Kolls J.K., *et al.*, *Am. J. Physiol.* **268** (1995), L991–998.
192. Terebuth P.D., *et al.*, *Am. J. Pathol.* **140** (1992), 649–657.
193. Nill M.R., *et al.*, *J. Leuk. Biol.* **58** (1995), 563–574.
194. Mori S., *et al.*, *Int. Immunol.* **6** (1994), 149–156.
195. Goto F., *et al.*, *Br.J.Exp.Path.* **70** (1989), 597–606.
196. Hangai M., *et al.*, *Invest. Ophthalmol. Vis. Sci.* **36** (1995), 571–578.
197. Ivey C.L., *et al.*, *J. Clin. Invest.* **95** (1995), 2720–2728.
198. Williams F.M. *et al.*, *Br. J. Pharmacol.* **111** (1994), 1123–1128.
199. Matsumoto T., *et al.*, *Lab. Invest.* **77** (1997), 119–125.

200. Sakanashi Y., *et al.*, *J. Leuk. Biol.* **56** (1994), 741–750.

201. D'Angio C.T. *et al.*, *Am. J. Physiol.* **12** (1995), L826–L831.

202. Wu X., Dolecki G.J., Sherry B., Zagorski J. and Lefkowith J.B. *J. Immunol.* **158** (1997), 3917–3924.

203. Matsukawa A., *et al.*, *Clin. Exp. Immunol.* **93** (1993), 206–211.

204. Matsukawa A., *et al.*, *J. Immunol.* **154** (1995), 5418–5425.

205. Matsukawa A., Yoshimura T., Miyamoto K., Ohkawara S. and Yoshinaga M., *Lab. Invest.* **76** (1997), 629–638.

206. Jordan M., *et al.*, *J. Immunol.* **154** (1995), 4081–4090.

207. Tilg H., *et al.*, *Blood* **83** (1994), 113–118.

208. Dai W.J., *et al.*, *J. Immunol.* **158** (1997), 5297–5304.

209. Thomas J., Gangappa S., Kanangat S. and Rouse B.T., *J. Immunol.* **158** (1997), 1383–1391.

210. Mosmann T.R. and Coffman R.L., *Ann. Rev. Immunol.* **7** (1989), 145–173.

211. Romagnani S., *Ann. Rev. Immunol.* **12** (1994), 227–257.

212. Romani L., Puccetti P. and Bistoni F., *Chem. Immunol.* **63** (1996), 115–137.

213. Romani L., *et al.*, *Res Immunol* **147** (1996), 512–518.

214. Romani L., Mencacci A., Tonnetti L., *et al.*, *Eur. J. Immunol.* **22** (1994), 909–913.

215. Puccetti P., Romani L. and Bistoni F., *Trends Microbiol.* **3** (1995), 237–240.

216. Fresno M., Kopf M. and Rivas L., *Immunol. Today* **18** (1997), 56–58.

217. Kudo C., *et al.*, *J. Immunol.* **150** (1993), 3728–3738.

218. Kudo C., *et al.*, *J. Immunol.* **150** (1993), 3739–3746.

219. Kudo C., *et al.*, *J. Immunol.* **147** (1991), 2196–2201.

220. Tamura M., *et al.*, *J. Immunol.* **153** (1994), 1301–1308.

221. Midorikawa Y., Yamashita T., and Sendo F., *Cancer Res.* **50** (1990), 6243–6247

222. Tanaka E. and Sendo F., *Int. J. Cancer* **54** (1993), 131–136.

223. Gosselin E.J., *et al.*, *J. Immunol.* **151** (1993), 1482–1490.

224. Stoppacciaro A., *et al. J. Exp. Med.* **178** (1993), 151–161.

225. Colombo M.P., *et al.*, *Am. J. Pathol.* **148** (1996), 473–483.

226. Fink G.W. and Norman J.G., *J. Surg. Res.* **63** (1996), 369–373.

227. Hubner G., *et al.*, *Cytokine* **8** (1996), 548–556.

228. Bartholdi D. and Schwab M.E., *Eur. J. Neurosci.* **9** (1997), 1422–1438.

229. Carrington J.L., *et al.*, *J. Cell. Biol.* **107** (1988), 1969–1975.

CHAPTER 6

NEUTROPHILS AND APOPTOSIS

NF Fanning, HP Redmond[1] and D Bouchier-Hayes

1. Introduction

Apoptosis or programmed cell death is a morphologically distinct mode of
eukaryotic cell death. It occurs through the activation of a cell-intrinsic suicide
programme which can be modulated by many exogenous signals. Apoptosis is
fundamentally different from degenerative cell death or necrosis. It
characteristically affects scattered single cells, not groups of contiguous cells
as in necrosis. The dying cell undergoes a relatively ordered form of cell death
characterised by cell shrinkage, cellular crenation, cytoplasmic and chromatin
condensation and internucleosomal DNA fragmentation(1–4). The orderly
cleavage of DNA by endonucleases is characteristic of apoptosis and produces
a ladder pattern of DNA fragmentation on standard DNA electrophoresis, which
has been used by many investigators to identify and confirm programmed cell
death (5,6). Changes in membrane glycosylation and lipid profiles, and
alteration in expression of surface receptors of apoptotic cells have also been
observed during the apoptotic process (7–11). Apoptotic cells are rapidly
phagocytosed and degraded by tissue macrophages without an inflammatory
response. This mechanism prevents the release of the cytotoxic contents of
apoptotic proinflammatory cells and limits the possibility of neighbouring host
cell injury. The apoptotic process differs significantly to cell death by necrosis

[1]Correspondence to: HP Redmond; Professor of surgery, University Hospital Cork, Cork, Ireland,
Ph: 00 353 21 546400; Fax: 00 353 21 343307; e-mail: redmondp@ iol.ie

or lysis where cells release their contents into the surrounding tissues and perpetuate the local inflammatory response.

Apoptosis is responsible for the deletion of cells in normal tissues and complements cell proliferation in normal tissue homeostasis. It occurs in processes as diverse as embryological remodelling, inflammation, immune tolerance and neoplasia (1,5,12). Apoptosis plays an essential role in the functional requirements of the immune system (12,13). It is responsible for self-tolerance by deleting auto-reactive T cells in the thymus, for selection of B cell clones in lymphoid germinal centres during hormonal immune response (14), and deletion of effete cells such as senescent neutrophils and megakaryocytes (15,16). Apoptosis of neutrophils and macrophages is essential for normal resolution of inflammation. Dysregulated apoptosis is associated with diseases such as cancer, autoimmunity, AIDS, allergic disorders and neurodegenerative diseases (17–20).

2. Fate of Extravasated Neutrophils: Necrosis or Apoptosis?

The neutrophil remains the key pro-inflammatory cell activated in the initial cell mediated host response to a septic insult. Injury results in a rapid systemic neutrophilia and these cell are responsible for mediating the first line of host immune defence. Neutrophils are released from the bone marrow as terminally differentiated cells incapable of further division, with the half-life of circulating neutrophils in the region of only seven hours (21). The fate of extravasated neutrophils at inflamed sites was first eluded to by the seminal observations of Elie Metchnikoff in the late 19th century (22). Using vital microscopy, Metchnikoff observed that neutrophils were removed from the inflamed site by being ingested while still intact by macrophages. This fundamental observation spawned the study into the destiny of the inflammatory neutrophil.

Histological and radiolabelled neutrophil studies in patients and animals have revealed that the majority of extravasated neutrophils never leave the inflamed site, with most cells dying *in situ* (23,24). Although neutrophil necrosis and disintegration has been observed at inflamed sites, with vasculitis being a prime example (25), the weight of evidence is against neutrophil necrosis as the 'physiological' means of cell clearance from resolving inflamed sites. Histological studies have shown that apoptosis and phagocytic clearance by macrophages of extravasated neutrophils occurs in inflammation of the joint (26), lung (27), gut (28), and kidney (29). A recent careful time course study of resolving acute lung inflammation revealed that apoptosis is the major clearance mechanism of extravasated neutrophils at this site (30). Hughes et al. using radiolabelling techniques to track the fate of neutrophils accumulating within the glomerular microvasculature following experimentally induced injury, showed that the majority of recruited neutrophils rather than migrating into tissues, apparently detach from damaged vessel walls and return to the blood stream before meeting their fate elsewhere, presumably the liver and spleen (31). Even in the situation where neutrophils remain sequestered in the vessel lumen, approximately one quarter of recruited neutrophils meet their fate *in situ*, undergoing apoptosis and then engulfment by intravascular macrophages, particularly in glomerular vessels occluded by thrombus (31). It appears, therefore, that neutrophils that are trapped in inflamed sites and are unable to return to the blood preferentially undergo apoptosis and clearance by macrophages.

3. Neutrophil Apoptosis Limits Neutrophil-Induced Tissue Injury

The neutrophil contains powerful oxidative (cytotoxic reactive oxygen species and reactive nitrogen species) and non-oxidative processes, (degradative granule enzymes, chemotactic proteins, toxic cationic proteins), which are critical in the defense against infection (32). Uncontrolled release of these toxic contents during necrosis may exacerbate local tissue injury and promote persistence of leukocyte influx. Apoptosis limits the phlogistic potential of neutrophils by a number of mechanisms. First, apoptotic neutrophils become isolated from the inflammatory milieu, losing their ability to respond to receptor-mediated activating stimuli by mechanisms that include down-regulation of cell-surface receptors (10,33). Second, apoptotic neutrophils are functionally effete with a number of neutrophil phlogistic functions downregulated, including, chemotaxis, phagocytosis, granule release, and the respiratory burst

(33). Third, macrophage phagocytosis of apoptotic neutrophils prevents release of its autotoxic contents (15). If professional phagocytosis is blocked *in vitro*, apoptotic neutrophils eventually disintegrate, releasing their toxic contents (34). Fourth, uptake of apoptotic neutrophils fail to stimulate macrophage release of proinflammatory mediators (35). These mechanisms act to limit tissue injury and promote the resolution of inflammation.

4. Regulation and Mechanisms of Neutrophil Apoptosis

The regulation of apoptosis is complex and presently is incompletely understood. Apoptosis represents an active gene-directed mechanism, which is controlled by intrinsic cell-specific genetic factors and the death programme can be modulated by exogenous "survival" factors. Neutrophil apoptotic mechanisms are only beginning to be elucidated. Intrinsic factors involved in regulating and mediating the neutrophil's exquisite susceptibility to undergo apoptosis include, expression of the death factor receptor Fas, expression of the corresponding death factor (Fas ligand) which transduces the death signal to its receptor, and the paucity of expression of the anti-apoptotic bcl-2 family of proto-oncogenes. Extracellular factors also regulate the susceptibility of cells to undergo programmed cell death. The concept that cells are programmed to commit suicide unless they receive signals for survival was first expounded by Raff (36). The neutrophil is a cell self-programmed to die, but its longevity can be extended by "survival" factors present in the inflammatory milieu. Removal of these "survival" factors may be a common signal for neutrophils to apoptose.

4.1 *Intrinsic genetic regulation*

Of prime importance in transducing the death signal in neutrophils is the Fas-Fas ligand system. Activated neutrophils intrinsically express the death factor receptor known as Fas/Apo-1 (CD95). Fas is a type I cell surface glycoprotein of the tumour necrosis factor (TNF)/nerve growth factor receptor superfamily

(37). It transduces the intracellular apoptotic death signal in Fas positive cells, through ligation of Fas by Fas agonist antibodies or its specific ligand (11,38,39). Fas is ubiquitously expressed on various tissues with abundant expression in the thymus, heart, liver, and kidney (40). Fas is also expressed by activated proinflammatory cells, such as lymphocytes, macrophages and neutrophils but is only functional in these cells when they are activated during an immune response. Expression of functional Fas on activated leukocytes targets these cells for destruction, limiting the immune response.

Fas ligand (FasL) is a type II cell surface glycoprotein related to TNF. It is predominantly expressed on activated T lymphocytes and natural killer (NK) cells. Its expression on T cells is not constitutive and is short lived. FasL acts as a death effector molecule of cytotoxic T cells and is deployed to kill Fas-bearing target cells (41). The role of Fas-FasL system in phagocytes has been less characterised. Fas is expressed on activated neutrophils, monocytes, and eosinophils. Constitutive FasL expression, however, appears to be restricted to mature neutrophils (42,43). These three types of phagocytes demonstrate differential sensitivity to Fas-induced apoptosis, with neutrophils most sensitive, and eosinophils least sensitive. The constitutive expression of Fas and FasL on mature neutrophils raises the possibility that the Fas system plays a fundamental, but not exclusive, role in the regulation of spontaneous neutrophil apoptosis (43). Neutrophils may be irretrievably committed to autocrine death induced by Fas/FasL interaction on the cell surface.

Proteolysis of membrane-bound FasL by metalloproteinases produces soluble FasL (sFasL) (44). The soluble form of human FasL is functional, unlike soluble mouse FasL. Activated T cells and neutrophils have been shown to be capable of secreting a soluble FasL and may function in a paracrine pathway to mediate cell death via a Fas dependent mechanism (43). Tanaka et al (44) have suggested that systemic sFasL may play a role in the induction of inappropriate tissue injury. Failure of neutrophil apoptosis could, in theory, increase FasL release and exacerbation of tissue injury at sites of inflammation.

While it is clear that the Fas/FasL pathway plays an important role in spontaneous and activated neutrophil apoptosis, the precise intracellular pathway of Fas signalling in neutrophils is unknown. Experiments performed in the yeast two-hybrid screening method, a powerful technique to determine protein-protein interactions, has led to the identification of a number of death effectors and regulator proteins linked to the Fas receptor (45). These proteins include FAP-1, RIP, Daxx and FADD and play an important role in transducing the Fas death signal in specific cell types (46–50). Fas accessory proteins, however, have yet to be identified in neutrophils, but could conceivably play regulatory roles in neutrophil programmed cell death.

Downstream events leading to neutrophil apoptosis following Fas signalling are beginning to be deciphered. The role of reactive oxygen intermediate (ROI) products in neutrophil apoptosis has been explored. Bacterial ingestion may induce neutrophil apoptosis via an oxygen dependent mechanism (51), but the role of the Fas pathway in this is unknown. In addition, the antioxidants taurine, n-acetylcysteine and gluthatione, attenuate sodium arsenite induced neutrophil apoptosis and are cytoprotective for endothelial cells (52,53), though their role in the inhibition of Fas-mediated apoptosis is unproven. It appears, however, that Fas-induced neutrophil apoptosis may indeed be mediated, in part, by endogenous ROI products. By comparing rates of apoptosis in neutrophils isolated from normal donors and from patients with chronic granulomatous disease (CGD), a hereditary defect in ROI production, Kasahara et al (54) found that both spontaneous and Fas-induced apoptosis was much slower in CGD neutrophils than that seen in normal neutrophils. Addition of catalase inhibited both spontaneous and Fas-mediated apoptosis in normal neutrophils, while addition of hydrogen peroxide increased both spontaneous and Fas mediated apoptosis in CGD neutrophils in proportion to that seen in normal neutrophils. This suggests that ROI are important mediators in neutrophils and may have a role in effecting the Fas-mediated signal transduction pathway.

Other mechanisms are likely to be involved in Fas-induced neutrophil apoptosis. The neutrophil's apoptotic response to intracellular calcium ($[Ca^{2+}]_i$) fluxes differs to other cell types. Minor increases in $[Ca^{2+}]_i$ inhibits programmed cell death in neutrophils, but induces apoptosis in lymphocyte cell lines (55,56). We have recently demonstrated that Fas activation results in a rapid downregulation of $[Ca^{2+}]_i$ leading to apoptosis (unpublished data). The non-toxic amino-acid taurine appears to exert its anti-apoptotic effect by attenuating the Fas induced decrease in $[Ca^{2+}]_i$ (unpublished data). Other studies have shown that the selective tyrosine kinase inhibitors herbimycin A and genistein, suppress

Fas-induced apoptosis in neutrophils suggesting a role for tyrosine kinase activity in Fas-mediated signal transduction (57,58). The role of ceramide, an important intracellular messenger of the Fas death pathway in several cell types, in Fas-mediated neutrophil apoptosis is undetermined (43).

The intrinsic susceptibility of a cell to undergo apoptosis is determined by members of the proto-oncogene bcl-2 gene family. The prototypic regulator of cell death is bcl-2. This has been shown to prolong cellular survival by blocking programmed cell death and sets the basic apoptotic resistance threshold of cells (59). Iwai et al have shown that there is marked variation among leukocytes regarding bcl-2 expression with lymphocytes expressing bcl-2 intensely, monocytes less so, and neutrophils essentially not at all (60). The relative susceptibility of monocytes and neutrophils to Fas-induced apoptosis has been attributed to the degree of expression of bcl-2 by these cells (42,60).

4.2 *Extrinsic regulation*

Extracellular factors also regulate the neutrophils susceptibility to undergo programmed cell death. Removal of "survival" factors may be a common pathway to apoptosis. Neutrophil apoptosis can be modulated by a variety of inflammatory mediators. Inhibition of apoptosis and prolongation of the functional life span of neutrophils occurs with lipopolysaccharide (LPS), glucocorticoids, granulocyte colony stimulating factor (G-CSF), granulocyte-macrophage colony stimulating factor (GM-CSF), and interleukin-2 (IL-2) (43,61–63). Conflicting data has been reported on the role of IL-6, C5a, TNF-α and FMLP in neutrophil apoptosis (43,62–67). Platelets also appear to be able to modulate neutrophil apoptosis by inhibiting this process but the mechanism for this is currently unknown (68).

The mechanisms by which "survival" factors mediate their anti-apoptotic mechanism in neutrophils is largely unknown. Both proinflammatory cytokines and glucocorticoids suppress Fas-induced apoptosis in normal neutrophils, suggesting they suppress neutrophil apoptosis via inhibition of a component of the Fas death programme, however, it is unlikely to be mediated by simple downregulation of cell-surface Fas expression(43). Recently intracellular acidification has been shown to precede, and may be causally related to neutrophil apoptosis, with G-CSF delaying programmed cell death in neutrophils by up-regulating the vacuolar H^+-ATPase (69).

Lipopolysaccharide (LPS) also delays neutrophil apoptosis. This appears, at least in part, to be as a consequence of adhesion molecule engagement and the subsequent process of endothelial transmigration. LPS treated neutrophils showed increased expression of the β_2 integrin CD11b, and decreased expression of L-selectin (70). Ligation of CD11b resulted in delayed apoptosis. In contrast, ligation of L-selectin resulted in induced apoptosis. Integrin engagement with ICAM on endothelial cells initiates an intracellular signalling pathway in neutrophils that is mediated via tyrosine kinases and serine-threonine kinase dependent pathways. This in turn results in increased $[Ca^{2+}]_i$ (71). L-selectin engagement induces tyrosine phosphorylation and activation of MAP kinase and potentiates oxidative burst activity (72,73). This suggests that adhesion molecules play a modulatory role in the expression of neutrophil programmed cell death.

5. Phagocytic Recognition Mechanisms of Apoptotic Neutrophils

Phagocyte recognition mechanisms of apoptotic neutrophils have been looked at *in vitro*. The rapid phagocytosis of apoptotic bodies before they lyse is of critical importance in preventing inflammation and injury in the surrounding tissues (9,74). Recognition by adjacent cells of apoptotic bodies occurs by multiple overlapping mechanisms. Savill et al proposed that macrophage recognition of apoptotic neutrophils occurs by at least two distinct mechanism (74). First, recognition of exposed phosphatidylserine moieties on apoptotic cells by a macrophage phosphatidylserine receptor, which has yet to be characterised (75). Phosphatidylserine exposure on apoptotic cells is a universal early event in apoptosis, and may be closely linked to mitochondrial permeability transition, a stage marking the "point of no return" for an apoptotic cell (76). Second, a putative thrombospondin binding moiety on apoptotic neutrophils, is recognised by the multifunctional secreted glycoprotein thrombospondin 1, which bridges the neutrophil to the $\alpha_v\beta_3$ (vitronectin) integrin/CD36 receptor complex on the macrophage. It appears that different populations of macrophages utilise distinct recognition mechanisms (either the phosphatidylserine or the $\alpha_v\beta_3$/thrombospondin/CD36 recognition mechanisms) to identify neutrophils undergoing apoptosis (77).

"Semi-professional" phagocytes, including glomerular mesangial cells and fibroblasts, may also recognise apoptotic neutrophils. Mesangial cells can ingest apoptotic neutrophils by a CD36-independent $\alpha_v\beta$/thrombospondin 1-mediated mechanism (29,78). Mesangial cells are less efficient phagocytes than macrophages, but could play an important role if the apoptotic neutrophil load in the mesangium exceeds the phagocytic capacity of available macrophages (28). Fibroblasts can selectively phagocytose apoptotic neutrophils and recognition involves two distinct mechanisms: $\alpha_v\beta$/thrombospondin/CD36 recognition mechanism as in macrophage ingestion of neutrophils and also an unique mechanism utilising a mannose-fucose specific lectin (75). The interaction between macrophage and fibroblast apoptosis of neutrophils is of great interest as fibroblasts are implicated in tissue scarring.

Macrophage-mediated phagocytosis of apoptotic neutrophils is regulated by both pro- and anti-inflammatory cytokines. A variety of external factors have been shown to increase recognition of apoptotic neutrophils by macrophages and include, as may be expected, the cytokines involved in tissue repair (transforming growth factor β, platelet derived growth factor). Interestingly, the cytokines involved in the initiation of inflammation (interferon-γ, TNF-α, IL-1β), and GM-CSF also increase apoptotic neutrophil recognition. These proinflammatory cytokines may form part of a negative feedback loop preparing the macrophage for the later removal of unwanted neutrophils once the initial inflammatory stimulus has been negated (74).

6. Conclusions

Alteration in physiological cell death contributes to a number of human diseases including, viral infections, the systemmic inflammatory response syndrome, and ischaemia-reperfusion injury. Neutrophils, mediators of the first line of host defense, are constitutivly programmed to apoptose, but the death programme can be modulated by exogenous inflammatory mediators. Apoptosis leading to phagocytosis by macrophages is the preferred mechanism for clearing neutrophils from inflamed sites, and acts to limit tissue injury and promote resolution of the inflammatory response. A better understanding of neutrophil apoptosis may provide important insight into the regulation of the inflammatory process and may suggest paradigms for therapeutic interventions.

7. References

1. Wyllie A.H., Kerr J.F.R., Currie A.R., *Int. Rev. Cytol.* **68** (1980), 251–30.
2. Searle J., Kerr J.F.R., Bishop C.J., *Pathol. Annu.* **17** (1982), 229–259.
3. Wyllie A.H., *Cancer Metatstasis Rev.* **11** (1992), 95–128.
4. Arends M.J., Wyllie A.H., *Int. Rev. Exp. Pathol.* **32** (1991), 223–254.
5. Duvall E., Wyllie A.H., *Immunol. Today* **7** (1986), 115–119.
6. Afranas'ev V.N., *et al., FEBS. Lett.* **194** (1986), 347–350.
7. Duvall E., Wyllie A.H., Morris R.G., *Immunology* **56** (1985), 531–538.
8. Morris R.G., *et al., Am. J. Pathol.* **115** (1984), 426–436.
9. Fadok V.A., *et al., J. Immunol.* **148** (1992), 2207–2216.
10. Dransfield I., *et al., J. Immunol.* **153** (1994), 1254–1263.
11. Dransfield I., *et al., Blood.* **8** (1995), 3264–3273.
12. Cohen J.J., *Adv. Immunol.* **50** (1991), 55–85.
13. Golstein P., Ojcius D.M., Young JD.-E., *Immunol. Rev.* **121** (1991), 29–65.
14. Liu Y.J., *et al., Nature.* **342** (1989), 929–931.
15. Savill J.S., *et al., J. Clin. Invest.* **83** (1989), 865–875.
16. Radley J.M., Haller C.J., *Br. J. Haematol.* **53** (1983), 227–287.
17. Thompson C.B., *Science.* **267** (1995), 1456–1462.
18. Arends M.J., Wyllie A.H., *Int. Rev. Exp. Pathol.* **32** (1991), 223–254.
19. Simon H.U., Blaser K., *Immunol. Today* **16** (1995), 53–55.
20. Barr P.J., Tomie L.D., *Biotechnology.* **12** (1995), 487–493.
21. Dancey J.T., Deubelbeiss K.A., Harker L.A., Finch C.A., *J. Clin. Invest.* **58** (1976), 706–711.
22. Metchnikoff E., Lecture VII in *lectures on the comparative pathology of inflammation*, eds. Starling F.A., Starling E.H. (Kegan, Paul, Trench, and Trubner, London, 1893), 107–131.

23. Hurley J.V., in *Acute Inflammation*, ed. Hurley J.V. (Churchill Livingstone, London, 1983), 109–117.

24. Haslett C., Henson P.M., in *The Molecular and Cellular Biology of Wound Repair*, eds. Clake R.A.F. and Henson P.M. (Plenum Publishing CORP., New York, 1988), 185–211.

25. Gammon R., *Clin. Rheum. Dis.* **8** (1982), 397–413.

26. Savill J.S., *et al.*, *J. Clin. Invest.* **83** (1989), 865–867.

27. Grigg J., *et al.*, *Lancet.* **338** (1991), 720–722.

28. Savill J.S., *Clin. Sci.* **83** (1992), 649–655.

29. Savill J.S., *et al.*, *Kidney Int.* **42** (1992), 924–936.

30. Cox G.J., Crossley J., Xing Z., *Am. J. Respir Cell Mol. Biol.* **12** (1995), 232–237.

31. Hughes J., *et al.*, *Am. J. Pathol.* **150** (1997), 223–234.

32. Smith J., *J. Leukoc. Biol.* **56** (1994), 672–686.

33. Whyte M.K.B., *et al.*, *J. Immunol.* **150** (1993), 5124–5134.

34. Kar S., Ren Y., Savill J.S., Haslett C., *Clin. Sci.* **85** (1993), 27a.

35. Meagher L.C., *et al.*, *J. Leuko. Biol.* **52** (1992), 269–273.

36. Raff M.C., *et al.*, *Science.* **262** (1993), 695–700.

37. French L.E., Tschopp J., *Nature. Med.* **3** (1997), 387–389.

38. Nagata S., Golstein P., *Science.* **267** (1995), 1449–1456.

39. Chinnaiyan A.M., *et al.*, *Science.* **274** (1996), 990–992.

40. Watanabe-Fukunaga R., *et al.*, *J. Immunol.* **148** (1992), 1274–1279.

41. Lowin B., *et al.*, *Nature.* **370** (1994), 650–652.

42. Liles W.C., Klebanoff S.J., *J. Immunol.* **155** (1995), 3289–3291.

43. Liles W.C., *et al.*, *J .Exp. Med.* **184** (1996), 429– 440.

44. Tanaka M., *et al.*, *Nature Med.* **2** (1996), 317–322.

45. Fields S., Song O., *Nature.* **340** (1989), 245–246.

46. Yang X. *et al.*, *Cell.* **89** (1997), 1067–1076.

47. Stranger B.Z., *et al.*, *Cell* **81** (1995), 513–523.

48. Chinnaiyan A.M., O'Rourke K., Tewari M., Dixit V.M., *Cell.* **81** (1995), 505– 512.

49. Cleveland J.L., Ihle J.N., *Cell.* **81** (1995), 479–482.

50. Sato T.S., Irie S., Kitada S., Reed J.C., *Science.* **268** (1995), 411–415.

51. Watson R.W.G., *et al.*, *J. Immunol.* **156** (1996), 3986–3992.

52. Wang J.H., Redmond H.P., Watson R.W.G., Condron C., Bouchier-Hayes D., *Shock.* **6** (1996), 331–338.

53. Watson R.W.G., Redmond H.P., Wang J.H., Condron C., Bouchier-Hayes D., *J. Leuko. Biol.* **60** (1996), 625–632.

54. Kasahara Y., *et al.*, *Blood.* **89** (1997), 1748–1753.
55. McConkey D.J., *et al.*, *Arch. Biochem. Biophys.* **269** (1989), 365–370.
56. Whyte M.K., *et al.*, *J. Clin. Invest.* **92** (1993), 446–455.
57. Yousefi S., Green D.R., Blazer K., Simon H., *Proc. Natl. Acad. Sci. USA.* **91** (1994), 10868–10872.
58. Liles W.C.,Waltersdorph A.M., Klebanoff S.J., *Clin. Res.* **42** (1994), 148a.
59. Hockenbery D., *et al.*, *Nature.* **348** (1990), 334–336.
60. Iwai K., *et al.*, *Blood.* **84** (1994), 1201–1208.
61. Yamamoto C., *et al.*, *Infect. Immun.* **61** (1993) 1972–1979.
62. Brach M.A., *et al.*, *Blood.* **80** (1992), 2920–2924.
63. Pericle F., *et al.*, *Eur. J. Immunol.* **24** (1994), 440–444.
64. Lee A., *et al.*, *FASB. J.* **3** (1989), A1344.
65. Takeda Y., *et al.*, *Int. Immunol.* **5** (1993), 691–694.
66. Calotta F., Polentarutti N., Montovani A., *Blood.* **80** (1992), 2012–2020.
67. Afford S.C., *et al.*, *J. Biol. Chem.* **267** (1992), 21612–21616.
68. Andonegui G., *et al.*, *J. Immunol.* **158** (1997), 3372–3377.
69. Gottlieb R.A., *et al.*, *Proc. Natl. Acad. Sci. USA.* **92** (1995), 5965–5968.
70. Watson R.W.G., et al., *J. Immunol.* **158** (1997), 945–953.
71. Clark E.A., Brugge J.S., *Science.* **268** (1995), 233–239.
72. Waddell T.K., *et al.*, *J. Biol. Chem.* **270** (1995), 15403–15411.
73. Waddell T.K., *et al.*, *J. Biol. Chem.* **269** (1994), 18485–18491.
74. Savill J., *et al.*, *Immunol. Today.* **14** (1993), 131–136.
75. Hall SE., *et al.*, *J. Immunol.* **153** (1994), 3218–3227.
76. Castedo M., *et al*, *J. Immunol.* **157** (1996), 512–521.
77. Fadok V.A., *et al.*, *J. Immunol.* **149** (1992), 4029–4035.
78. Savill J.S., *et al.*, *J. Leuk. Biol.* **61** (1997), 375–380.

CHAPTER 7

NEUTROPHIL MIGRATION AND METHODS FOR ITS *IN VITRO* STUDY

Antal Rot[1]

1. Introduction

Almost all cells, independently of being classified as either mobile or sessile, are capable of performing locomotion. However, for no other cell type the ability to migrate constitutes such an important functional attribute as it is for leukocytes, in particular neutrophils, which are the fastest moving leukocyte type. After being passively carried by blood to the sites of their exit, neutrophils, like other blood-borne leukocytes, leave the circulation, move across the vessel wall, enter the tissues and migrate towards the foci of their (fatal) attraction. Only in the tissues, at diverse extravascular sites, can neutrophils fulfill their homeostatic and inflammatory roles. During a lifetime the body may get assaulted by a multitude of primitive and vicious organisms (viruses, bacteria, parasites and humans with firearms, etc.). Without the ability to move and orientate during migration, leukocytes would not be able to deliver the "cargo" of their complex effector functions to the site of injury. Such a defect would leave our organism devoid of its ability to mount innate and acquired immune responses, eliminate infections and heal the inflicted wounds. Considering the paramount importance of this cellular response, our understanding of the

[1] Novartis Forschungsinstitut, Brunner Strasse 59, A-1235 Vienna, Austria, Tel: 43-1-86634-234; Fax: 43-1-86634-354; E-mail: antal.rot@pharma.novartis.com

mechanism of directed leukocyte locomotion is still rather limited. The egress of leukocytes from blood in response to inflammatory stimuli was observed and described over a century ago by Cohnheim (1), Metchnikoff (2) and Leber (3) who, each through their individual insights, contributed to the establishment of a still largely valid concept linking leukocyte emigration to inflammation and the host defense. These "founding fathers" of the leukocyte migration theory also bestowed on us the belief that leukocyte emigration from blood and migration in the tissues is driven by the gradients of molecules perceived and followed by leukocytes. Such directional cell migration induced by gradients of soluble molecules is called chemotaxis, whereas the molecules themselves are called chemoattractants or chemotaxins.

Neutrophil chemotaxis is a complex process which entails repeating phases of (a) the attractant binding to specific cell surface receptors, (b) signal transduction via complex second messenger pathways, (c) conformational changes of cytoplasmic contractile elements leading to polarized behavior, including (d) development of morphological asymmetry, (e) coordinated cell attachment to the surface at the front end and detachment at the trailing end, (f) generation of motile force- all finally resulting in continuous leukocyte movement (5). Some molecular aspects of this process have also been discussed in Chapter 1.

The study of the mechanism of neutrophil chemotaxis contributed greatly to the understanding of chemotaxis of different types of cells. Also, because of the many common characteristics of directed migration of eukaryotic cells the knowledge derived from studying e.g. slime mold chemotaxis, may and has been, with few reservations, projected onto neutrophil chemotaxis. Moreover, the locomotion of all different leukocyte types, which may be attracted by different chemotactic molecules, shares a multitude of common features. For this reason, some of the aspects of migration of different leukocytes are discussed here and conclusions, where relevant, extrapolated to neutrophil migration.

The recent breakthroughs in biochemical separation techniques and recombinant technology, combined with widely available user-friendly *in vitro* assays for measuring cell locomotion, led to the discovery of numerous new chemoattractants. These include, factors produced by microorganisms, factors generated in the blood from serum proteins and secreted by platelets, derived from extracellular matrix, produced by leukocytes themselves, endothelial cells, smooth muscle cells, fibroblasts, different epithelial cells, etc.

As discussed in detail below, the currently available *in vitro* migration assays do not allow for the measurement of all the relevant parameters of neutrophil chemotaxis and, at the same time, give rise to numerous experimental artefacts. In addition, alternative mechanisms of *in vitro* neutrophil migration exist which can be delineated from chemotaxis only with the help of additional assays. Therefore, it is possible that chemotactic activity of molecules, which do not influence the direction of leukocyte locomotion but stimulate other leukocyte responses (e.g. high rate random locomotion or secretion of true chemoattractants), has been credulously described in the literature. One can suspect that the list of molecules which fulfill the stringent criteria of a leukocyte chemoattractant is actually much shorter than the one compiled based on published literature. In the hierarchy of attractants the members of the numerous and still growing family of chemotactic cytokines (chemokines) occupy a special place (4). The interest in the unique features of chemokines is largely responsible for the renaissance which leukocyte chemotaxis studies enjoy today. Unlike the majority of chemoattractants which affect a broad spectrum of leukocyte types, different chemokines induce the migration of distinct leukocyte types, e.g. IL-8 is an attractant for neutrophils but not monocytes, whereas MCP-1 is *vice versa*. Many inflammatory or homeostatic stimuli can induce chemokine production by a broad variety of cells. In addition, chemokines can be preformed, stored by cells, e.g. platelets and endothelial cells, and rapidly released upon demand. It is hard to envisage an inflammatory disease where one or several chemokines would not contribute to its pathogenesis. The differences in cell source, potency and target cell population of chemokines are some of the most important sources of the variability and pleomorphic appearance of cellular exudates in different locations and in different stages and types of inflammatory diseases.

The contemporary interest in neutrophil chemotaxis is due to the fact that today, just like hundred years ago, this *in vitro* phenomenon is thought to emulate the events of *in vivo* neutrophil emigration whereas chemoattractants are considered to be its driving force. However, in contrast to *in vitro* chemotaxis, neutrophil emigration and migration *in vivo* is complicated by several factors unrelated to chemoattraction. The *in vivo* situation is perplexed by (a) the involvement of vascular tone and lateral shear stress of blood flow, (b) expression and activation of specific adhesion molecules by the endothelial, mesenchymal and epithelial cells, (c) presence of three dimensional matrices rather than two dimensional surfaces, etc. Also, due to the abundance of cell populations other than responding neutrophils there is a possibility of either relay amplification of chemotatic signals or inactivation of chemotactic factors. Numerous non-chemotactic molecules can cause neutrophil emigration in different *in vivo* experimental models, possibly, by inducing the production of leukotrienes, chemokines or other attractants which, in turn, are ultimately responsible for the emigration of neutrophils. Due to these circumstances, it is often not clear if the elicited *in vivo* neutrophil emigration happens in response to injected factors or by other, indirect mechanisms. Therefore, neutrophil chemotaxis, like many other basic cell responses, is best studied as isolated from other biological phenomena as possible, namely, *in vitro*. In fact, almost all our current knowledge on neutrophil chemotaxis is derived from different *in vitro* methods of measurement of cell locomotion. However, as much as it is problematic to study neutrophil chemotaxis *in vivo*, it is difficult to extrapolate the knowledge derived from the studies of *in vitro* chemotaxis to the *in vivo* conditions. It is not even entirely clear if neutrophil chemotaxis, as we know it from the *in vitro* studies, takes place at all *in vivo* and what role it may play under different physiological and pathological circumstances. Therefore, all our knowledge on neutrophil chemotaxis which has derived from *in vitro* studies should be viewed only as a distant approximation of the relevant *in vivo* situation.

Despite the significant practical and theoretical contributions of the early leukocyte chemotaxis studies (6–8), meaning of most of the historical chemotaxis experiments is difficult to translate into modern terms. This is mainly due to the different emphasis and considerations of the primeval chemotaxis studies and also because the early investigators, who scrutinized *in vitro* leukocyte chemotaxis with great enthusiasm and devotion, lacked the well defined attractants, pure leukocyte populations and reproducible methods for measuring chemotaxis. Modern researchers have a multitude of pure molecules with apparent pro-migratory activities. Human neutrophils, due to their preponderance in blood have always been relatively easy to obtain in large numbers and to study *in vitro*. Conversely, only the modern methods of leukocyte purification, which use gradient centrifugation (9) elutriation (10–12) fluorescence activated (13,14) or magnetic (15,16) sorting procedures or a combination of several methods, can yield viable, ample populations of pure leukocytes of all types and subtypes, even those present in the blood in very low numbers, e.g. eosinophils and basophils (17). The methodology of measurement of leukocyte chemotaxis also witnessed seminal achievements, most notably the development and widespread use of chemotactic chambers based on the Boyden-type design (18,19). However, the uncertainties about what type of migratory cell responses are measured using different *in vitro* methods, including the Boyden-type chamber, what are the important parameters of the chemotactic response and what are their *in vivo* relevance remain unresolved. The following discussion gives an overview of the different methods for *in vitro* study of leukocyte chemotaxis and how they may be employed to study different parameters of migration and used to differentiate chemotaxis from other mechanisms of leukocyte migration. For more detailed information on the techniques and procedures the reader is referred to the original publications and for a more comprehensive bibliography — to the available reviews (20,21).

2. Methods for Measurement of Neutrophil Chemotaxis

The technique of visual **time-lapse microscopic analysis** of locomoting leukocytes was probably the most important methodological contribution to chemotaxis studies devised during the first half of this century (22). Various methods which allow to trace the movement of leukocytes on sequential photographic-, cinematographic-, video- or computer- recordings obtained under a microscope, are still used today (23–26). Although the time-lapse microscopy studies of leukocyte chemotaxis are time-consuming and permit simultaneous observation of only few selected leukocytes, they remain among the very few existing methods allowing for direct observation of leukocyte locomotion and recording of its parameters. A very important conceptual description was made from the time-lapse experiments which asserted that chemoattractants can enhance unidirectional leukocyte locomotion by both increasing its rate (velocity) and providing for persistence of its direction (23). Unfortunately, it is very cumbersome to acquire a careful attractant dose-leukocyte migration response curve and to obtain statistically valid information about the responses of a whole population of leukocytes rather than its few individual members. For successful time-lapse microscopy studies and also using other methods for measuring *in vitro* leukocyte chemotaxis it is crucially important to induce stable chemoattractant gradients and maintain them over prolonged periods of time. In early studies this task was achieved, with a limited degree of success, either by using bacterial clumps, damaged cells or impregnating surfaces or microscopic particles such as starch or Sephadex beads with attractants which were leaked from them during the assay (24,27). This hurdle has been overcome by the design of special devices in which gradients can be formed; the best known of them is the "**Zigmond-chamber**" (28). This apparatus is basically a transparent slide with two deep parallel chambers separated by a shallow bridge (Figure 7.1).

A modification of the Zigmond chamber is the "**Dunn-chamber**" in which a central well is surrounded by an annular bridge, encompassed, in turn, by a

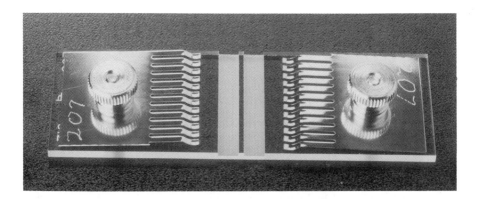

Figure 7.1.   Zigmond chamber for study leukocyte migration and polarization. Courtesy of R. Goodwin, NeuroProbe, Cabin John, MD, USA.

concentric moat-shaped outer well (29). In both chambers a cross-bridge attractant gradient is established by placing over the bridge a coverslip with leukocytes attached to it cell-side-down while filling medium in one chamber and attractant into the other. Chemotactic gradients remain relatively stable across the bridge for prolonged periods of time and the locomotory behavior of leukocytes in response to it can be observed in time-lapse studies. In addition, the Zigmond-chamber has found its use as an assembly for observation of the morphological changes in leukocytes upon attractant stimulation. Such studies yielded a notion that following attractant stimulation and before commencing locomotion, leukocytes very rapidly change shape first from spherical to irregular; later a polar dorso-ventral orientation of the leukocytes develops (28). This observation prompted the introduction of several "minimalistic" methods for measuring "chemotaxis" where the change in leukocyte shape and not cell movement itself was measured in response to chemoattractants (30). Curiously, when leukocytes are stimulated by a gradient of a chemoattractant the change in shape develops unidirectionally: the majority of cells extend their cytoplasm in the direction of the gradient. This observation inspired the establishment of the so called leukocyte **orientation assay** where the number of cells with pseudopod-like extension in the direction of the gradient is compared to the number of cells with pseudopod being extended in the opposite direction (30,31). In addition to morphological observation under the microscope, shape change can be detected by using either computerized morphometry, turbidimetric reading in spectrophotometer or by FACS analysis of forward versus side scatter of leukocytes (31–36). The morphological cell changes during leukocyte migration can also be observed in the process of studying leukocyte **chemotaxis into glass capillaries**. In this method capillary tubes which contain the putative chemoattractant are placed in the dish containing the leukocyte suspension and their migration into the capillaries is studied (7). The modifications of the *in vitro* method, where thin capillaries are used and various biophysical parameters are tightly controlled, allow for careful study of the attractant effects on a migratory response and morphological changes of an isolated single leukocyte (37–39). Another method which allows to study the changes of leukocyte morphology in the process of their locomotion is the measurement of leukocyte **migration under agarose** (26,40–42). For this assay, which has its roots in the methodology used for studying inhibition of leukocyte migration, agarose plates are pre-poured and upon hardening series of triplicate wells are carefully punched in. The leukocyte suspension is placed in each of the middle wells, where leukocytes then have a "choice" of migrating either in the direction of the well containing attractant or in the diametrically opposite direction towards the equidistant well filled with a buffer control. The assay can be evaluated by e.g. epidiascopic projection and enlargement of the area around the middle well and measurement and comparison of the distance which leukocytes migrate under the influence of the tested attractant and buffer control, respectively. In this assay the leukocytes actually migrate under the agarose on the two dimensional surface of the Petri dish, and the agarose gel serves the purpose of retarding the diffusion of the tested attractants. This method allows for the study of a response to several different chemoattractant gradients set up simultaneously (42). In contrast to the migration under agarose, methods for studying leukocyte **migration into gels** and sponges which can be prepared from different extracellular matrix proteins provide the possibility to examine leukocyte locomotion in three dimensional matrices. The migratory leukocyte behavior under these *in vitro* assay conditions is thought to resemble the *in vivo* migratory cell responses in the extravascular tissues (43–45). Also, the use of the three dimensional protein gels allows for the observation of the migration of different subtypes of leukocytes including lymphocytes which, unless stimulated, show a low level of adhesion to non-biological matrices (46). Also, a device has been designed to directly view, capture on videotape and quantify the different parameters of leukocyte migration in collagen gels (47). This method combines the advantages of time lapse studies with the ability to investigate cell locomotion in three dimensional gels and often reveals additional facets of leukocyte responses to attractants.

3. Boyden-Type Chamber

The new era of *in vitro* studies of leukocyte migration started with S. Boyden's description of a method to ascertain *in vitro* leukocyte chemotaxis using a device of new design (18). The **Boyden-type chamber technique,** because of its ease, reproducibility and ability to demonstrate migration in response to the broadest possible spectrum of molecules, became the most popular method for measuring cell migration *in vitro*. The numerous variants of Boyden chamber hardly resemble the first prototype (Figure 7.2), but are nevertheless based on the same main principle.

Typically, the Boyden-type chamber consists of cell containing (upper) and attractant containing (lower) compartments which are separated by a permeable membrane. Upon assembly of the chamber, the attractant gradient is formed across the membrane which is detected and followed by the migrating leukocytes. Either a thick membrane, a mesh of cellulose ester fiber (18), or a thin membrane, polycarbonate nuclepore sheet with uniform, randomly distributed pores (48), can be used. In the case of a thick filter, the distance which the cells migrate into the filter is defined either for the representative population of all the cells in the filter (49–51) or for one or a couple of leukocytes which moved the longest distance: the leading front method (49,52). Alternatively, the number of cells which migrated all the way through the filter is determined (53). In the case of a thin membrane, the cells migrate through the pores and their number is defined by counting them on the lower surface of the filter either by eye, image analyzer (54) or densitometry (55). Alternatively, it is possible to measure one of the cell associated physicochemical (56), immunological (57), or biochemical (58–61) markers in the lower compartment of the chamber. Also, for easy automated counting of the migrated leukocytes the cells could be labeled either with radioactive (62) or fluorescent markers, which appear to have no influence on leukocyte migration and can be used for marking the leukocytes before their migration (63,64). Other fluorescent dyes detect specific leukocyte sub-populations and are used for labeling leukocytes after the assay (65). Among the numerous modifications of the Boyden chamber, the **48-well chamber** (19) is one of the most successful ones. Due to the small well volume, the chamber's attractant and cell requirement is minimal and the fast assembly allows for the simultaneous use of several chambers (66). Both nuclepore (19) and Millipore (67) filters can be used for studying chemotaxis of all leukocyte types (68–70). The trans-well type culture dishes can also be used for estimating leukocyte migration based on the Boyden-type chamber principle (64). Both trans-wells and disposable **96-well chemotactic chambers**

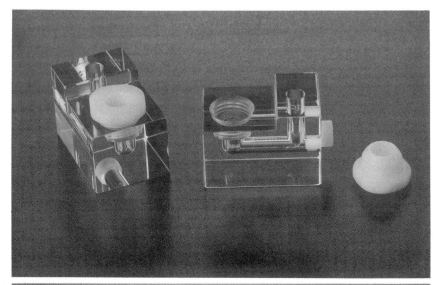

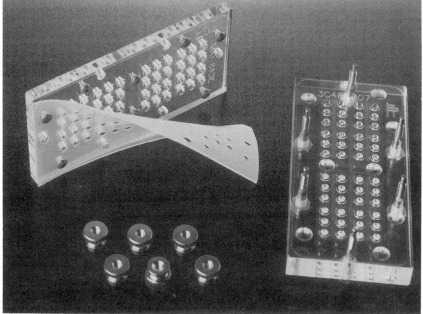

Figure 7.2.　The original Boyden chambers (upper photograph) and 48-well modification of Boyden chamber (lower photograph). Courtesy of R. Goodwin, NeuroProbe, Cabin John, MD, USA.

of novel design (Figure 7.3) allow the study of leukocyte migration through confluent monolayers of endothelial, epithelial or mesenchymal cells (71,72).

Despite the fact that *in vitro* grown cells seldom reflect the functional make-up of their *in vivo* counterparts, such complex transmigration experiments represent the first steps in the direction of better *in vitro* emulation of *in vivo* circumstances where leukocytes are required to cross complex barriers of matrices and cells. Boyden-type chambers played an important role in making the measurement of leukocyte migration a routine accessible to a great number of basic and clinical researchers. However, while making the study of leukocyte migration easy, this method completely obscures many of the important characteristics and parameters of leukocyte migration e.g. rate of locomotion or number and angle of leukocyte turns. Also, as discussed in detail below, it does not distinguish between different types of leukocyte migration. In addition,

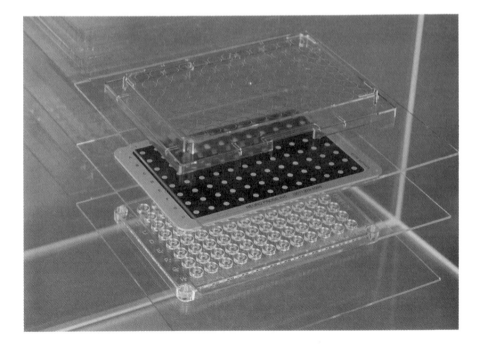

Figure 7.3.   Disposable 96-well chamber. Courtesy of R. Goodwin, NeuroProbe, Cabin John, MD, USA.

the Boyden-type chamber is not ideal, neither for simulation of the *in vivo* chemotaxis in the extravascular tissues nor for strict control of *in vitro* physicochemical and biological parameters (21). However, surprisingly the transendothelial emigration step might be mimicked rather well in the Boyden-type polycarbonate filter assay (73).

4. Different Forms of *in vitro* Leukocyte Migration

4.1 *Chemokinesis and chemotaxis*

Chemotaxis is only one of several distinct forms of *in vitro* leukocyte movement. Unstimulated leukocytes exhibit **spontaneous random migration** which is characterized by low velocity locomotion and random direction of turns. The higher velocity movement which is caused by stimulation of leukocytes by a defined molecule is called **chemokinesis** (74). Because its initial description put the emphasis on the speed and not on the direction of locomotion, leukocyte "chemokinesis", very confusingly, can be either random in its direction or contribute to the uni-directional gradient-driven "chemotactic" cell movement (75). This is due to the fact that the gradients of "chemotactic" molecules affect not only the direction of migration (by decreasing the angle and/or number of leukocyte turns) but, usually, also augment the rate of locomotion. Hence, according to the "classical" definition (74,75) all chemoattractants have "chemokinetic" effect. Importantly though, there are molecules which can activate the cells by various mechanisms and increase only the rate of leukocyte locomotion, but in a gradient setting have no impact at all on its direction. These molecules are the *bona fide* "chemokinetic" agents. Unfortunately, the intricacy of definitions can be further increased. The time lapse studies indicate that often the migration of individual leukocytes even in the absence of soluble gradients is "unidirectional". This higher velocity and, similar to chemotaxis, low number and angle of cell turns results in the migration of the leukocyte in the same direction in which it started the locomotion. This type of chemokinesis is called "**orthokinesis**". However, when the migratory trajectories of a whole leukocyte population are examined during orthokinesis in relationship to their environment, the overall migration can be clearly characterized as multidirectional. This contrasts with the gradient-induced chemotaxis where the sum of the individual leukocyte migration vectors is in the direction of the gradient. Orthokinesis can also be contrasted to "**klinokinesis**" (74), an archaic term used to characterize an increased frequency and angle of leukocyte turns induced by a tested substance. Both these forms of enhanced leukocyte movement occur either in the absence of a chemical gradient or under the influence of molecules which stimulate the locomotion (orthokinesis) or turning potential (klinokinesis) of leukocytes but cannot provide them with directional cues under gradient conditions. In the absence of gradient conditions, klinokinesis can be a part of leukocyte chemokinesis, but it is questionable if leukocyte klinokinesis exists in its pure, isolated form. In view of the considerable complexity of manifestations of enhanced *in vitro* leukocyte migration and the confusing nature of "classical" definitions, it is not surprising that the term "chemokinesis" has lately been used broadly to characterize the substance-induced increased-rate leukocyte locomotion with random direction. Thus, in practical, but not necessarily semantically correct terms, the increased migration of a leukocyte population can be called "chemokinesis" when the cell locomotion is unaffected by the abolishment of gradient conditions. This definition excludes the chemokinetic component of chemotaxis, i.e. uni-directional, gradient-induced leukocyte movement. Chemotaxis, in contrast to chemokinesis, implies that the leukocyte receives two signals from a gradient: (a) stimulation of its locomotion and (b) a cue in which direction the locomotion should happen.

The reliable discrimination between "chemotaxis" and different types of "chemokinesis" can only be achieved by the observation of the direction and the velocity of the gradient-induced leukocyte migration by direct viewing methods. However, a method based on the Boyden-type chamber assay has been extensively used to study chemokinesis and differentiate it from chemotaxis. This is accomplished by placing different concentrations of the tested substance (a) simultaneously in the top and bottom compartments (no gradient); or (b) together with the responding cells in the top compartment (negative gradient); and (c) in the bottom well only (positive gradient). The comparison of leukocyte migration under these different gradient conditions can reveal the nature of the pro-migratory molecule. This principle constitutes the basis of the so called **checkerboard assay**, described by Hirsch and Zigmond (76) which compares the effect of different concentrations of an attractant molecule in the absence of gradient conditions with that of several checkerboard combinations of positive and negative gradients of different steepness. Very unfortunately, the thick filter checkerboard assay is rarely performed and the "checkerboard correction" is almost never calculated. However, even when the correction is appropriately used, the Boyden chamber-based checkerboard analysis is not entirely immune from doubts regarding its ability to dissociate chemotaxis and chemokinesis (77). The checkerboard analysis is based on two fundamental assumptions:

a) the attractant gradient is uniform and linear; and
b) the migrating cells move in a continuous straight line with constant acceleration.

The first condition has not been proven to be fulfilled in the Boyden type assay and no one knows how the attractant gradients which form across the Millipore filter look like and how their development is influenced by adding leukocytes to the top compartment. The second condition simply cannot be fulfilled. This is because instead of crawling consistently forward, leukocytes engage in a "random walk", perpetually changing their velocity and angle of turns. Due to the latter fact it could be argued that when stimulated by a gradient of pure chemokinetic (orthokinetic) substance which has no effect on the angle of leukocyte turns, but increases only the rate of locomotion, the cells would migrate faster when they turn towards higher concentrations and slower when they turn towards lower concentrations of the agent (77). As a result, at the end of the test period the distribution of the cells would be biased in the direction of the gradient. Thus, the checkerboard assay should not be able to differentiate between the effects of chemotactic and chemokinetic substances (77). Also, due to the ability of leukocytes in the top compartment to consume, rapidly degrade or inactivate chemotaxins (78–80), the contribution of chemokinesis to the overall cell locomotion can be underestimated. An improvement which reduces the detected level of "background" migration and may be effective in dissociating chemokinetic from chemotactic effects calls for the use of the "sparse-pore" filter where the distance between the pores is increased (81,82). Such a filter reduces the chances of a leukocyte to cross the membrane in the process of random chemokinetic movement. However, despite all the numerous reservations and repeatedly voiced concerns (81,82) the standard ("ample-pore") polycarbonate-filter checkerboard assay remains as the method most widely used for the discrimination of chemotactic and chemokinetic activities of tested substances. Due to this fact and because the overwhelming majority of initially described novel chemotactic molecules have not been followed up by studies with direct viewing methods for measuring leukocyte migration, it is very likely that a significant part of the molecules known in the literature as chemoattractants are only chemokinetic agents. Unfortunately, this trend will probably continue in the future since the Boyden-type chamber checkerboard assay which employs polycarbonate filters is likely to stay as the most popular method for dissociating chemotaxis from chemokinesis. Also there are no easy ways to discriminate leukocyte chemotaxis from chemokinesis *in vivo*.

4.2 *Haptotaxis*

When motile cells are placed on a surface coated by a gradient of molecules to which they can adhere, cell populations redistribute from the sites with lower adhesive properties to the sites with higher ones. This phenomenon was described by Carter and called **haptotaxis** (83). Haptotaxis was shown to be an important mechanism of cell migration during embryogenesis (84,85) and *in vitro* tumor cell migration (86). Different pro-adhesive matrix proteins (87) and other molecules (88) were established as potent haptotactic agents. Some of these molecules have also been known to attract cells when in solution, suggesting that the same molecule, depending on the conditions of the assay, could behave as either a chemotactic or haptotactic agent. Probably due to this fact, the term haptotaxis had been used lately, with considerable corruption of the initial meaning, to characteize the unidirectional cell migration induced not only by pro-adhesive but also by other surface-bound molecules, including known attractants. This latter point is contrasts with genuine chemotaxis which, according to the classical definition, is caused by gradients of soluble attractants.

During "classical haptotaxis", which is induced by the immobilized adhesion gradients, the resulting unidirectional migration of the cell is due only to the directional cues received from the environment but not from the stimulation of the rate of cell locomotion. Conversely, during the haptotaxis induced by surface-immobilized attractants, both the directional cues and enhanced rate of movement may be conveyed. Despite this difference, the original and the new meanings of "haptotaxis" might not be so remote, since attractant molecules by virtue of their ability to activate integrins can rapidly induce cell adhesion to a variety of substrata.

Unlike bacteria, which swim in the process of their migration, leukocytes crawl on surfaces. In addition, the initially soluble leukocyte chemoattractants often bind to different *in vitro* and *in vivo* surfaces. Therefore, it has been considered plausible that not only tumor cells but also leukocytes recognize the gradients of the substrate-bound ligands and migrate along them, thus utilizing a haptotactic mechanism of locomotion. Since most of the conventional methods for studying leukocyte migration do not permit the differentiation between directed migration in response to soluble or surface-bound gradients of molecules, the contribution of haptotaxis to the overall attractant-induced *in vitro* leukocyte migration might have been underestimated. This is despite the fact that data consistent with leukocyte haptotaxis have been repeatedly observed under different experimental conditions (89–91). Simple Boyden-type chamber-based assays were developed which could distinguish between chemotaxis and haptotaxis (90,92). First, the chemotactic filters (either thick or thin) are exposed for short periods of time to the positive and negative gradients of attractant in the first chamber, then washed, blotted, air-dried and placed in a second chamber over the bottom wells which contain only buffer and no attractant. The resulting leukocyte migration is compared to that induced by soluble "chemotactic" gradients of the same attractant. The latter response, because attractant molecules can rapidly bind to the filter and haptotactic gradients can form during the assay, is actually the sum of haptotaxis and chemotaxis. Using such assays it was revealed that several "classical" chemoattractants, including C5a, chemokines IL-8 and RANTES and also some newly discovered "chemotactic" molecules e.g. phosphatidic acid and lysophasphatidic acid induce *in vitro* leukocyte migration primarily by a haptotactic mechanism and therefore, could be qualified as "haptoattractants" (90,92–94). Since the experimental conditions might define the *in vitro* behavior and mechanism of leukocyte response to an attractant molecule, a strict distinction between "chemoattractant" and "haptoattractant" is better avoided; all molecules which induce unidirectional *in vitro* migration could be called cumulatively "attractants". *In vivo*, or under pathophysiologically relevant *in vitro* conditions, several leukocyte attractants can be found not as soluble mediators but immobilized by different specific mechanisms on various biological surfaces where they exert their pro-migratory effect. Some, e.g. platelet activating factor (96) and a novel chemokine, fractalkine (96,97) known also as neurotactin (98), may be expressed on the membranes of the endothelial cells. Others, e.g. collagen fragments, may constitute an organic part of the modified extracellular matrix. Yet others, for example the majority of chemokines, can bind specifically to glycosaminoglycans which are present in the extracellular matrix, basal membrane and on different cell surfaces. The glycosaminoglycan-bound chemokines still retain their pro-migratory and pro-adhesive activity on leukocytes (99–101). The differential ability of different glycosaminoglycans and their fractions to specifically interact with different chemokines (102) provides a mechanism of specific localization of chemokines which determines the sites where these molecules can be retained and exert their proemigratory effect. Curiously, in the case of IL-8 the residues involved in specific *in vivo* binding to glycosaminoglycans and those required for non-specific *in vitro* immobilization on plastic surfaces are the same (73). These are primarily the charged residues of the C-terminal α-helix, a domain of the chemokine which serves for its localization and is not involved in binding to the specific leukocyte receptors (73,101). However, the engagement of this domain may modify the leukocyte responses to the chemokine. It was shown that heparan sulfate dramatically enhances the *in vitro* neutrophil migration induced by suboptimal concentrations of the neutrophil chemoattractant IL-8 (101). Analogously, the chemokine MIP-1β can induce lymphocyte adhesion to vascular cell adhesion molecule-1 only when immobilized on proteoglycan (103). The mechanism of enhancement of chemokine responses by the engagement of their C-terminus is not known. Theoretically, glycosaminoglycans can achieve this effect by either cross-linking the chemokines on their leukocyte surface receptors or by modifying the tertiary configuration of the chemokines in the process of their presentation which, in turn, may result in a better receptor fit. In other experimental systems heparin, heparan sulfate and other glycosaminoglycans can paradoxically function as biological chemokine antagonists by competing for IL-8 and other chemokines with the natural chemokine "presentation molecules". In addition to glycosaminoglycans, other molecules may immobilize and present chemokines on the endothelial cell surface: a prime candidate is a Duffy blood group antigen/ receptor for chemokines which is expressed by the venular endothelial cells (104) and can bind several chemokines (73). All these facts led to a recent important realization that leukocyte haptotaxis can be a significant form of *in vivo* leukocyte locomotion and can take place during both emigration and migration in the tissues. The haptotactic response of cells was characterized by Carter as "passive" and its repeated cycles of lamellipodium extension and uropod retraction was explained by him on the basis of thermodynamic behavior of three different phases: surface, cell and medium fluid (105). According to his initial hypothesis, cell and fluid "compete" for the surface which, due to the gradient of adhesive substance present on it, possess differential "wettability", which, determines the direction of the cell movement. It is safe to suggest now that, just like chemotaxis, haptotaxis is mediated by the recognition of different ligands by the specific cell surface receptors and involves spatially integrated signal transduction mechanisms. However, it is possible that in analogy to the findings with the tumor cells, molecules involved in signal transduction and regulation of the haptotactic migratory response of the leukocyte might differ from those which are used by cells during chemotaxis (106,107). It is not entirely clear if these distinctions of haptotactic from chemotactic stimulation are equally true for immobilized gradients of "adhesion" and "attractant" molecules. Additional differences in how chemoattractants and haptoattractants exert their effects on leukocyte migration are independent of the "adhesive" or "attractant" nature of the immobilized molecules. Theoretically, among different chemoattractants, which by definition freely diffuse in three dimensions, only those molecules with the highest affinity for their receptors should be able to associate with them and efficiently induce leukocyte migratory responses. Conversely, among haptoattractant molecules, which by definition are immobilized on surfaces, even those with low affinity for their receptors, have a good chance to associate with their receptors and provide directional queues during the crawling movement of leukocytes. Also, due to their immobilization, haptoattractants are expected to be present at the site of their production longer, whilst chemoattractants are more likely to be washed away.

4.3 *"Chemogenic" migration mechanism*

In addition to inducing enhanced leukocyte migration by chemotactic, haptotactic and chemokinetic mechanisms, accumulating evidence indicates that certain molecules can induce leukocyte migration indirectly, by stimulating the release from leukocytes of secondary mediators which, in turn, have a chemotactic or chemokinetic effect. Leukocytes constitute a very rich source of different attractants which can be either preformed or rapidly induced. Therefore, it is possible that leukocyte activators or secretagogues, i.e. molecules which have no chemotactic activity of their own, still induce directed *in vitro* leukocyte migration by a **chemo(attracto)genic mechanism**. Because the responses of a whole population of leukocytes are usually studied, almost all the assays of leukocyte migration, not only the Boyden-type, are prone to detect the response to "chemogenic" molecules and register it as either chemotactic, chemokinetic or haptotactic leukocyte migration. Long incubation periods of the migration assays and the use of media which augment random migration, for example, those with a high protein content increase the chance for "chemogenic" effects to take place. In addition, conditions of leukocyte isolation and storage which prime them and may induce the production of preformed mediators may also play a role in chemogenic migration. Despite the fact that it does not represent a separate mechanism of directed migration (leukocytes ultimately respond by either chemotaxis, haptotaxis or chemokinesis), it is important to differentiate the chemogenic migration from other mechanisms of leukocyte migration. The direct viewing methods or the thick filter Boyden-type chamber assay which allow the discrimination between chemotactic and chemokinetic mechanisms of cell migration, are helpless in differentiating molecules with chemotactic from those with chemogenic effects. This unfortunately is true for every method where the migratory responses of the whole population of leukocytes are studied whereby interaction of cells with each other can occur during the assay. Only the use of methods where the locomotory behavior of isolated leukocytes is studied (e.g. migration in micro-capillaries) can assure that no migration is observed in response to chemogenic molecules. However, to get a hint if a certain molecule is inducing leukocyte migration by direct or indirect (chemogenic) mechanisms three different Boyden-type chamber-based assays can be performed. First, the responding leukocytes can be stimulated by a pro-migratory molecule and their short-term culture supernatant tested in a migration assay in comparison with the stimulant alone. Even if no increase in migratory response is detected in this system, it is still possible that additional attractant is generated but is immediately "consumed" by the producing cells. Alternatively, cell adhesion to the substrate or each other may be required as a co-stimulus for the production of the secondary attractant; e.g. the requirement for the engagement of adhesion molecules was demonstrated for the induction of a secondary attractant produced by monocytes following their stimulation by RANTES (108). In a second type of experiments, the responding cells can be added together with test attractant to the bottom wells of the Boyden-type chamber. In the case of a chemogenic effect an increase in leukocyte migration should be observed in comparison with attractant alone. However, even if this assay is negative, a chemogenic effect cannot be excluded, because it is possible that the attractant produced does not readily diffuse from the bottom to the top of the lower compartment or is a haptoattractant. In both cases the secondary attractant molecule can be effective if produced by the leukocytes which release it while they pass through the filter. Finally, a chemogenic effect of a molecule can be detected in a "cell increment assay" (CIA) recently conceived by us. In the CIA migration to the test molecule is studied after the leukocytes have been added to the top wells of a Boyden-type chamber in different numbers. The higher the leukocyte input, the more of them will randomly migrate across the filter. If in response to chemogen an attractant is generated during the assay, the higher number of migrated leukocytes will produce more of the secondary attractant, resulting in a higher proportion of migrated leukocytes. If the leukocytes are responding only to the attractant placed in the bottom well and no chemogenic effect takes place, the relative number of migrated cells (percentage of total input) should remain constant, independent of the number of input leukocytes. Attractant molecules themselves can induce the secretion of additional attractants from the leukocytes which they target (109–112). Using CIA it is possible to show if an attractant molecule, in addition to its chemotactic activity, also exerts a chemogenic effect during the assay. For example, using CIA and other methods for dissecting chemotactic and chemogenic effects, we could recently demonstrate that the *in vitro* monocyte migration induced in the Boyden-type assay by the β-chemokine RANTES consists of both direct chemotactic and indirect chemogenic components (113). Undoubtedly there are many chemogenic molecules among the great number of the alleged chemoattractants described during the last couple of decades. There is a continuous debate in the literature whether the major inflammatory cytokines e.g. IL-1, TNF and growth factors e.g. GM-CSF and PDGF have a direct *in vitro* leukocyte chemotactic effect or not (114–130). Since almost all of these cytokines stimulate the production of chemoattractants in leukocytes, they may be inducing *in vitro* leukocyte migration via a chemogenic mechanism.

The chemogenic effect of attractants and other molecules may also play an important role *in vivo*. The first wave of leukocyte egress into the inflammatory site may be accompanied by the immediate production of additional attractants which contribute to the following waves of emigration of additional leukocytes. Molecules which induce the production of attractants by resident cells also lead to leukocyte emigration by chemogenic mechanism.

It is theoretically possible that the induction of the attractant receptor expression on the cells may enhance *in vitro* leukocyte migration. Such a "**receptorgenic**" mechanism has not yet been demonstrated, however circumstantial evidence indicates that this type of response might exist *in vitro*. For example, it was shown recently that IL-2 can upregulate the lymphocyte migratory responses to several C-C chemokines by inducing the expression of their receptors (131) A similar mechanism has been described for G-CSF which upregulates the expression of IL-8 receptors on neutrophils (132). Whilst it is feasible that during the long incubation period of the lymphocyte chemotaxis, IL-2 and other molecules with similar activity might have enough time to upregulate the expression of attractant receptors, it is less likely that such a mechanism can take place during the much shorter migration period of neutrophils.

4.4 *Alternative mechanisms of directional leukocyte migration*

According to current knowledge, the leukocyte recognition of the chemical signals in their environment may only result in their movement in the direction of the substance gradient (chemoattraction, "positive chemotaxis") but never in the direction opposite to the gradient source. This is in sharp contrast to bacteria where "**negative chemotaxis**" is prominent and several chemorepellent molecules have been described (133). Negative chemotaxis can also be observed in eukaryotic cells other than leukocytes. For example, semaphorins, a family of secreted and transmembrane eukaryotic chemorepellents has been described and may play a role in the establishment of axonal connections during brain development (134). CD100, a human member of this family of molecules was shown to be expressed by lymphocytes, monocytes and neutrophils and other cells in many different tissues. The known effects of CD100 on leukocytes are limited so far to the induction of B cell aggregation; its possible role in induction of negative leukocyte chemotaxis or, since CD100 is an integral membrane protein, haptotaxis, has not been investigated (135).

Gradients of some molecules, e.g. fibronectin, can also mediate unidirectional movement of leukocytes. This, the so-called **matrix driven translocation**, does not involve any active response from the cell itself, but is dependent on the interaction of matrix molecules, e.g. fibonectin with cell surface counterligands (136–138).

In addition to chemical signals which may be the driving force and provide directional cues for the leukocyte migration, leukocyte locomotion may be controlled by several other mechanisms; physical characteristics of the leukocyte environment can greatly influence the direction of leukocyte locomotion. These include the electromagnetic properties of the fields in which leukocytes are found or mechanical properties of the surfaces on which migration occurs. **Galvanotaxis**, the directional *in vitro* guidance of cell motility exerted by electrical fields either in the direction of the cathode or anode has been suggested to play a role in embryogenesis (139,140) and was demonstrated *in vitro* for several different cells, including leukocytes (141–145). Since the inflammatory foci are positively charged, it is possible that *in vivo* galvanotaxis-driven leukocyte migration can also take place and play a role in the inflammatory leukocyte recruitment. It is not clear what is the molecular mechanism which allows the cells to orient in electromagnetic fields and if their rate of locomotion or only orientation is affected.

If leukocytes meet parallel oriented physical barriers they are likely to change the direction of locomotion and migrate along such barriers (146–148). In such cases of **"contact guidance"** the migration happens along a particular axis rather than in one specific direction: the probability of a cell moving parallel to the axis of the barrier in either of the two diametrically opposite directions is equal (149). Though it has been suggested that cells do not "recognize" very well their physical environment and their contact guidance has been compared to the "groping around" of a short sighted man (146), cues derived from the physical contact with the surface on which they crawl may bias the direction of the leukocyte migration in response to chemotactic stimuli (148,149). *In vivo* leukocytes may also simultaneously receive directional cues from chemotactic stimulation and contact guidance where leukocyte chemotaxis may be influenced by the direction of fibers in the connective tissue or orientation of the cell processes.

5. Parameters of Leukocyte Chemotaxis

When leukocyte chemotaxis is measured various parameters of the locomotory response can be analyzed and compared with those in the absence of the stimulus. Because of the considerable confusion in terms used in the literature a short introduction to chemotaxis terminology is provided. As discussed above, different methods for measuring chemotaxis allow study of different sets of parameters of the chemotactic response. For example, the distance covered by either one cell or a whole population of leukocytes can be evaluated by direct viewing methods or using the Boyden type chamber with thick nitrocellulose

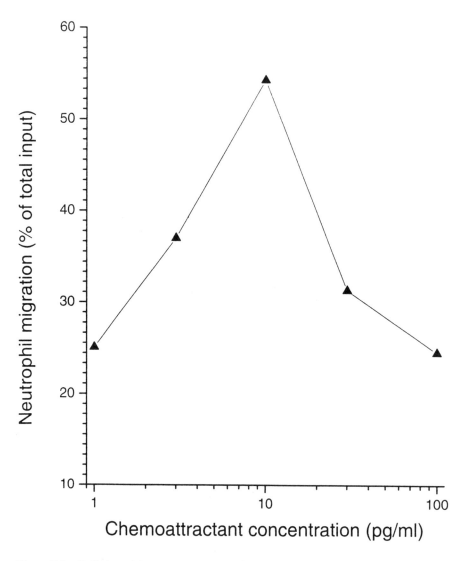

Figure 7.4.   Bell-shaped dose-response curve of in vitro neutrophil migration in Boyden-type chamber assay.

filters. Conversely, the number of cells responding to a particular attractant could be estimated most conveniently using the thin polycarbonate filter. Such parameters of migratory response as mean velocity of the leukocyte locomotion, number and angle of leukocyte turns can be obtained using only direct viewing methods. Similarly to many other cellular responses, the magnitude of chemotactic response differs depending on the concentrations of applied attractants. This is reflected in a dose-response curve which in the case of leukocyte chemotaxis is bell-shaped (Figure 7.4).

The lower level of migration induced by higher attractant concentrations is probably due to the desensitization of the cell surface attractant receptors. Curiously, when chemoattractants are injected *in vivo* in the preformed cavity, e.g. peritoneum, a bell-shaped curve is also observed. However, by increasing the attractant concentration we were not able to achieve the descending wing of the curve when chemoattractants were injected into peripheral sites e.g. skin (own unpublished observation).

Two important characteristics of chemotactic migration can be deduced from the attractant dose-response curve. These are the **efficacy**, or the magnitude of migratory response at the optimal attractant concentration and the **potency**, the attractant concentration which elicits optimal leukocyte migration. For example, a molecule which in the Boyden-type chamber induces the directional migration of a hundred percent of the input leukocytes is an efficacious attractant independent of whether this response is elicited by either high or low concentrations of the molecule. Conversely, an attractant can be called potent if it induces the directional leukocyte migration at low concentrations, even if the migration of only a few percent of input leukocytes is being induced or the leukocytes migrate only a short distance. Analogously, a chemoattractant which induces high velocity locomotion is efficacious, whereas the one which induces the increase of locomotion at low concentrations is a potent one, independent of the speed of migrating cells. The bell-shaped dose-response curve of the leukocyte chemotaxis clearly demonstrates that the same level of migration can be induced by either suboptimal or supraoptimal concentrations of the attractant. Therefore, it is crucial to test several different concentrations. The potency and efficacy are independent characteristics of the chemotactic response; both, despite wide individual differences in leukocyte chemotactic responses, can be used to identify of an attractant molecule (67). The potency of an attractant is thought to be primarily the function of its binding affinity to the cell surface receptor, whereas the efficacy may depend on several factors including the distribution of the chemoattractant receptors within the studied cell population or where on the agonist-antagonist scale a particular attractant can be found or how well the signal from an individual receptor can be transduced. Due to the differences in the execution of leukocyte chemotaxis assays by different investigators and in order to normalize inter-assay variables different types of "migration indices" have been introduced. These compare the migration elicited by a particular chemotactic molecule to that of a positive or a negative control, but usually do not tell more than the "unprocessed" data itself.

6. Concluding Remarks

The study of *in vitro* migration of neutrophils and other leukocyte types has recently experienced a rebirth with hundreds of new publications describing the chemotactic activity of dozens of novel molecules appearing yearly. Numerous methodological and conceptual pitfalls, which have been known and carefully considered in the past but largely forgotten recently, are awaiting the novice chemotaxis researcher. The easy accessibility of the methods to study leukocyte "chemotaxis", together with the lack of recent consensus on what leukocyte chemotaxis is and how it can and should be measured (and therefore lack of stringency of peer review) has resulted in a recent flood of molecules with apparent "chemotactic" activity for neutrophils and other leukocytes. It is not clear at all which ones are real chemoattractants and which ones are not. Also, in the past several years it has become clear that leukocytes, in addition to exhibiting chemotactic migration, may use different mechanisms of unidirectional *in vitro* locomotion. Several of these mechanistically very different leukocyte responses to directional molecular cues from the environment and methods which allow their study and discrimination from chemotaxis have been summarized in this chapter.

7. Acknowledgement

The careful reading of the manuscript and helpful comments by Dr. Henri Moore are gratefully acknowledged.

8. References

1. Cohnheim, J., *Virchows Arch. Path. Anat.* **40** (1867), 1–79.
2. Metchnikoff, E., *Lectures on comparative pathology of inflammation.* Dover Press, New York (1891, reprinted 1968).
3. Leber, T., *Fortschr. Med.* **6** (1888), 460–464.
4. Rollins, B.J., *Blood* **90** (1997), 909–928.
5. Lauffenburger D.A. and Horwitz A.F., *Cell* **84** (1996), 359–369.
6. Haris, H., *Physiol. Rev.*, **34** (1954), 529–562.
7. McCutcheon, M., *Physiol. Rev.* **26** (1946), 319–336.
8. Movat, H.Z., *The inflammatory reaction*, Elsevier, Amsterdam (1985).
9. Böyum, A., *Scand. J. Clin. Lab. Invest., Suppl.* **21** (1968), 77–89 .
10. De Mulder, P.H., *et al.*, *J. Immunol. Methods* **47** (1981), 31–38.
11. Berkow, R.L., *et al.*, *J. Lab. Clin. Med.* **102** (1983), 732–742.
12. Berger, C.L. and Edelson, R.L., *J. Inves. Dermatol.*, **73** (1979), 231–235.
13. McCarthy, K.F., Hale M.L. and Fehnel P.L., *Cytometry* **8** (1987), 296–305.
14. Goddeeris, B.M. *et al.*, *J. Immunol. Methods* **89** (1986), 165–173.
15. Miltenyi, S., *et al.*, *Cytometry* **11** (1990), 231–238.
16. Zahler, S., *et al.*, *J. Immunol. Methods* 200 (1997), 173–179.
17. Hansel, T.T., *et al.*, *J. Immunol. Methods* **145** (1991), 105–110.
18. Boyden, S., *J. Exp. Med.,* **115** (1962), 453–466.
19. Falk, W., Goodwin, R.H., and Leonard, E.J., *J. Immunol. Methods* **33** (1980), 239–247 .
20. Wilkinson, P.C., *J. Immunol. Methods* **51** (1982), 133–148.
21. Bignold, L.P., *J. Immunol. Methods* **108** (1988), 1–18.
22. De Bruyn, P.P.H., *Anat. Rec.* **95** (1946) 177–191.
23. Allan, R.B. and Wilkinson, P.C., *Exp. Cell. Res.* **111** (1978), 191–203.
24. Ramsey, W.S., *Exp. Cell. Res.* **70** (1972). 129–139.
25. Cheung, A.T., *et al.*, *J. Leukoc. Biol.* **41** (1987), 481–491.
26. Pedersen, J.O., *et al.*, *J. Immunol. Methods* **109** (1988), 131–137.

27. Wilkinson, P.C. and Allan R.B., In *Leukocyte chemotaxis: methods, physiology and clinical implications*. Raven Press, NY, pp 1–24, (1978).

28. Zigmond, S.H., *J. Cell Biol.* **75** (1977), 606–616.

29. Zicha, D., Dunn, G.A. and Brown, A.F., *J. Cell Sci.* **99** (1991), 769–775.

30. Haston, W.S. and Shields, J.M., *J. Immunol. Methods* **81** (1985), 229–237.

31. Harkin, D.G., Gadd, S.J. and Bignold, L.P., *Biol. Cell* **79** (1993), 251–257.

32. Keller, H.U., Fedier A. and Rohner, R., *J. Leukoc. Biol.* **58** (1995), 519–525.

33. Coates,T.D., *et al.*, *J. Cell Biol.* **117** (1992), 765–774.

34. Zhang, J., *et al.*, *Biol. Cell* **84** (1995) 147–53.

35. Sklar, L. A., Oades, Z.G. and Finney, D.A., *J. Immunol.* **133** (1984), 1483–1487.

36. Jadwin, D.F., Smith C.W. and Meadows T.R., *Am. J. Clin. Pathol.* **76** (1981), 395–402.

37. Skalak, R., Skierczynski, B.A., Wung S.L., Chien S. and Usami, S., *Blood Cells* **19** (1993), 389–397.

38. Skierczynski, B.A., Usami, S., Chien, S. and Skalak, R., *J. Biomech. Eng.* **115** (1993), 503–509.

39. Vereycken, V., Bucherer, C., Lacombe, C. and Lelievre, J.C., *J. Mal. Vasc.* **20** (1995), 113–116.

40. Nelson, R.D., Quie, P.G. and Simmons, R.L., *J. Immunol.* **115** (1975), 1650–1656.

41. Krauss, A.H., Nieves, A.L., Spada, C.S. and Woodward, D.F., *J. Leukocyte Biol.*, **55** (1994), 201–208.

42. Foxman, E.F., Campbell, J.J. and Butcher, E.C., *J. Cell. Biol.* **139** (1997), 1349–1360.

43. Islam, L.N., McKay, I.C. and Wilkinson, P.C., *J. Immunol. Methods* **85** (1985) 137–151.

44. Moghe, P.V., Nelson. R.D. and Tranquillo, R.T., *J. Immunol. Methods* **180** (1995), 193–211.

45. Loike, J.D., *et al.*, *J. Exp. Med.*, **181** (1995), 1763–1772.

46. Wilkinson, P.C., *J. Immunol. Methods* **76** (1985), 105–120.

47. Haddox, J. L., Pfister, R. R. and Sommers, C. I., *J. Immunol. Methods* **141** (1991), 41–52.

48. Horwitz, D. A. and Garrett, M. A., *J. Immunol.* **106** (1971), 649–655.

49. Swanson, M.J. and Becker, E.L., *J. Immunol. Methods* **13** (1976), 191–197.

50. Maderazo, E.G. and Woronick, C.L., *Clin. Immunol. Immunopathol.* **11**, (1979) 196–211.

51. Jensen, P. and Kharazmi, A., *J. Immunol. Methods* **144** (1991), 43–48.

52. Zigmond, S.H. and Hirsch, J.G., *J. Exp. Med.* **137** (1973), 387–410.
53. Thomsen, M.K. and Jensen, A.L., *Vet. Immunol. Immunopathol.* **29** (1991), 197–211.
54. Minkin, C., Bannon, D. J. Jr, Pokress, S. and Melnick, M., *J. Immunol. Methods* **78** (1985), 307–321.
55. Mrowietz, U. and Jürgens, G.A., *J. Biochem. Biophys. Methods* **30** (1995), 49–58.
56. Watanabe, K., Kinoshita, S. and Nakagawa, H., *J. Pharmacol. Methods* **22** (1989), 13–18.
57. Tekstra, J. and Tuk, C.W., Beelen, R.H., *Immunbiol.* **195** (1996), 491–498.
58. Creamer, H.R., Gabler, W.L. and Bullock, W.W., *Inflammation* **7** (1983), 321–329.
59. McCafferty, A.C. and Cree, I.A., *Cytokine* **6** (1994), 450–453.
60. Pelz, G., Schettler, A. and Tschesche, H., *Eur. J. Clin. Chem. Clin. Biochem.* **31** (1993), 651–656.
61. Junger, W.G., Cardoza, T. A., Liu, F. C., Hoyt, D. B. and Goodwin, R., *J. Immunol. Methods* **160** (1993), 73–79.
62. Galin, J.I., Clark, R.A., Kimball, H.R., *J. Immunol.* **110** (1973), 233–240.
63. Denholm, E.M. and Stankus, G.P., *Cytometry* **19** (1995), 366–369.
64. Schratzberger, P., Kahler, C.M. and Wiedermann, C.J., *Ann. Hematol.* **72** (1996), 23–27.
65. McCrone, E.L., Lucey, D.R. and Weller, P.F., *J. Immunol. Methods.* **114** (1988), 79–88.
66. Rot, A., *et al.*, *Proc. Natl. Acad. Sci. U.S.A.* **88** (1987), 7967–7971.
67. Richards, K.L. and McCullough, J., *Immunol. Commun.* **13** (1984), 49–62.
68. Harvath, L., Falk, W. and Leonard, E.J., *J. Immunol. Methods* **37** (1980), 39–45.
69. Leonard, E.J., *et al.*, *J. Immunol.* **144** (1990), 1323–1330.
70. Foster, C.A., Mandak, B., Krömer, E., and Rot, A., *Ann. N.Y. Acad. Sci.* **657** (1992), 397–404.
71. Mohle, R., Moore, M.A., Nachman, R.L., Rafii, S., *Blood* **89** (1997), 72–80 .
72. Molossi, S., Elices, M., Arrhenius, T. and Rabinovitch, M., *J. Cell. Physiol.* **164** (1995), 620–633.
73. Middleton J., *et al.*, *Cell* **91** (1997), 385–395.
74. Keller, H.U., *et al.*, *Clin. Exp. Immunol.* **27** (1977), 377–380.
75. Wilkinson, P.C, *J. Immunol. Methods* **110** (1988), 143–144.
76. Zigmond, S.H. and Hirsch, J.G., *J. Exp. Med.* **137** (1973), 387–410.
77. Rhodes, J.M., *J. Immunol. Methods* **49** (1982), 235–236.

78. Clark, R.A., *J. Immunol.* **129** (1982), 2725–2728.
79. Yuli, I. and Snyderman, R., *J. Biol. Chem.* **261** (1986), 4902–4908.
80. Yoshimura, T., Rot, A., and Leonard, E.J. *Biochem. Biophys. Res. Comm.* **138** (1986), 66–71.
81. Bignold, L.P., *J. Immunol. Methods* **105** (1987), 275–80.
82. Rice, J. E. and Bignold, L.P., *J. Immunol. Methods* **149** (1992), 121–125.
83. Carter, S.B. *Nature* **208** (1965), 1183–1187.
84. Winklbauer, R., Nagel, M., Selchow, A. and Wacker, S., *Int. J. Dev. Biol.* **40** (1996), 305–311.
85. Winklbauer, R. and Nagel, M., *Dev. Biol.* **148** (1991) 573–589.
86. Grimstad, I. A., *Exp. Cell Res.* **173** (1987) 515–523.
87. McCarthy, J.B. and Furcht, L.T., *J. Cell Biol.* **98** (1984) 1474–1480.
88. Wang, J.M., *et al.*, *Biochem. Biophys. Res. Com.* **169** (1990) 165–170.
89. Dierich, M.P., Wilhelmi, D. and Till, G. *Nature* **270** (1977) 351–352.
90. Webster, R.O., Zanolari, B. and Henson, P.M. *Exp. Cell Res.* **129** (1980) 55–62.
91. Wilkinson, P.C. and Allan, R.B. *Exp. Cell Res.* **117** (1978) 403–412.
92. Rot, A. *Eur. J. Immunol.* **23** (1993), 303–306.
93. Wiedermann, C. J., *et al.*, *Curr. Biol.* **3** (1993), 735–742.
94. Zhou, D., Luini, W., Bernasconi, S., *et al.* *J. Biol. Chem.* **270** (1996), 22549–25556.
95. Zimmerman, G. A., *et al.*, *Adv. Exp. Med. Biol.,* **416** (1996), 297–304.
96. Bazan, J.F., *et al.*, *Nature*, **385** (1997), 640–644.
97. Imai, T., *et al.*, *Cell* **91** (1997), 521–530.
98. Pan Y., *et al.*, *Nature* **387** (1997), 611–617.
99. Rot, A., *Immunol. Today* **13** (1992), 291–294.
100. Tanaka, Y., Adams, D.H. and Shaw, S., *Immunol. Today* **14** (1993), 111–115.
101. Webb, L.M.C., Ehrengruber, M.U., Clark-Lewis, I., Baggiolini, M. and Rot. A. *Proc. Natl. Acad. Sci. USA.* **90** (1993), 7158–7162.
102. Witt, D. P. and Lander, A. D., *Curr. Biol.* **4** (1994), 394–400.
103. Tanaka, Y., *et al.*, *Nature* **361** (1993), 79–82.
104. Hadley, T.J., *et al.*, *J. Clin. Invest.* **94** (1994), 985–991.
105. Carter, S.B., *Nature*, **213** (1967), 256–260.
106. Aznavoorian, S., Stracke, M.L., Parsons, J.; McClanahan, J. And Liotta, L. A. *J. Biol. Chem.,* **271** (1996), 3247–3254.
107. Wiedermann, C.J., *et al.*, *J. Leukoc. Biol.* **58** (1995), 438–44.
108. Weyrich, A.S., *et al.*, *J. Clin. Invest.* **97** (1996),1525–1534 .
109. Cassatella, M.A., *et al.*, *J. Immunol.* **148** (1992), 3216–3220.

110. Cassatella, M.A., *et al.*, *Eur-J-Immunol.* **27** (1997), 111–115.
111. Cassatella, M.A., *Immunol. Today* **16** (1995) 21–26.
112. Ember, J. A., Sanderson, S.D., Hugli, T.E. and Morgan, E.L., *Am. J. Pathol.* **144** (1994) 393–403.
113. Rot, A. and Hub, E. In *Biology of the chemokine RANTES.* ed. Krensky, A.M, R.G. Landes Company, Austin, Texas, pp 35–54 (1995).
114. Bignold, L.P., Ferante, A. and Haynes, D.R. *Int. Arch. All. Appl. Immunol.* **91** (1990), 1–7.
115. Yoshimura, T., Matsushima, K., Oppenheim, J.J. and Leonard, E.J, *J. Immunol.* **139** (1987), 788–793.
116. Thomsen, M.K. and Thomsen, H.K., *Vet. Immunol. Immunopathol.* **26** (1990), 385–393.
117. Faccioli, L.H. , Souza,G.E., Cunha, F.Q., Poole S. And Ferreira, S.H., *Agents Actions*, **30** (1990), 344–349.
118. Sayers, T.J., *et al.*, *J. Immunol.* **141** (1988), 1670–1677.
119. Hunninghake, G.W., Glazier, J, Monick, M.M. and Dinarello, C.A., *Am. Rev. Respir. Dis.* **135** (1987), 66–71.
120. Wang, J.M., Walter, S. and Mantovani, A., *Immunology.* 71 (1990), 364–367.
121. Mrowietz, U., Schroder, J.M. and Christophers, E . *Biochem. Biophys. Res. Commun.* **153** (1988) 1223–1228.
122. Kharazmi, A., Nielsen, H. and Bendtzen, K., *Immunobiology.* **177** (1988), 363–370.
123. Newman, I. and Wilkinson, P.C., *Immunology*, **66** (1989), 318–320.
124. Graves, D.T., Grotendorst, G.R., Antoniades, H.N., Schwartz, C.J. and Valente, A.J., *Exp. Cell Res.* **180** (1989), 497–503.
125. Shure, D., Senior, R.M., Griffin, G.L. and Deuel, T.F., *Biochem. Biophys. Res. Commun.* **186** (1992), 1510–1514.
126. Noso, N., *et al.*, *J. Immunol.* **156** (1996), 1946–19453.
127. Bittleman, D.B., Erger, R.A. and Casale, T.B., *Inflamm. Res.* **45** (1996), 89–95.
128. Wang, J.M., Colella, S., Allavena, P. and Mantovani., A. *Immunology*, **60** (1987), 439–144.
129. Kownatzki, E., Liehl, E., Aschauer, H. and Uhrich, S. *Immunopharmacology,* **19** (1990), 139–143.
130. McCain, R.W., Dessypris, E.N. and Christman, J.W., *Am. J. Respir. Cell Mol. Biol.* **8** (1993) 28–34.
131. Loetscher, P. , Seitz, M., Baggiolini, M. and Moser, B., *J. Exp. Med.,* **184** (1996), 569–577.

132. Lloyd , A.R., *et al.*, *J. Biol. Chem.* **270** (1995), 28188–28192.
133. Benov, L. and Fridovich, I., *Proc. Natl. Acad. Sci. USA.* **93** (1996), 4999–5002.
134. Kolodkin, A.L., Matthes, D.J. and Goodman, C.S. *Cell* **75** (1993),1389–1399.
135. Hall, K.T., *et al.*, *Proc. Natl. Acad. Sci. USA.* **93** (1996), 11780–11785.
136. Godfrey, H.P., Frenz, D.A., Canfield, L.S., Akiyama, S.K. and Newman, S.A., *J. Immunol.* **143** (1989), 3691–3696.
137. Newman, S.A., Frenz, D.A., Tomasek, J.J. and Rabuzzi, D.D., *Science* **228** (1985), 885–889.
138. Newman, S.A., Frenz, D.A., Hasegawa, E. and Akiyama, S.K., *Proc. Natl. Acad. Sci. U.S.A.* **84** (1987), 4791–4795.
139. Thiery, J.P., *Cell Differ.*, **15** (1984), 1–15.
140. Nuccitelli, R. and Erickson, C.A., *Exp. Cell Res.* **147** (1983), 195–201.
141. Robinson, K.R., *J. Cell Biol.* **101** (1985), 2023–2027.
142. Gruler, H., *Blood Cell.* **19** (1993), 91–113.
143. Nishimura, K.Y., Isseroff, R.R. and Nuccitelli, R., *J. Cell Sci.* **109** (1996), 199–207.
144. Franke, K. and Gruler, H., *Eur. Biophys. J.*, **18** (1990), 335–346.
145. Franke, K. and Gruler, H., *Z. Naturforsch. C.*, **49** (1994), 244–249.
146. Matthes, T. and Gruler, H., *Eur. Biophys. J.*, **15** (1988), 343–357.
147. Wilkinson, P.C. and Lackie, J.M. *Exp. Cell Res.* 145 (1983), 255–264.
148. Wilkinson, P.C., Shields, J.M. and Haston, W.S. *Exp. Cell. Res.* **140** (1982), 55–62.
149. Mandeville, J.T., Lawson, M.A. and Maxfield, F.R., *J. Leukoc. Biol.* **61** (1997), 188–200.

CHAPTER 8

DIAGNOSTIC EVALUATION OF NEUTROPHIL FUNCTION

Gabriel Virella[1]

1. Introduction

Neutrophils and other polymorphonuclear leukocytes are "wandering" cells, constantly circulating around the vascular network, able to recognize foreign matter by a wide variety of immunological and non-immunological mechanisms. Their main biological characteristics have been discussed in other chapters of this book and have also recently been summarized elsewhere (1). However, it is important to briefly review some of the major points in neutrophil physiology which have a direct impact on the diagnostic evaluation of their function. As a starting point one needs to recall that the effective participation of neutrophils in an anti-infectious response depends on their ability to respond to chemotactic signals, migrate to an infected tissue, ingest the pathogenic agent, and destroy it after ingestion.

1.1 Chemotaxis and migration to the extravascular compartment

The migration of neutrophils out of the intravascular compartment is an extremely regulated phenomenon, which depends on the sequential expression

[1]Correspondence: Gabriel Virella, M.D., Ph.D., Department of Microbiology and Immunology, Medical University of South Carolina, 171 Ashley Avenue, Charleston, S.C. 29425, E-mail: virellag@musc.edu

of a number of cell adhesion molecules, both in neutrophils and in endothelial cells (2,3). In normal conditions, the interaction between leukocytes and endothelial cells is rather loose and involves a family of molecules known as selectins, which are constitutively expressed on endothelial cells, and glycoproteins expressed on the leukocyte cell membrane. These interactions cause the slowing down ("rolling") of leukocytes along the vessel wall, but do not lead to firm adhesion of leukocytes to endothelial cells.

Several chemotactic stimuli, some of bacterial origin (such as f-methionine-leucine-phenylalanine (f-met-leu-phe), some released or activated as a result of monocyte and lymphocyte activation (including proteases which may activate the complement system, leukotriene B4, and chemokines such as IL-8, monocyte chemotactic protein-1, and RANTES), and some generated as a by-product of complement activation (C5a), are involved in the recruitment of leukocytes to the extravascular space. It must be also noted that many of these chemotactic factors are also activating stimuli for neutrophils.

After receiving a chemotactic stimulus, the neutrophil undergoes changes in the cell membrane which are characteristic of the activated state. The membrane becomes "ruffled" and several membrane adherence molecules become upregulated. Among those cell adhesion molecules (CAMs) expressed by activated neutrophils, the integrins of the CD11/CD18 complex, which include CD11a [the a chain of LFA (leukocyte function antigen)-1], CD11b molecule (the C3bi receptor or CR3, also known as Mac-1), CD11c (also known as protein p150,95), and CD18 [the β chain of LFA (leukocyte function antigen)-1] deserve special atention.

Indeed, the upregulation of these CAMs mediates a variety of physiological changes. The neutrophils become able to interact with each other, forming aggregates, or to interact with endothelial cells, particularly when those cells have also upregulated CAMs which serve as receptors for those expressed by activated neutrophils. For example, CD11a (LFA-1) and CD11b interact with molecules of the immunoglobulin gene family, such as ICAM-1, ICAM-2 and VCAM-1, expressed by endothelial cells. This interaction has a fundamental role in promoting the migration of neutrophils into the extravascular compartment. This aspect is discussed in details in chapter 3.

The transmigration of neutrophils involves interaction with a fourth cell adhesion molecule — the platelet endothelial cell adhesion molecule 1 (PECAM-1) — which is expressed at the intercellular junctions between endothelial cells. The interaction of leukocytes with PECAM-1 mediates the process of diapedesis, by which leukocytes squeeze through the endothelial cell junctions into the extravascular compartment. The diapedesis process involves the locomotor apparatus of the neutrophils, a contractile actin-myosin system stabilized by polymerized microtubules. Its activation is essential for the neutrophil to move to the extravascular space and for several other functions, including phagocytosis (4).

1.2 *Phagocytosis and intracellular killing*

Once neutrophils reach the source of chemotactic stimuli, the responsible material will be ingested, and if it happens to be a live microorganism, it will be killed after ingestion. Several recognition systems appear to be involved in the phagocytosis step, the best defined of which are the reactions of two types of Fcγ receptors, FcγRII and FcγRIII, with the Fc fragment of opsonizing antibodies of the IgG isotype and the interaction of complement receptors, particularly CR1 and CR3, with C3b and C3bi (5,6). However, neutrophils are also able to ingest non-opsonized particles, such as microorganisms with polysaccharide-rich outer layers, latex beads, silicone, asbestos fibers, etc.

Intracellular killing depends on two sets of events. On one hand, fusion of phagosomes, containing ingested organisms, and lysosomes results in the delivery of a variety of enzymes into the phagolysosome, including lysozyme, cationic proteins, lactoferrin, and several proteases (1). On the other hand, the engagement of Fc receptor (7) signals delivered by a variety of PMN activating stimuli, ranging from f-met-leu-phe to C5a (8), are known to activate the assembly of NADPH oxidase, leading to the generation of highly toxic oxygen reactive products and by-products, a phenomenon which is described as the "respiratory burst".

NADPH oxidase is a molecular complex located on the cell membrane, constituted by Cytochrome B, an heterodimer formed by two polypeptide chains

(91 Kd and 22 Kd, respectively), and two cytosolic proteins (p47 and p67), one of which (p47) is a substrate for protein kinase C (8–11). After the cell is activated p47 is phosphorylated, becomes associated with p67 (and possibly with a third protein, p21^{rac}), and the phosphorylated complex binds to cytochrome B in the phagosome membrane. At that point an active oxidase has been assembled, and its activity results in the transfer of a single electron from NADPH to oxygen, generating superoxide (O_2^-), which is delivered to the phagosome. Superoxide is quickly converted to H_2O_2, which through myeloperoxidase can be peroxidated and led to form hypochlorous acid and other halide ion derivatives. Superoxide, peroxide, hypochlorite and other halide ion derivatives are toxic to the engulfed microorganisms, and are believed to be the most significant microbicidal compounds generated by the neutrophil (11). For more detailed information, see chapter 2.

2. Evaluation of Neutrophil Function

Phagocytosis by neutrophils can be depressed as a result of a reduction in cell numbers or as a result of a functional defect. Quantitative defects, which can be primary or secondary, are by far the most frequent neutrophil defects (12) and are easy to detect through a complete blood count with differential, which is always the first step in the investigation of a possible phagocytic defect. Some specific defects, such as the abnormally large lysosomes present in the neutrophils of patients with Chediak-Higashi Syndrome (13) can be recognized in stained peripheral blood smears, and special myeloperoxidase cytochemical staining procedures can be used to detect myeloperoxidase defects (14). In the presence of normal neutrophil counts with normal morphology, a wide range of primary and secondary abnormalities remains, because functional defects affecting every stage of the phagocytic response have been reported and have to be evaluated by different tests. The choice of tests can be frustrating, given the many different alternatives that are often described for testing the same basic function, as well as the lack of reference techniques sufficiently standardized to yield reproducible results in different laboratories.

2.1 Blood collection and neutrophil separation

In general, neutrophil function studies are carried out with isolated neutrophils. With the exception of the expression of surface markers (CD18/CD11 complex and others), which can be upregulated during isolation (15), and can, therefore, be more accurately estimated by flow cytometry with a small volume of whole blood, all other functional parameters seem to be more accurately estimated with isolated neutrophils. In our experience, citrate-or heparin-anticoagulated venous blood yields large numbers of functionally intact neutrophils. Similar observations with regard to heparin have been published by Bateman et al. (16), who also reported that EDTA-collected blood yielded functionally unresponsive neutrophils. On the other hand, others have reported that heparin interferes with chemotaxis (17), so we have used exclusively blood collected in citrate for several years. It is important to use endotoxin-free buffers in the isolation procedure, to avoid inadvertent activation (18).

Even more important is to observe some well established rules about PMN isolation, summarized by Metcalf et al. (19), and to keep in mind that the half life of neutrophils is 7 hours (20), which means that it is essential to isolate and test neutrophils as soon as possible after blood collection. It also means that results of functional tests obtained in reference or commercial laboratories are unlikely to be reliable, even if blood is refrigerated and delivered overnight. While short term refrigeration (up to 4 hr. at 4°C) has no adverse effects on most neutrophil function tests, exposure to cold temperatures for as short a period as 1.5 hours has an adverse effect on random locomotion and chemotaxis (21).

Several approaches have been used to isolate neutrophils. Centrifugal elutriation has been heralded as a procedure able to yield large amounts of highly purified neutrophils (21), but it is usually performed in blood banks, where the equipment is usually available; therefore, using this technique in laboratories engaged in diagnostic testing is unusual. Cells separated by one of many protocols based on differential sedimentation are most often used in diagnostic laboratories. A comparison of several density gradient separation techniques for neutrophils was carried out by Venaille et al. (22), who concluded that all techniques yielded pure and active polymorphonuclear leukocytes, but

Percoll sedimentation caused the least degree of pre-activation during separation.

In our laboratory, neutrophils are separated from venous blood by dextran sedimentation (0.6% Dextran T500) at 37°C, followed by centrifugation on Ficoll-Paque. The cell pellet is immediately washed (2x) with Hanks BSS (HBSS), and contaminated red cells are lysed by addition of distilled water to the cell pellet resuspended in HBSS (3 parts distilled water to each part of resuspended pellet). The purity of neutrophil suspensions has been shown to impact on chemotaxis and chemiluminescence assays, and the elimination of contaminant red cells by hypotonic shock does not appear to have an adverse effect on neutrophil functions (21). This question was analyzed in a more systematic manner by Thorson et al. (23) who recommended to keep the time of exposure to hypotonic conditions under 30 s, although even after 100 s the percentage of damaged neutrophils (determined by flow cytometry) was only of 2.04 ± 1.8%. In our personal protocol, we have timed the hypotonic shock at 60 s, at the end of which we add enough hypertonic NaCl and HBSS to bring the suspension to isotonic molarity, and immediately centrifuge the cells. The neutrophil cell pellet obtained after red cell lysis is resuspended in Tyrodes buffer with Ca^{2+}, Mg^{2+} and immediately tested. Because all these steps are time-consuming, it is important to start the NBT test as soon as possible after blood collection. In our laboratory the test is set up in the hour following blood drawing and all procedures other than dextran sedimentation are carried out at room temperature. Although different laboratories may use different protocols to obtain adequately pure and functionally intact neutrophil populations, it is important for each laboratory to use a given protocol consistently, to insure the reproducibility of the assay.

2.2 *Tests for adherence*

The adherence of activated phagocytic cells to endothelial surfaces is critical for the migration of these cells to infectious foci. Specialized tests to measure adherence of resting neutrophils to plastic, for example Metcalf et al. (19), and to test the aggregation and adherence of neutrophils activated in response to stimuli such as $C5a_{desarg}$ (a non-chemotactic derivative of C5a) have been described (24). More recently, methods to measure the interaction between neutrophils and activated endothelial cells have been reported (25). However, for diagnostic purposes this property is evaluated indirectly, by determining the expression of the different components of the CD11/CD18 complex which mediate adhesion by flow cytometry (26,27).

2.3 Chemotaxis assays

Some methodological aspects of chemotaxis are also discussed in chapter 7. The migration of phagocytes in response to chemotactic stimuli can be studied *in vitro* using two basic techniques: migration in soft agarose towards a chemoattractant, or migration in chemotactic chambers, such as the Boyden chamber or several of its variations, including 24, 48 and 96 well microchamber assemblies with inserted filters which has been used by several groups (28–30). Both types of techniques are difficult to reproduce and standardize, but in general, migration in chemotactic chambers is the most widely used approach.

The basic principle of a chemotactic chamber is to have two compartments separated by a membrane whose pores are tight enough to represent a relative obstacle to the passive diffusion of PMN leukocytes from one chamber to the other, but are large enough to allow the active movement of these cells from the chamber where they are placed to the chamber where a chemotactic factor is introduced. A study of the performance of a variety of filter inserts available for 24 multi-well double chamber systems has demonstrated that polyethylene terephthalate membranes with 3 µm pore yield the best results in chemotaxis assays. Finally, some groups have used combinations of filters, the filter to the side of the chamber receiving neutrophils being of larger pore (5–8 µm) than the filter facing the compartment where the chemotactic factor is applied (0.22–0.3 µm). In these procedures chemotaxis is usually evaluated by determining, directly or indirectly, the number of neutrophils reaching the filter proximal to the chemotactic factor (31,32).

Several chemotactic factors have been used, particularly the tetrapeptide f-met-leu-phe, C5a, IL-8, leukotriene B4 and PAF (33–35). After incubation for an adequate time, the chambers are disassembled and three types of parameters can be measured: (1) the number of neutrophils migrated into the filters, (2) the distance of migration by the leading front of cells into the filter, and (3) the number of neutrophils that reach the chamber containing the chemotactic factor.

The enumeration of neutrophils migrated into the filters can be done manually or by microscopic examination after staining of the filters (36). This procedure is the one classically used to measure the distance of migration of the leading front of cells into the filter, which some claim to be a more accurate measurement than just the number of cells in the filter (35,36).

A variety of methods for more objective quantitation of chemotaxis have been published. Usually the methods are based on estimating indirectly the number of neutrophils that reach the chamber containing the chemotactic factor. This can be achieved in a variety of ways. Originally, ^{51}Cr-labeled neutrophils were used and counting radioactivity on the chamber that contained the chemotactic factor at the beginning of the assay after adequate incubation would give an indication of the number of migrated leukocytes (19). Several alternatives to the use of radiolabeled cells have been published, including the measurement of the levels of activity of a neutrophil enzyme (such as elastase, myeloperoxidase or lactic dehydrogenase) after lysing (usually with triton X) the migrated cells (29,31,37), measurement of ATP level of migrated cells by bioluminescence (38), and labeling the migrated cells with a fluorescent dye (calcein AM) and then measuring the total fluorescence in the suspension of migrated neutrophils (30).

Quantitative approaches for estimating the number of neutrophils imbedded in the filter have also been published, such as computerized image analysis (39–41). A method which determines the sum of the numbers of neutrophils imbedded in the filter and migrated to the side of the membrane proximal to the chemotactic factor was developed by Lejeune et al. (42) where nonmigrated cells in the upper compartment are discarded and both the membrane and the cells in the lower compartment are disrupted with triton X, and the enzymatic activity of lactic dehydrogenase released by lysed cells is determined.

These techniques are mainly used in research, to characterize chemotactic compounds or to evaluate the effects of compounds which may inhibit chemotaxis. Clinically, most cases of impaired chemotaxis seem to be secondary to lack of expression of adhesion molecules which is easily determined by flow cytometry. Only in cases of Job's Syndrome (Hyper-IgE Syndrome) have there been reports of an isolated chemotactic defect, which affects primarily monocytes but also neutrophils (43,44).

2.4 *Ingestion assays*

Ingestion tests are relatively simple to perform and reproduce. They are usually based on incubating PMN with opsonized particles or microorganisms, and after an adequate incubation, determining either the number of ingested particles or a phagocytic index (the simpler approach when the results of the test are scored by microscopic examination):

$$\text{Phagocytic index} = \frac{\text{No. of cells with ingested particles}}{\text{Total no. of cells}} \times 100.$$

Several types of particles have been used, including latex, zymosan, live or killed *C. albicans* and [^{51}Cr]-labeled IgG-coated red cells (19). All these particles or organisms will activate complement by either one of the pathways and will become coated with C3 if incubated with an adequate source of complement. Organisms such as *C. albicans* can be easily visualized by staining cytospin slides with Giemsa stain (21). The easiest particles to visualize once ingested are fluorescent latex beads; their use considerably simplifies the assay, particularly if performed in a flow cytometer (45). Flow cytometry has also been used to measure the ingestion of fluorescent-labeled bacteria (46,47). Another approach is to use radiolabeled bacteria, such as [^{14}C] or [^{3}H] labeled *S. aureus* as the probe for ingestion. However, most of these assays have the potential problem of not distinguishing between ingested particles and cell-associated particles.

Several approaches have been proposed to distinguish between cell-associated and ingested bacteria. One consists of using radiolabeled *S. aureus* and eliminating the non-ingested bacteria by treatment of the neutrophil suspension with lysostaphin. Under these circumstances the number of ingested bacteria can be calculated directly from the readings of neutrophil-associated radioactivity obtained on a scintillation counter (19,48). One alternative approach consists of measuring the uptake of isotopic labels added to the neutrophil-bacteria suspension after an incubation period (usually 30 min.) which should allow the ingestion of a significant number of organisms. Only the non-ingested organisms would incorporate the isotope, and by comparing the total incorporation by two identical suspensions of the organism in question, to one of which neutrophils are added, one can calculate the proportion of ingested organisms at the time of labeling (49,50).

A third approach consists of adding acridine orange to neutrophil suspensions incubated in the presence of opsonized *Candida albicans*. As phagocytosis progresses, there is an increase in red fluorescence in neutrophils, due to the denaturation of the ingested *C. albicans* DNA, which can be measured by flow cytometry (51). Cantinieaux et al. (47) proposed a simpler alternative which does not require sequential fluorescence measurements, consisting of quenching the fraction of membrane-adherent *S. aureus* by adding trypan blue to the neutrophils suspension. Then, a simple reading at a specific time will give an indication of how many organisms have been ingested. A similar approach can be used to eliminate the interference of membrane bound fluorescent microspheres with the measurement of phagocytosis. In this case, fluorescence quenching can be obtained by adding ethidium bromide to the neutrophil-florescent particle mixture after adequate time to allow particle ingestion has elapsed. Ethydium bromide will quench the emission of fluorescence by extracellular particles, but because this compound will not penetrate the membrane of a living cell, the fluorescence of ingested particles will not be affected (52).

All these tests are relatively laborious and require skilled personnel. Since methods such as the nitroblue tetrazolium reduction test using opsonized particles test both for ingestion and for the ability to mount a respiratory burst, ingestion tests tend not to be used for diagnostic purposes.

2.5 Degranulation tests

When the contents of cytoplasmic granules are released into a phagosome, there is always some leakage of their contents into the extracellular fluid. The tests to study degranulation involve ingestion of opsonized particles followed by quantitation of enzymes released by neutrophils, such as myeloperoxidase, lysozyme, β-glucuronidase, and lactoferrin. These tests have also limited diagnostic application, because pure degranulation defects are extremely rare.

2.6 *Measurement of the oxidative burst*

From the diagnostic point of view, the measurement of the oxidative burst is the most commonly used approach for the study of neutrophil function. This is due to the fact that chronic granulomatous disease is the most common primary deficiency of neutrophil function, and any of the NBT assays is considerably easier to perform than a killing assay.

The first assays to measure the oxidative burst that were successfully applied to the diagnosis of chronic granulomatous disease were nitroblue tetrazolium (NBT) reduction assays performed on a microscope slide, counting the number of neutrophils that reduced NBT after ingesting opsonized particles (19). However, microscopic assays are difficult to perform objectively and with adequate precision, so they have been largely abandoned and replaced by more objective techniques to measure the oxidative burst. Whether or not the several proposed techniques give equivalent results was questioned by Matsuda et al. (53), but their conclusions were invalidated by the fact that they used totally different stimuli in the techniques they tried to compare. To this date, this question has not been satisfactorily resolved with a properly conceived and executed study.

2.6.1 Chemiluminescence

The chemiluminescence assay is based on the fact that the superoxide ion is unstable, and that its dissociation can be measured either directly or indirectly after addition of luminol that is activated during superoxide dissociation (54). Opsonized zymosan is commonly utilized to induce the respiratory burst (55). Using opsonized fluorescein isothiocyanate-conjugated yeast particles, an assay has been devised that allows measurement of the respiratory burst by chemiluminescence and determination of the number of ingested yeast particles by fluorescence microscopy in the same sample (Sandgren et al., 1991). The chemiluminescence assays are extremely sensitive and provide a direct quantitation of the oxidative burst, but have as a major drawback the requirement for special and costly instrumentation which may not be available in a diagnostic laboratory.

2.6.2 Reduction of cytochrome C

The reduction of the cytochrome C can be used to measure superoxide release because this pigment, when reduced by superoxide, will change its light absorbance properties. The change in color of cytochrome C can be measured with a conventional spectrophotometer (19) or with a microplate reader (56). The main drawbacks of the assay are its relatively low sensitivity and difficulties in reproducibility. However, the performance of the assay can be reportedly improved using fluorinated microtiter plates (to minimize adherence-related activation of neutrophils) and dual wavelength readings on a microplate reader (56) .

2.6.3 Fluorescence assays

Several techniques for the measurement of the superoxide burst are based on the oxidation of intracellular 2', 7'-dichlorofluorescein diacetate (non-fluorescent) which results in the formation of 2', 7' -dichlorofluorescein (highly fluorescent). An alternative method that use dihydrorhodamine 123 as substrate has been heralded by virtue of the better signal-to-noise ratio obtained with this dye (57).

In most assays the respiratory burst is induced with phorbol myristate acetate, which induces phosphorylation of protein kinase C (58,59), but it can also be induced by ingestion of opsonized bacteria (60). The numbers of fluorescent cells and fluorescence intensity of activated and non-activated PMN suspensions from patients and suitable controls can be determined by flow cytometry (59). In patients with primary defects of NADPH enzymatic complex, both the mean fluorescence intensity and the numbers of fluorescent cells after stimulation are considerably lower than those determined in normal, healthy volunteers. Using opsonized particles as stimuli, an abnormal result can reflect both a defect in ingestion or a defect in NADPH oxidase. However, phagocytosis is associated with light scattering changes which allow to discriminate between the two possibilities (61). These techniques have been widely used in a large number of studies and are well suited for the diagnostic laboratory equipped with modern flow cytometers.

2.6.4 Nitroblue tetrazolium (NBT) reduction tests

Tests based on NBT reduction are the most commonly used for the evaluation of neutrophil function. The principle of the tests is simple. Oxidized NBT, colorless to pale yellow in solution, is transformed by reduction into blue formazan. The test usually involves incubation of purified neutrophils, NBT, and a stimulus known to activate the respiratory burst. Two types of stimuli can be used: (1) opsonized particles, which need to be ingested to stimulate the burst. In this way the test examines both the ability to ingest and the ability to produce a respiratory burst; (2) diffusible activators, such as phorbol esters. These compounds diffuse into the cell and activate protein kinase C, which in turn activates the NADPH-cytochrome B system and induce the respiratory burst directly, bypassing the ingestion step. Using phorbols the test examines the functional integrity of the NADPH enzymatic activity, but does not give any information concerning the physiological activation of this enzymatic complex as a consequence of the ingestion of opsonized particles.

There are many different variants of quantitative NBT assays. The classical quantitative technique involves the extraction of intracellular NBT with N-N-dimethylformamide and measurement of its absorbance at 515 nm (which corresponds to the absorbance peak of reduced NBT). This modality of the NBT test is extremely sensitive and accurate but is difficult to perform because the reagents used to extract the dye from the cells are highly toxic (19).

An alternative are tube tests in which the PMN are simultaneously exposed to opsonized particles and NBT, and the change of color of the supernatant from pale yellow to gray or purple (as a result of the spillage of oxidizing products during phagocytosis) is measured. This assay, however, is not very sensitive because it relies on the spillage of active oxygen radicals rather than relying on intracellular NBT reduction.

More recently, with the introduction of kinetic colorimeters, it has been possible to develop assays in which the color change of NBT can be measured without need to extract the dye from the cells or to separate the cells from the supernatant (62,63). We have about a decade of experience with such an assay which has proven to be reliable and very suitable for diagnostic work (62). With this test, the lack of NADPH oxidase activity associated with chronic granulomatous disease is obvious because of the lack of color development in the wells where patient's neutrophils are exposed separately to IgG-coated beads and phorbol myristate acetate (Fig. 1).

Oez et al. (64) described an alternative colorimetric procedure using 3-(4,5-dimethylthiazol-2-yl)-2,5-diphenyl-tetrazolium bromide (MTT) as the reduction substrate, measuring the color corresponding to the generation of formazan in an EIA reader at 560 and 630 nm. However, this procedure has several additional steps which we did not find necessary in our procedure.

Another alternative for the objective measurement of NBT reduction was proposed by Fattorossi et al. (65). These authors labeled neutrophils with fluorescein-tagged concanavalin A, which binds non-specifically to several membrane proteins expressed on the neutrophil membrane without delivering a significant activation signal. The generation of formazan as a consequence of the reduction of NBT is associated with the quenching of the concanavalin A-associated fluorescence. Hence, a reduction in the fluorescence emitted by tagged neutrophils is indicative of a normal respiratory burst.

Testing the NBT reduction response to IgG and C3 opsonized particles (IgG-coated beads and opsonized zymosan are adequate choices) and to phorbol myristate acetate (PMA) in every patient has the advantage that one single test may distinguish between NADPH defects and ingestion defects. While all stimuli should be ineffective when NADPH activity cannot be generated, patients with impaired phagocytosis (such as those with CD11/CD18

DIAGRAMATIC REPRESENTATION OF THE PROCOL USED FOR THE QUANTITATIVE NBT ASSAY

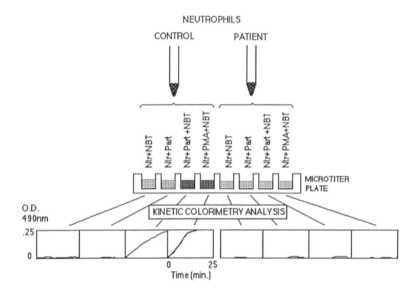

Figure 8.1.   Diagrammatic representation of the protocol for a quantitative NBT assay carried out by kinetic colorimetry. Neutrophils are isolated from a patient and a normal control and incubated separately in a microtiter plate with NBT (to check for spontaneous activation of neutrophils), with opsonized particles (to check for interference of cells and particles with the colorimetric assay), and with opsonized particles and phorbol myristate acetate (PMA) in the presence of NBT (to check for the induction of the respiratory burst). A kinetic colorimeter is used to monitor changes in O.D. due to the reduction of NBT over a 25-minute period, and the results are expressed diagrammatically and as an average of the variation of the O.D./unit of time. The graphic depiction of the results obtained with neutrophils from a normal control and from a patient with chronic granulomatous disease are reproduced in the lower part of the diagram (reproduced with permission from "Introduction to Medical Immunology (Virella, G., Ed.), Marcel Dekker, NY, 1998).

deficiency) yield negative results with opsonized zymosan, variable results with IgG-coated particles, and normal results with PMA (5).

2.6.5 Killing assays

Killing assays are certainly the gold standard for evaluation of neutrophil function. Performed in physiological conditions, these assays test for both ingestion and killing of microorganisms. This ability can be tested using a variety of viable bacteria and fungi that are mixed with PMN in the presence of normal human serum (a source of opsonins) and after a given time, the PMN are lysed and the number of viable organisms is determined (66). This procedure measures total killing (intracellular and extracellular). It is possible to determine strict intracellular killing using *Staphylococcus aureus* and staphylolysin to lyse extracellular bacteria (19). Other authors have proposed complex protocols in which after overnight incubation of PMN and bacteria, non-ingested bacteria are removed and the number of intracellular viable bacteria released by hypotonic shock is determined at three different time points (immediately after washing off noningested bacteria, 60 min. later and 120 min. later) to determine a ratio between the number of ingested bacteria at time zero and those that remain live after 60 and 120 minutes (67). To avoid proliferation of any remaining extracellular bacteria, some investigators add gentamicin to the medium where the final incubation of PMN with ingested bacteria takes place (35).

Several alternative killing assays which do not require culture have been developed. Some rely on counting live vs. dead *C. albicans* after incubation with neutrophils by methylene blue dye exclusion (68) or by differential Giemsa stain (69). Others rely on the detection of incorporated radiolabeled nucleotides by intracellular live bacteria (21). Alternatively, the inhibition of incorporation of nutrients, such as [^{3}H] glucose, by PMN suspensions to which *C. albicans* is added, can be used as an index of killing (70).

In general, bactericidal assays are difficult and cumbersome, and require close support from a microbiology laboratory, and for this reason the assays based on detection of the oxidative burst, which indirectly reflect the killing ability of neutrophils, or alternative and simpler approaches to the evaluation of intracellular killing based on the differential uptake of dyes (such as acridine orange) between live and dead bacteria, are more widely used.

One clinical entity in which killing assays may be more informative than NBT reduction assays is the Chediak-Higashi Syndrome. Neutrophils from patients with this syndrome are able to ingest microorganisms, but the cytoplasmic granules tend to coalesce into giant secondary lysosomes, with reduced enzymatic contents, that are inconsistently delivered to the phagosome. As a consequence, intracellular killing is slow and inefficient (71).

3. Conclusions

From the clinical point of view, the vast majority of phagocytic deficiencies are of a quantitative nature, secondary to the administration of cytotoxic drugs or to unexpected bone marrow depression caused by a wider variety of drugs. Those defects are easy to detect on a routine hemogram with differential and do not require special tests for confirmation. Secondary deficiencies in chemotaxis and other neutrophil functions have been repeatedly reported by different groups, but the impact of the characterization of those deficiencies in the management of the affected patients is virtually nonexistent. Thus, diagnostic laboratories seldom perform evaluations of secondary functional neutrophil deficiencies. Most of the diagnostic tests for neutrophil functions are carried out as part of the investigation of a suspected primary immunodeficiency. All primary neutrophil function deficiencies are rare, but chronic granulomatous disease (CGD) is certainly the most commonly seen. Thus, the neutrophil function tests most widely available are those that allow to diagnose or rule out CGD. While killing assays are certainly the gold standard, most diagnostic laboratories are ill suited to perform them. Hence, tests based on the detection of the respiratory burst after adequate stimulation are favored. The precise choice of test is most likely to depend on what equipment and expertise are available than on any real advantages of one method over another, although some methods have been abandoned either for their lack of sensitivity, lack of precision, or excessive complexity.

Acknowledgements

The author wishes to express his gratitude to Ms. Alva Mullins for her excellent editorial assistance and to Ms. Candace Ennockson, who critically revised the manuscript.

4. References

1. Virella, G. (1997). Diagnostic evaluation of phagocytic function. In "Introduction to Medical Immunology" (Virella, G., Ed.), Marcel Dekker, N.Y.
2. Abelda, S.M., Smith, C.W. and Ward, P.A. (1994). Adhesion molecules and inflammatory injury. Faseb J., 8: 504–512.
3. Collins, T. (1995). Adehesion molecules in leukocyte emigration. Sci. Amer. Medicine, 2: 28–37.
4. Todd, R.F. and Freyer, D.R. (1988). The CD11/CD18 leukocyte glycoprotein deficiency. Hematol./Oncol. Clin. N. Amer., 2: 13–31.
5. Arnaout, M.A., Dana, N., Pitt, J. and Todd, R.F. (1985). Deficiency of two human leukocyte surface membrane glycoproteins (Mo–1 and LFA-1). Fed. Proc., 44: 2664–2670.
6. Boackle, R. (1998). The complement system. In "Introduction to Medical Immunology" (Virella, G., Ed.), Marcel Dekker, N.Y.
7. Stromheier, G.R., Brunkorst, B.A., Seetoo, K.F. et al. (1995). Role of the Fc gamma R subclasses FcgRII and FcgRIII in the activation of human neutrophils by low and high valency immune complexes. J. Leukoc. Biol., 58: 415–422.
8. Thrasher, A.J., Keep, N.H., Wientjes, F. et al. (1994). Chronic granulomatous disease. Biochim. Biophys. Acta, 1227: 1–24.
9. Smith, R.M. and Curnutte, J.T. (1991). Molecular basis of chronic granulomatous disease. Blood, 77: 673–684.
10. Umeki, S. (1994). Mechanisms for the activation/electron transfer of neutrophil NADPH-oxidase complex and molecular pathology of chronic granulomatous disease. Ann. Hematol., 68: 267–277.
11. Pallister, C.J. and Hancock, J.T. (1995). Phagocytic NADPH oxidase and its role in chronic granulomatous disease. Brit. J. Biomed. Sci., 52: 149–156.
12. Boxer, L.A. and Blackwood, R.A. (1996). Leukocyte disorders: quantitative and qualitative disorders of the neutrophil, Part 1. Ped. in Review, 17: 19–28.

13. White, C.J. and Gallin, J.I. (1986). Phagocyte defects. Clin. Immunol. Immunopath., 40: 50–61.
14. Ottonello, L. Dapino, P., Pastorino, G. et al. (1995). Neutrophil dysfunction and increased susceptibility to infection. Eur. J. Clin. Invest., 25: 687–692.
15. Macey, M.G., Jiang, X.P., Veys, P. et al. (1992). Expression of functional antigens on neutrophils. Effect of preparation. J. Immunol. Methods, 149: 37–42.
16. Bateman, J., Parida, S.K. and Nash, G.B. (1993). Neutrophil integrin assay for clinical studies. Cell Biochem. Funct., 11: 87–91.
17. Freischlag, J.A., Colburn, M.D., Quninones-Baldrich, W.J. and Moore, W.S. Alteration of neutrophil (PMN) function by heparin, dexamethasone, and enalapril. J. Surg. Res., 52: 523–529.
18. Guthrie, L.A., McPhail, L.C., Henson, P.M. and Johnston, R.B. (1984). Priming of neutrophils for enhanced release of oxygen metabolites by bacterial lipopolysaccharide. Evidence for increased activity of the superoxide-producing enzyme. J. Exp. Med., 160: 1656–1671.
19. Metcalf, J.A., Gallin, J.I., Nauseef, W.M. and Root, R.K. (1986). Laboratory manual of neutrophil function, Raven Press, N.Y.
20. Price, T.H., Ochs, H.D., Geshoni-Baruch, R. et al., (1994). *In vitro* neutrophil and lymphocyte function studies in a patient with leukocyte adhesion deficiency type II. Blood, 84: 2635–1639.
21. Glasser, L. and Fiederlein, R.L. (1990). The effect of various cell separation procedures on assays of neutrophil function. Amer. J. Clin. Path., 93: 662–669
22. Venaille, T.J., Misso, N.L., Phillips, M.J. et al. (1994). Effects of different gradient separation techniques on neutrophil function. Scand. J. Clin. Lab. Invest., 54: 385–391.
23. Thorson, L.M., Turkalj, A., Hung, J.C. (1995). *In vitro* evaluation of neutrophil viability after exposure to a hypotonic medium. Nucl. Med. Commun. 16: 615–620, 1995.
24. Bellavite, P., Chirumbolo, S. Mansoldo, C., Gandini, G. and Driu, P. (1992). Simultaneous assay for oxidative metabolism and adhesion of human neutrophils evidence for correlations and dissociations of the two responses. J. Leukoc. Biol., 51: 329–335.
25. Gozalez-Alvaro, I., Carmona, L., Diaz-Gonzalez, F. et al. (1996). Aceclofenac, a new nonsteroidal antiinflammatory drug, decreases the expression and function of some adhesion molecules on human neutrophils. J. Rheumatol., 23: 723–729.
26. Boxer, L.A. and Blackwood, R.A. (1996). Leukocyte disorders: quantitative and qualitative disorders of the neutrophil, Part 2. Ped. in Review, 17: 47–50.

27. McEvoy, L.T., Zakem-Cloud, H. and Tosi, M.F. (1996). Total content of CR3 (CD11b/CD18) and LFA-1 (CD11a/CD18) in neonatal neutrophils: relationship to gestational age. Blood, 87: 3929–3933.

28. Falk, W., Goodwin, R.H. and Leonard, E.J. (1980). A 48-well micro chemotaxis assembly for rapid and accurate measurement of leukocyte migration. J. Immunol. Meth., 33: 239–247.

29. Junger WG, Cardoza, T.A., Liu, F.C. et al. (1993). Improved rapid photometric assay for quantitative measurement of PMN migration. J. Immunol. Methods, 160: 73–79.

30. Sunder-Plassmann, G., Hoffbauer, R., Sengoelge, G. et al. (1996). Quantification of leukocyte migration: improvement of a method. Immunol. Invest., 25: 49–63.

31. Somersalo, K., Salo, O.P., Bjorksten, F. et al. (1990). A simplified Boyden chamber assay for neutrophil chemotaxis based on quantitation of myeloperoxidase. Anal. Biochem., 185: 238–242.

32. Rossman, J.E., Caty, M.G., Rich, G.A. et al. (1996). Neutrophil activation and chemotaxis after *in vitro* treatment with perfluorocarbon. J. Pediatr. Surg., 31: 1147–1150.

33. Elsner, J., Roesler, J., Emmendorffer, A. et al. (1992). Altered function and surface marker expression of neutrophils induced by rhG-GSF treatment in severe congenital neutropenia. Eur. J. Haematol., 48: 10–19.

34. Hasslen, S.R., Nelson, R.D., Ahrenholz, D.H. et al. (1993). Thermal injury, the inflammatory process, and wound dressing reduce human neutrophil chemotaxis to four attractants. J. Burn Care Rehabil., 14: 303–309.

35. Itälä, M., Vainio, O. and Remes, K. (1996). Functional abnormalities in granulocytes predict susceptibility to bacterial infections in chronic lymphocytic leukemia. Eur. J. Haematol., 57: 46–53.

36. Zigmond, S.H. and Hirsch, J.G. (1973). Leukocyte locomotion and chemotaxis. New methods for evaluation, and demonstration of a cell-derived chemotactic factor. J. exp. Med., 137: 387–410.

37. Pelz, G., Schettler, A. and Tschesche, H. (1993). Granulocyte chemotaxis measured in a Boyden chamber assay by quantification of neutrophil elastase. Eur. J. Chem. Clin. Biochem., 31: 651–656.

38. Partsch, G. and Schwarzer, C. (1991). An indirect bioluminescence method for the quantitative measurement of polumorphonuclear cell chemotaxis. J. Biolumin. Chemilumin., 6: 159–167.

39. Jensen, P. and Kharazmi, A. (1991). Computer-assisted image analysis of human neutrophil chemotaxis *in vitro*. J. Immunol. Methods, 144: 43–48.

40. Coates, T.D. (1992). An integrated system for quantitation of chemotaxis using a 48-well millipore filter assay. Comput. Methods Porgrams Biomed., 38: 177–192.

41. Storgaard, M., West, M.J., Nielsen. S.L. et al. (1995). Quantification of neutrophil chemotaxis: a comparison of stereological and 51Cr-labelling methods. APMIS, 103: 185–192.

42. Lejeune, M., Sariban. E., Canitinieaux, B. et al. (1996). Granulocyte functions in children with cancer are differentially sensitive to the toxic effect of chemotherapy. Pediatr. Res., 39: 835–842.

43. Nielsen, H., Valerius, N.H., Valerius, N.H. et al. (1986). Selective defect of phagocyte responsiveness to N-f-Met-Leu-Phe in a familial syndrome of recurrent cold abscesses. J. Infect. Dis., 153: 1184–1186.

44. Jeppson, J.D., Jaffe, H.S. and Hill, H.R. (1991). Use of recombinant human interferon gamma to enhance neutrophil chemotactic responses in Job's syndrome of hyperimmunoglobulinemia E and recurrent infections. J. Pediatr., 118: 383–387.

45. Dunn, P.A. and Tyrer, H.W. (1981). Quantitation of neutrophil phagocytosis, using fluorescent latex beads. Correlation of microscopy and flow cytometry. J. Lab. Clin. Med., 98: 374–381.

46. Bassoe, C.F., Laerum, O.D., Solberg, C.O. and Haneberg, B. (1983). Phagocytosis of bacteria by human leukocytes measured by flow cytometry. Proc. Soc. Exp. Biol. Med., 82: 253–259.

47. Cantinieaux, B., Hariga, C., Courtoy, P. et al. (1989). *Staphylococcus aureus* phagocytosis. A new cytofluorometric method using FITC and formaldehyde. J. Immunol. Meth., 121: 203–208, 1989.

48. Gabka, C.J., Benhaim, P., Mathes, S.J. et al. (1995). An experimental model to determine the effect of irradiated tissue on neutrophil function. Plastic & Reconstr. Surg., 96: 1676–1688.

49. Verhoef, J., Peterson, P.K. and Quie, P.G. (1977). Kinetics of staphylococcal opsonization, attachment, ingestion and killing by human polymorphonuclear leukocytes: a quantitative assay using [3H]thymidine labeled bacteria. J. Immunol. Meth., 14: 303–311.

50. Yamamura, M., Boler, J. and Valdimarson, H. (1977). Phagocytosis measured as inhibition of uridine uptake by Candida albicans. J. Immunol. Meth., 14: 19–24.

51. Wilson, R.M., Galvin, A.M., Robins, R.A. et al. (1985). A flow cytometric method for the measurement of phagocytosis by polymorphonuclear leucocytes. J. Immunol. Meth., 76: 247–253.

52. Simms, H.H. and D'Amico, R. (1994). Polymorphonuclear leukocyte dysregulation during the systemic inflammatory response syndrome. Blood, 83: 1398–1407.

53. Matsuda, J., Tsukamoto, M., Sitoh, N. et al. (1993). Polymorphonuclear leukocyte function tests: a comparison of cytochrome C reduction and flow cytometric analysis. Brit. J. Biomed. Sci., 50: 60–63.

54. Bondestam, M., Håkansson, L., Foucard, T. and Venge, P. (1986). Defects in polymorphonuclear neutrophil function and susceptibility to infection in children. Scand. J. Clin. Lab. Invest., 46: 685–694.

55. Robinson, P. Wakefield, D., Breit, S.N. et al. (1984). Chemiluminescent response to pathogenic organisms: normal human polymorphonuclear leukocytes. Infec. Immun., 43: 744–752.

56. Chapman-Kirkland, E.S., Wasvary, J.S. and Seligmann, B.E. (1991). Superoxide anion production from human neutrophils measured with an improved kinetic and endpoint assay. J. Immunol. Meth., 142: 95–104.

57. Rothe, G., Emmendörffer, A., Oser, A. et al. (1991). Flow cytometric measurement of the respiratory activity of phagocytes using dihydrorhodamine 123. J. Immunol., 138: 133–135.

58. Bass, D.A., Parce, J.W., Dechatelet, L.R. et al. (1983). Flow cytometric studies of oxidative product formation by neutrophils: a graded response to membrane stimulation. J. Immunol., 130: 1910–1917.

59. Epling, C.L., Stites, D.P., McHugh, T.M. et al. (1992). Neutrophil function screening in patients with chronic granulomatous disease by a flow cytometic method. Cytometry, 13: 615–620.

60. Szejda, P., Parce, J.W., Seeds, M.S. et al. (1984). Flow cytometric quantitation of oxidative product formation by polymorphonuclear leukocytes during phagocytosis. J. Immunol., 133: 3303–3307.

61. Casado, J.A., Merino, J., Cid, J. et al. (1993). Simultaneous evaluation of phagocytosis and FcγR-mediated oxidative burst in human monocytes by a simple flow cytometric method. J. Immunol. Meth., 159: 173–176.

62. Virella, G., Thompson, T. and Haskill-Stroud, R. (1990). A new quantitative nitroblue tetrazolium reduction assay based on kinetic colorimetry. J. Clin. Lab. Anal., 4: 86–89.

63. Piva, E., DeToni, S., Caenazzo, A. et al. (1995). Neutrophil NADPH oxidase activity in chronic myeloproliferative and myelodysplastic diseases by microscopic and photometric assays. Acat Haematol., 94: 16–22.

64. Oez, S., Platzer, E. and Welte, K. (1990). A quantitative colorimetric method to evaluate the functional state of human polymorphonuclear leukocytes. Blut, 60: 97–102.

65. Fattorossi, A., Nisini, R., Le Moli, S. et al. (1990). Flow cytometric evaluation of nitroblue tetrazolium (NBT) reduction in human polymorphonuclear leukocytes. Cytometry, 11: 907–912.

66. Quie, P.G., White, J.G., Holmes, B. et al. (1967). *In vitro* bactericidal capacity of human polymorphonuclear leukocytes: diminished activity in chronic granulomatous disease of childhood. J. Clin. Invest., 46: 668–679.

67. Waterlot, Y., Canitinieaux, B., Hariga, C. et al. (1985). Impaired phagocytic ability of neutrophils of patients receiving haemodialysis: the critical role of iron overload. Brit. Med. J., 291: 501–504.

68. Lehrer, R.I. and Cline, M.J. (1969). Interaction of *Candida albicans* with human leukocytes and serum. J. Bacteriol., 98: 996–1004.

69. Leherer, R.I. (1970). Measurement of candidicidal activity of specific leukocyte types in mixed cell populations. I. Normal, myeloperoxidase-deficient, and chronic granulomatous disease neutrophils. Infect. Immun., 2: 42–47.

70. Djeu, J.Y., Parapanissios, A., Halkias, D. and Friedman, H. A rapid [³H] glucose incorporation assay for determination of lymhoid cell-mediated inhibition of *Candida albicans* growth. J. Immunol. Meth., 92: 73–77, 1986.

71. Boxer, L.A., Albertini, D.F., Bahener, R.L. et al. (1979). Impaired microtubule assembly and polymorphonuclear leukocyte function in the Chediak-Higashi syndrome correctable by ascorbic acid. Br. J. Haematol., 43: 207–213.

CHAPTER 9

NEUTROPHILS IN VIRAL INFECTIONS

Robert L. Roberts[1]

The containment and killing of bacteria are the major functions of neutrophils in host defense. After penetrating the body, factors released by the bacteria themselves or generated by complement breakdown and by other inflammatory cells attract great numbers of neutrophils to the site of the bacterial invasion. As soon as the bacteria attach to the surface receptors on the neutrophil, they are rapidly sequestered into phagolysomes and then killed by release of toxins from the granules and the production of oxygen radicals.

The role of neutrophils in viral infections is much less apparent. Although neutrophils can be induced to inactivate viruses *in vitro*, it is difficult to determine how important this anti-viral activity is *in vivo*. In rhinoviral infections of the upper respiratory tract, or the "common cold," most of the discomfort of the patient appears to be due to the great influx of neutrophils into the nasal secretions and not injury to the nasal epithelium by the virus itself. Many other viruses are capable of activating neutrophils *in vitro*, which may account for the exaggerated inflammatory response in some viral infections if this activation also occurs *in vivo*.

Viruses may also inhibit neutrophil function, and hence, their ability to contain bacterial infections. The influenza A virus may depress many phagocytic activities, making their host more susceptible to bacterial superinfections which

[1]Robert L. Roberts, MD, PhD, Associate Professor of Pediatrics, Division of Immunology/ Allergy, UCLA School of Medicine, Los Angeles, CA 90095, Phone (310) 825-6777/825-6481, Fax (310) 206-5843

was the most common cause of death in past influenza epidemics. Inhibition of neutrophil function may also play an important part role in the present day AIDS epidemics. Although the neutrophil may not be infected by the human immunodeficiency virus (HIV), many defects in neutrophil function have been reported in HIV patients. A large percentage of HIV-infected patients will develop anti-neutrophil antibodies which can destroy neutrophils or inhibit their function. Oxidant stress due to low-levels of the anti-oxidant glutathione, inhibitory HIV proteins and abnormalities in cytokine production may also inhibit neutrophil function. This loss of neutrophil surveillance for bacteria and fungal pathogens makes the patient more susceptible to these microorganisms, and further contributes to their immune deficiency. Impairment in neutrophil function may be even of greater importance in HIV-infected children who are a greater risk for more common bacterial infections than adult patients. This may also account in part for the observation that children can become much more ill more quickly than adults even when their CD4 counts are relatively high.

In this chapter the various interactions between neutrophils and viruses will be discussed. We will also examine the role of neutrophils in specific viral infections including influenza and HIV. By understanding these interactions between neutrophils and viruses, we can hopefully devise better therapeutic strategies for the benefit of patients.

1. Inhibition of Viruses By Neutrophils

Neutrophils are able to inactivate or inhibit viral replication by a number of mechanisms as shown in Table 1. Despite these *in vitro* studies, most patients with neutropenia or impairment of neutrophil function, as in chronic granulomatous disease (CGD), are not particularly susceptible to severe viral infections. This observation may be due to the fact that other cell populations in these patients, such as monocytes, NK cells, and T lymphocytes, also are able to inhibit viruses more effectively than neutrophils. Normal antibody production is also a strong deterrent to viral infections although neutrophils may play a role in antibody-mediated killing of virally-infected cells. However,

Table 9.1   Inhibition of viruses by neutrophils

Mechanisms	Viruses	Selected References
Ingestion and inactivation by cationic granular proteins	Vaccina Herpes	1, 2, 3, 4
Release of cytokines that attract other cells	Rhinovirus Influenza	5, 6
Release of oxygen intermediates	Herpes Influenza Vaccina	7, 8, 9
Antibody-dependent cellular cytotoxicity	Herpes Varicella Influenza HIV	10, 11, 12, 13
Complement-mediated cytotoxicity	Herpes RSV	14
Collectin-mediated phagocytosis	Influenza	15, 16

the anti-viral properties of neutrophils may become of greater significance in patients whose lymphocytes and monocytes are decreased or functionally impaired as occurs in AIDS patients.

When neutrophils encounter bacteria, the usual response is phagocytosis which is greatly facilitated by antibody or complement components binding to the bacteria. Viruses may enter neutrophils by phagocytosis but also by other mechanisms such as fusion with membrane proteins and endocytosis. If entry of the virus activates the neutrophil, then the virus is more likely to be destroyed by the release of granule proteins such as defensins and generation of reactive oxygen intermediates. The granule protein defensin will inhibit HIV replication *in vitro*, and lactoferrin, an iron-binding cationic protein, can inhibit adsorption and penetration of HIV and CMV in cell culture. (17,18).

If entry of the virus does not activate the neutrophil, then the neutrophil may actually act as a reservoir for the virus, allowing it to escape inactivation by other means. Viruses that have been found within neutrophils include vaccinia, herpes simplex, influenzae, CMV, adenovirus, and HIV (19). In CMV infection the virus is more readily cultured from neutrophils than from monocytes although both may contain the virus (20,21). This implies that monocytes may be better at inactivating the virus. Neutrophils may also be a major reservoir for hepatitis B virus (22).

Neutrophils produce a number of cytokines that have anti-viral effects themselves or that attract other cells with anti-viral properties (23). This would include interleukin (IL)-1 which activates T cells and NK cells, IL-8 that also attracts T cells, interferon-a that activates NK cells, and tumor necrosis factor (TNF)-a that activates T and NK cells. These other cells may then generate more cytokines, such as interferon-gamma, which have also antiviral properties.

1.1 *Viral inactivation by oxygen intermediates*

Oxygen intermediates generated by neutrophils will inactivate viruses *in vitro* but its clinical significance has not been proven. Poliovirus and vaccinia virus exposed to the combination of hydrogen peroxide, myeloperoxidase, and halide (which would generate hypophalous acid) were inactivated *in vitro* (24). It has been demonstrated that neutrophils from CGD patients are less able to destroy herpes or vaccina virus as compared to normal controls (27,8). Our laboratory also found that neutrophils from CGD patients were unable to inhibit the replication of herpes simplex virus despite stimulation with phorbol myristate acetate which greatly stimulates inhibition by neutrophils from normal controls (25). The production of oxygen intermediates also appears to play a role in impairing the infectivity of HIV using a T cell line as targets (26).

1.2 *Antibody and complement induced viral inactivation*

Neutrophils are able to lyse virally-infected cells by antibody-dependent cellular cytotoxicity (ADCC) as has been demonstrated using target cells infected with herpes-simplex, varicella-zoster, influenzae, and HIV (27,28,29,30,31,32,33). ADCC of HIV-infected targets may also be enhanced by cytokines such as granulocyte-colony stimulating factor G-CSF and granulocyte-macrophage colony stimulating factor GM-CSF using neutrophils from normal controls and as well as from HIV patients (34). The activation and fixation of complement to virally-infected cells will greatly increase the ability of neutrophils to kill the infected cell. Complement cells will fix to RSV-infected cells in the absence of specific antibody (35,36,37) and will stimulate lysis by neutrophils. A newly described group of collagenous lectins, named collectins, found in blood and pulmonary fluid, will induce aggregation of influenza A virus (IAV) particles. This aggregation will stimulate binding of IAV to neutrophils as well as prevent inhibition of neutrophils function by IAV (15,16).

2. Activation of Neutrophils by Viruses

Viruses are capable of stimulating various neutrophil functions, as shown in Table 2. The stimulation may occur through direct binding of the virus to the neutrophil, increased adherence of the neutrophil to virally-infected cells, or release of the cytokines by virally-infected cells. In some viral infections much of the inflammatory response is due to the activation of neutrophils, as is the case with rhinovirus infections which cause upper respiratory tract infections.

2.1 *Activation by binding of virus*

Sendai and myxovirus (strain of IAV) can bind directly to neutrophils in the absence of antibody. Oxidative burst activity will occur within one minute after binding, resulting in generation of reactive oxygen intermediates (55,56). However, this oxidative burst activity is "atypical" compared with other stimuli in that only hydrogen peroxide is released from the cell. The mechanism for the anomaly will be discussed later in the section on IAV.

Opsonization of the virus with antibody or complement may enhance binding to neutrophils. This may result in activation of the neutrophil through its Fc or complement receptors which initiates a number of neutrophil activities including phagocytosis and generation of oxygen intermediates (57,58). In the case of HSV-1, opsonization of viral particles with complement alone will increase

Table 9.2   Activation of neutrophils by viruses

Neutrophil Function	Virus	Selected References
Adherence to infected cells	Adenovirus Measles Polio RSV Rhinovirus	38, 39
Phagocytosis	Adenovirus Coxsachie CMV Herpes simplex Influenzae Measles Mumps Polio	40–46
Oxidative burst	Adenovirus Hepatitis B Influenzae Japanese encephalitis RSV Sendai	47–54

binding but HSV-specific antibody must be present to activate phagocytosis of the virus (59).

2.2 *Adherence of neutrophils to infected cells*

Viral infection of endothelial or fibroblasts *in vitro* will enhance adherence of neutrophils to these cells as shown in Table 2. If these neutrophils are activated, injury or death of the infected endothelial cells may occur (60,61). This adherence to infected cells by neutrophils may be enhanced by the presence of virus-specific antibody as is the case for RSV-infected cells but is not required for herpes simplex-infected cells (39,62). Complement will also fix to RSV-infected cells and this also will increase the adherence of neutrophils even in the absence of specific antibody (39).

2.3 *Activation of oxidative burst activity*

Several *in vitro* and *in vivo* studies indicate that oxidative burst activity in neutrophils may be activated directly by viruses or in viral infections. Direct binding of virus particles may initiate an oxidative burst as previously noted, possibly by direct binding to surface glycoproteins on the neutrophil (51,52,53). Oxidative metabolism may also be activated following phagocytosis of viral particles or binding to Fc or complement receptors if specific viral antibody is present.

In clinical studies it has been observed that neutrophils from the peripheral blood of patients with influenzae or adenoviral infections have elevated resting levels of oxidative metabolism (48,49). This could be due to the direct activation of the neutrophils by virus although the release of inflammatory cytokines such as interferon-gamma could also increase this activity. Many abnormalities in oxidative burst activity in neutrophils and monocytes from HIV patients have been described as will be discussed later.

3. Neutrophil Functions Inhibited by Viruses

There has long been an association between viral infections and neutrophil dysfunction. As previously noted most patients in the major influenzae epidemics died from bacterial pneumonia which was likely due to impairment of their neutrophils' capacity to fight bacteria. Table 3 lists some of the neutrophils functions impaired by virus, with influenzae being listed in every category. Patients with CMV and rubeola infections are also at much greater risk from dying from bacterial infections that is blamed in part on inhibition of neutrophil function (19,70,76,77).

Neutrophil and monocyte function are also impaired in HIV infection (78). This may be due to the direct effect of the virus, abnormality in cytokine production, formation of anti-neutrophil antibodies, or depletion of endogenous

Table 9.3   **Neutrophil functions inhibited by viruses**

Function	Viruses	Selected References
Chemotaxis	CMV Influenza Rubeola (measles) RSV HIV Herpes simplex	63–67
Phagocytosis	Hepatitis B Influenzae Mumps	68, 69
Cytotoxicity, Killing	CMV Hepatitis B Influenzae HIV Para influenza	67, 70, 71, 72
Oxidative Burst	Influenzae HIV CMV	73, 74, 75

oxygen scavengers such as glutathione. This inhibition of phagocytic cells further increases the patients' susceptibility to bacterial and fungal infections.

Viruses may also cause neutropenia due to impairment of neutrophil maturation in bone marrow. Parvovirus may cause anemia, thrombocytopenia, and neutropenia, which is of particular concern in patients already immunologically compromised by HIV infection or chemotherapy for cancer (79,80,81). Other viruses that commonly cause neutropenia in children include RSV, varicella, influenza A and B, measles, mumps, roseola, and rubella (82,83,84). The neutropenia will often develop in the first 48 hours of the illness and may last up to 8 days. The neutropenia may be due to the virus-induced redistribution of the neutrophils from the circulating to the marginating pool, and usually does not put the child at great risk for serious infection. Other viruses such as Epstein-Barr, hepatitis, and HIV may cause a more protracted neutropenia due to infection of the hematopoietic stem cells or formation of immune complexed that bind to neutrophils, causing them to be sequestered in the spleen (85,86).

4. Neutrophils and Influenza A Virus

Many viruses may exert inhibitory effects on neutrophil function as previously noted, but effects of influenza A virus (IAV) on neutrophils is unique and also of great medical significance. The clinical importance is due to the thousands of deaths from bacterial pneumonia that occur every year following a bout of flu due to IAV. The interactions between virus and neutrophil is unique due to the ability of the virus to activate the cell in an abnormal fashion. These interactions have been examined extensively by Abramson, Tauber and others, and a listing of some of the interactions are shown in Table 4 (6,70,87).

The IAV has hemagglutinin molecules on its surface that bind to specific residues on glycoproteins on neutrophil membranes including CD43 (88,89). Desialation of the neutrophil by neurominidase treatment which alters these binding sites will inhibit IAV binding and activation (or deactivation) of the neutrophil by the virus. Crosslinking of these bound viruses by antibody enhances the ability of the virus to activate the neutrophil (87).

The exposure to the virus will cause a marked inhibition of phosphorylation of multiple membrane and cytosolic proteins that are part of the activation process that occurs following stimulation with such agents as N-formyl methionyl-leucylphenylalanine (FMLP) (90,91,92). This would suggest that IAV is altering G-protein function in the neutrophil. Binding of IAV to the neutrophil also results in a rise in intracellular calcium that is independent of extracellular calcium unlike stimulation with FMLP which is dependent on extracellular calcium (6,93).

IAV also stimulates the production of hydrogen peroxide from neutrophils but this occurs without the concominant release of superoxide anion as occurs with other activators of oxidative burst activity (94,95). More extensive studies indicate that this stimuation of respiratory burst activity by IAV occurs at an intracellular location rather than at the membrane as would be the normal response (6,56,70,73). Thus, all of the superoxide anion which is generated

Table 9.4   Influenza a virus (IAV) effects on neutrophils

• Unopsonized IAV stimulates aberrant oxidative burst on binding to neutrophil

• Impairs fusion of primary and secondary granules with cell membrane

• Inhibits lysosome-phagosome fusion

• Decreases G-protein function in the activation process

• Interferes with G-protein phosphorylation

• Inhibits neutrophil chemotaxis

• Greatly increases binding (>500 times) of neutrophils to IAV-infected epithelium cells

• Interferes with neutrophil cytoskeletal protein function

• Stimulates intracellular calcium mobilization

• Stimulates neutrophil membrane depolarization

---

first has been converted to hydrogen peroxide by the time it was released from the cell or had been scavenged by the cell components. Stimuation of neutrophils with IAV does not result in extracellular release of granule contents as would occur with stimulation with agents such as FMLP (94).

These aberrations in activation that occur with IAV make neutrophil resistant to activation by other stimuli, thus, making it much less effective in its normal host defense functions such as chemotaxis and bacterial killing. IAV causes similar defects in non-oxidative neutrophil functions using cells from patients with CGD, suggesting the defects are not dependent on the abnormal release of oxygen intermediates. Inhibition of fusion of primary and secondary granules with the plasma membrane occurs with exposure to the IAV may account for defects in chemotaxis and other functions (95,96,97,98).

Some of the abnormalities in neutrophil activation that occurs with IAV may be partially prevented by priming the neutrophils with GM-CSF and G-CSF (99,100). This suggests that cytokines such as GM-CSF and G-CSF may be useful in overcoming the inhibition of neutrophil function that occurs in patients infected with IAV, and would have the added benefit of increasing the neutrophil number and enhancing neutrophil function.

5. Neutrophils and HIV

The devastating effects of HIV infection on the immune system by destruction of CD4 lymphocytes is compounded by many impairments of neutrophil function that have been reported in this disease. Children infected with HIV are particularly vulnerable to bacterial infections as their naive immune systems have not developed the repertoire of antibodies needed to combat the more common bacterial infections. The death rates from bacterial infections in AIDS patients are also higher in less developed parts of the world where antibiotics are not as accessible as was the case in the pre-antibiotic era when thousands of patients died from bacterial pneumonia during the influenzae epidemics secondary to inhibition of their neutrophils by the influenza virus. The number of neutrophils is also decreased in many HIV patients due to anti-neutrophil antibodies present in many of these patients, myleodysplastic changes in the marrow, and some of the anti-retroviral drugs. In this section we will discuss some of the abnormalities in neutrophil function found in HIV patients, the mechanisms responsible for these abnormalities, and the role of neutrophils in the progression of HIV infection.

5.1 *Myelodysplastic changes in HIV infection*

Several reports have indicated that the myeloid precursor cells in the marrow of AIDS patients may be infected with HIV, leading to inhibition of myelopoeisis (101,102). HIV-RNA is present in the myeloid precursor cells from bone marrow aspirates of AIDS patients which may alter their differentiation (103). Donahue, *et al* reported that bone marrow progenitor cells for monocytes maybe infected *in vitro* with HIV (104). Infections of myeloid progenitor cells by HIV was shown more directly by Folks *et al* who showed that purified CD34[+] cells from human bone marrow could be infected with HIV-1 (105). Abnormalities in the myeloid stromal cells have also been reported in the marrow of HIV patients which may also contribute to the myelodysplastic changes (106).

5.2 *HIV infection of neutrophils*

Although neutrophils lack the CD4 receptor which is the usual route of entry of HIV, there is evidence that neutrophils in the peripheral blood of AIDS patients carry the virus. Spear, *et al.* found that 2 out of 10 patients he studied had neutrophils that contained HIV DNA copies detected by chemilumnescense, and that the number of DNA copies was much less in the neutrophils as compared to the patients lymphocytes (107). The presence of the HIV DNA in the neutrophils may come about by infection of the myeloid precursor cells as noted above, and the infected neutrophils would likely have a decreased life span and abnormal function in the peripheral blood (108,109). There is also evidence that neutrophils may be infected by direct fusion of the HIV envelope will the cell membrane (110,111).

In later studies (1993), Gabrilovich, *et al* was able to detect HIV DNA by polymerase chain reaction (PCR) in the neutrophils of 30% of his HIV-patients (112). Detection of the HIV DNA in neutrophils was more common in symptomatic (47%) than in asymptomatic (18%) patients, and also more common in patients with recurrent bacterial pneumonias and *Pneumocystis carinili* pneumonia. The detectable HIV DNA was also more common in patients with neutropenia and with low CD4/CD8 ratios (113). They suggested that infection of the neutrophils in these patients leads to impairment in neutrophil function.

5.3 *Anti-neutrophil antibodies in HIV infection*

Neutropenia occurs in 20 to 40% of AIDS patients and, in addition to faulty myelopoiesis, this neutropenia may be due to autoimmune antibodies to neutrophils or to the deposition of immune complexes on the neutrophil surface (114,115). Although granulocyte-associated immunoglobulins that are not specifically bound may occur in over 20% of asymptomatic HIV-infected subjects (116), neutrophil-specific antibody also occur in many patients (117). Stroncek, *et al*, (118) studied 100 HIV-infected patients, and found granulocyte antibodies in 66% of the samples by granulocyte immunoflouresence (GIF) and in 21% of the samples by granulocyte agglutination (GA). Further testing showed some of the GIF positive samples were due to the presence of immune complexes on the neutrophils. However, those sera samples positive by GA were due to antibodies directed against neutrophils themselves. The presence of these autoimmune antibodies may contribute to neutropenia in some patients.

5.4 *Neutrophil chemotaxis in HIV infection*

Neutrophil chemotaxis is reported by several investigators to be markedly depressed although the mechanism underlying this defect is unclear. Defects in adult homosexual males with presumed HIV infection were noted as early as 1984, before the virus itself was identified (119). This finding was thought to account for the increased number of bacterial infections in these patients and was confirmed in later studies (120,121). Lazzarin, *et al*, reported also that neutrophil chemotaxis was defective in HIV infected adult males regardless of how they acquired the infection (122). In 1990 Roillides, *et al,* found neutrophil chemotaxis in defective in HIV infected children and was more profound in children with more advanced disease (123). They also reported this defect was partially corrected by incubation in GM-CSF. In a longitudinal study of HIV-infected males neutrophil chemotaxis was inhibited 19% compared to normal controls and this inhibition increased to 32% after 3 years in follow-up studies in this same group of patients (124). Phagocytosis of neutrophils and monocytes has also been reported to be depressed in AIDS patients using *Staphylococcus aureus* as the target cell (125).

5.5 *Abnormalities in respiratory burst activity*

The production of ROI by neutrophils is necessary for killing of many bacteria and fungi to which HIV patients are susceptible, but excess production of ROI can damage host tissue as occurs in autoimmune disease. Unfortunately, HIV patients are at risk for both infections and autoimmune disease. In an early paper (126) nitroblue tetrazolium (NBT) reduction, a measure of ROI production, was increased in patients in the early stages of HIV disease but decreased in patients with advanced AIDS. In 1993, Pitrak (127) reported that superoxide production was decreased in HIV patients, and that the impairment in superoxide production was more pronounced in patients with lower CD4 cell counts. However, Bandres, *et al*, using a flow cytometric technique to measure ROI release, found greater ROI production in neutrophils from HIV patients as compared to controls (128). This finding of greater production of ROI with neutrophils from HIV patients was confirmed in 1995, also using a flow cytometric method (129). Laursen, *et al*, using chemiluminescence to measure ROI production, found lower responses in HIV patients who previously had had *Pneumocytis carinii* pneumomonia but not in patients with less advanced disease (130). Our laboratory reported decreased superoxide production in neutrophils and monocytes from HIV infected children and adults using the cytochrome C reduction technique in a 2 hour assay (74). Production of hydrogen peroxide was also decreased in HIV patients in this study that measured production for 90 minutes.

Thus, many abnormalities in the respiratory burst activity of neutrophils and monocytes from HIV infected patients have been reported but the findings are sometimes conflicting. Some investigator report that neutrophils from HIV patient are in a more primed state and have a greater respiratory burst activity while other have found the ability of neutrophils to generate ROI in HIV patients is decreased compared to that of controls. Although some of these differences may be due to differences in technique or the population studied, another explanation might be that neutrophils in these patients do tend to be exposed to more stimuli, such as chronic fungus or parasitic infections, that would place them in more activated state, requiring less provocation to initiate a respiratory burst. However, HIV patients also have decreased levels of glutathione in their plasma and white cells, which acts as an antioxidant to protect neutrophils from their own ROI.

Thus, the respiratory burst may be more easily initiated in HIV patients, but production of ROI cannot be as sustained as long as that of controls possibly due to the impairment to the neutrophils themselves by their own ROI. This inability of neutrophils to protect themselves may also be reflected by the accelerated rate of apoptosis in neutrophils from HIV patients as demonstrated by various techniques (131). The percentage of neutrophils undergoing apoptosis was 2 to 3 fold higher at 3 to 18 hours after isolation in the HIV group. Apoptosis could be greatly reduced in the patients cells if they were incubated in G-CSF.

5.6 *Neutrophil cytotoxicity in HIV infection*

The defects in neutrophil motility and ROI production noted in HIV patients make it not surprising that defects in neutrophil cytotoxicity are also found in HIV patients. Neutrophils from AIDS patients were significantly slower in killing *Staphylococcus aureas* as compared to normal controls in a study performed at the NIH (132). Roillides, *et al*, also reported a defect in *S. aureas* killing using neutrophils from HIV-infected children (67). He later reported that neutrophils from HIV-infected children were also impaired in their ability to kill *Aspergillas fimigatus*, and that this defect could be partially corrected with G-CSF (133). A defect in killing another fungi, candida, was reported to occur in adult AIDS patients which was attributed to impairment of non-oxidative killing mechanisms (134).

Antibody-dependent cellular cytotoxicity (ADCC) is a mechanism for killing HIV-infected lymphocytes as well as other cells, and defects in ADCC have been found in HIV patients. Neutrophils from HIV patients were reported to be defective in ADCC using herpes infected cells and chicken erythrocytes as target cells (135,136). Our laboratory reported that the ADCC of neutrophils from HIV-infected children was defective compared to age-matched controls using an HIV-coated cells as our target (137). In a later study we reported that some of the defects in ADCC in neutrophils from HIV patients could be corrected by N-aectyl-cysteine, which restores the anti-oxidant glutathione found to be decreased in HIV patients (13). Thus, cytokines such as G-CSF and anti-oxidants may play a role in improving the defective neutrophil cytotoxicity found in HIV-infected patients.

6. Conclusion

The interactions between neutrophils and virus is complex and its clinical significance is still not fully understood. Although neutrophils can be shown to inhibit or destroy viruses *in vitro*, we are not certain how important these anti-viral mechanism are *in vivo*.

The ability of viruses to inhibit neutrophils, however, is better documented and can be of upmost importance in epidemics of viral disease. Influenza still continues to take its toll, due in large part to its ability to make the patient much more susceptible to life-threatening bacterial infections. The modern epidemic, HIV infection, also results in depression of neutrophil function, which is particularly devastating in children and in underdeveloped countries where antibiotics are much less available. Neutrophils are, however, able to kill HIV-infected cells in the presence of antibodies by ADCC. Neutrophil-mediated ADCC may become of greater importance if anti-HIV vaccine lead to production of antibodies more effecient in HIV-infected cells.

References

1. Lehrer, R.I., *et al.*, *J. Virol.* **54** (1985), 467.
2. Van Strijp, J.A.G., *et al.*, *J. Gen. Virol.* **71** (1990), 1205–1209.
3. Lehrer, R.I. and Ganz T., *Blood* **76** (1990), 2169–2181.
4. Levy, O., *Eur. J. Haematol.* **56** (1996), 263–277.
5. Turner, R.B., *Pediatr. Infect. Dis. J.* **9** (1990), 832–835.
6. Hartshorn, K.L., Karnad, A.B., Tauber, A.I., *J. Leuk. Biol.* **47** (1990), 176–186.
7. McFarlane, P.S., Speers, A.L., Sommerville, R.G., *Lancet* **1** (1967), 408.
8. Jones, J.R., *Pediatr. Res.* **16** (1982), 525.
9. Henricks, P.A.J., van der Tol, M.E., Verhoef, J., *Scand. J. Immunol.* **22** (1985), 721–725.
10. Oleske, J. M., *et al*, *Clin. Exp. Immunol.* **27** (1977), 446.
11. Siebens, H., Trevethia, S.S., Babior, B.M., *Blood* **54** (1979), 88.
12. Grewal, A.S., Carpio, M., Babiuk, L.A., *Can. J. Microbiol.* **26** (1980), 427–435.
13. Roberts, R.L., Aroda, V.R., Ank, B.J., *J. Infect. Dis.* **172** (1995), 1492–502.
14. Grewal, A.S., Rouse, B.T., Babiuk, L.A., *J. Immunol.* **124** (1980), 312.
15. Benne, C.A., *et al.*, *European Journal of Immunology* **4** (1997), 886–90.
16. Lu, J., *Bioessays* **6** (1997), 509–18.
17. Nakashima, H., Yamamoto, N., Masuda, M., Fujii, N.,
18. Harmsen, M.C., *et al.*, *J. Infect. Dis.* **172** (1995), 380–388.

19. Faden, H. and Ogra, P., *Pediatr. Infect. Dis.* **5** (1986), 86–92.
20. Dankner, W.M., *et al.*, *J. Infect. Dis.* **161** (1990), 31–36.
21. Rice, G.P.A., Schrier, R.D., Oldstone, M.B.A., *Proc. Natl. Acad. Sci. USA* **81** (1984), 6134–6138.
22. Hoar, D.I., Bowen, T., Matheson, D., Poon, M.C., *Blood* **66** (1985), 1251–1253.
23. in *Human Cytokines: Their Role in Disease and Therapy*, ed. Aggarwal, B.B. and Puri, R.K. (Blackwell Science, Massachusetts, 1995),
24. Belding, M.E., Klebanoff, S.J., Ray, C.G., *Science* **167** (1970), 195.
25. Roberts, R.L., Ank, B.J., Stiehm, E.R., *Pediatr. Res.* **36** (1994), 792–798.
26. Ennen, J. and Kurth, R., *Immunology* **78** (1993), 171–176.
27. Oleske, J.M., *et al.*, *Clin. Exp. Immunol.* **27** (1977), 446.
28. Siebens, H., Trevethia, S.S., Babior, B.M., *Blood* **54** (1979), 88.
29. Smith, J.W. and Sheppard, A.M., *Infect. Immun.* **36** (1982), 685.
30. Wardley, R.C., Rouse, B.T., Babiuk, L.A., *J. Reticuloendothel. Soc.* **19** (1976), 323.
31. Grewal, A.S., Rouse, B.T., Babiuk, L.A., *Infect. Immun.* **15** (1977), 698.
32. Hashimoto, G., Wright, P.F., Karzon, D.T., *Infect. Immun.* **42** (1983), 214.
33. Hashimoto, G., Wright, P.F., Karzon, D.T., *J. Infect. Dis.* **148** (1983), 785.
34. Baldwin, G.C., *et al.*, *Blood* **74** (1989), 1673–1677.
35. Kaul, T. N., *et al.*, *Clin. Exp. Immunol.* **56** (1984), 501.
36. Kaul, T.N., Welliver, R.C., Ogra, P.L., *J. Med. Virol.* **9** (1982), 149.
37. Cines, D.B., *et al.*, *J. Clin. Invest.* **69** (1982), 123.
38. MacGregor, R.R., *et al.*, *J. Clin. Invest.* **65** (1980), 1469.
39. Faden, H., Hong, J.J., Ogra, P.L., *J. Virol.* **52** (1984), 16.
40. Sommerville, R.G. and MacFarlane, P.S., *Lancet* **1** (1963), 911.
41. Sommerville, R.G., *Prog. Med. Virol.* **10** (1968), 398.
42. Kovac, E., *et al.*, *Life Sci.* **2** (1963), 901.
43. Rinaldo, C.R., Balck, P.H., Hirsch, M., *J. Infect. Di.s* **136** (1977), 667.
44. Boand, A.V., Kern, J.E., Hansen, R.J., *J. Immunol.* **79** (1957), 416.
45. Abramson, J.S., Lyles, D.S., Heller, K.A., *J. Clin. Invest.* **69** (1982), 1393.
46. Padawar, J., *J. Reticuloendothel. Soc.* (1971), 923.
47. Rosenbaum, M.J., *et al.*, *Proc. Soc. Exp. Biol. Med.* **146** (1974), 868.
48. Sieber, O.F., Wilska, M.L., Riggin, R., *Pediatrics* **58** (1976), 122.
49. Hellum, K.B. and Solberg, C.O., *Lancet* **1** (1971), 1181.
50. Vierucci, A., *et al.*, *Pediatr. Res.* **17** (1983), 814.
51. Mills, E.L., *et al.*, *Infect. Immun.* **32** (1981), 1200.
52. Peterhans, E., *Biochem. Biophys. Res. Commun.* **91** (1979), 383.

53. Peterhans, E., *Virology* **105** (1980), 445.
54. Faden, H., *et al.*, *Blood* **58** (1981), 221.
55. Wheele,r J.G., *et al.*, *J. Leuk. Biol.* **47** (1990), 332–343.
56. Kazhdan, M., White, M.R., Tauber, A.I., Hartshorn, K.L., *J. Leuk. Biol.* **56** (1994), 59–64.
57. Ehlenberger, A.G. and Nussenzweig, V., *J. Exp. Med.* **145** (1983), 357–371.
58. Van Strijp ,J.A.G., *Arch. Virol.* **104** (1989), 287–298.
59. Van Strijp, J.A.G., Van Kessel, K.P.M., van der Tol, M.E., Verhoef, J., *J. Clin. Invest.* **84** (1989), 107–112.
60. Boeke, D.J., *et al.*, *J. Exp. Med.* **134 (Suppl)** (1971), 330–336.
61. Gower, R.G., *et al.*, *J. Allergy Clin. Immunol.* **62** (1978), 222–228.
62. Capsoni, F., *et al.*, *Scand. J. Immunol.* **36** (1992), 541–546.
63. Tannous, R., Meyers, M.G., *N. Engl. J. Med.* **300** (1979), 1345–1349.
64. Rinaldo, C.R., Stossel, T.P., Black, P.H., Hirsch, M.S., *Clin. Immunol. Immunopathol.* **12** (1979), 331–334.
65. Abramson, J.S., Lyles, D.S., Heller, K.A., Bass, D.A., *Infect. Immun.* **37** (1982), 794–799.
66. McMhesney, M.B. and Oldstone, M.B., *Adv. Immunol.* **45** (1989), 335–380.
67. Roilides, E., *et al.*, *J. Pediatr.* **117** (1990), 531–540.
68. Maggiore, G., *et al.*, *Am. J. Dis. Child* **137** (1983), 768–770.
69. Abramson, J.S., *et al.*, *J. Clin. Invest.* **9** (1982), 1393–1397.
70. Abramson, J.S. and Wheeler J.G., *Pediatr. Infect. Dis. J.* **13** (1994), 643–652.
71. Davies, D.H., McCarthy, A.R., Keen, K.L., *Vet. Microbiol.* **12** (1986), 147–159.
72. Jakab, G.J., Warr, G.A., Sannes, P.L., *Infect. Immun.* **27** (1980), 960–968.
73. Ertürk, M., Jennings, R., Oxley, K.M., Hastings, M.J.G., *Med. Microbiol. Immunol.* **178** (1989), 199–209.
74. Chen, T.P., *et al.*, *Pediatr. Res.* **34** (1993), 544–550.
75. Winston, D.J., Stevens, P, Lin C.H., Gale, R.P., *Clin. Res.* **29** (1981), 398.
76. Abramson, J.S. and Mills, E.L., *Reviews of Infectious Diseases* **10** (1988), 326–341
77. Hartshorn, K.L., Daignault, D., Tauber, A.I., in *Inflammation: Basic Principles and Clinical Correlates, Second Edition*, ed. Gallin, J.I., Goldstein, I.M., Snyderman, R. (Raven, New York, 1992), 1017–1031.
78. Shyur, S. and Hill, H.R., in *Immunology of HIV Infection*, ed. Gupta S. (Plenum, New York, 1996), 377–386.
79. Brown, K.E. and Young, N.S., *Blood Reviews* **9** (1995), 176–182.
80. Pont, J., *et al.*, *British J. Haematology* **80** (1992), 160–165.

81. McClain, K., Estrov, Z., Chen, H., Mahoney, Jr.D.H., *British J. Haematology* **85** (1993), 57–62.
82. Boxer, L.A. and Blackwood, R.A., *Pediatrics in Review* **17** (1996), 19–28, 47–50.
83. Sievers, E.L. and Dale, D.C., *Blood Reviews* **10** (1996), 95–100.
84. Kaplan, C., Morinet, F., Cartron, J., *Seminars in Hematology* **29** (1992), 34–44.
85. Sammons, W.A.H. and Medearis, Jr.D.N., *Pediatr. Inf. Dis. J.* **7** (1988), 887–888.
86. Klaassen, R.J.L., *et al.*, *British J. Haematology* **77** (1991), 398–402.
87. Daigneault, D.E., *et al.*, *Blood* **80** (1992), 3227–3234.
88. Hartshorn, K.L., *et al.*, *J. Immunol.* **154** (1995), 3952–3960.
89. Rothwell, S.W. and Wright, D.G., *J. Immunol.* **152** (1994), 2358.
90. Caldwell, S.E., Cassidy, L.F., Abramson, J.S., *J. Immunol.* **140** (1988), 3560–3567.
91. Hartshorn, K.L., *et al.*, *Blood* **75** (1990), 218–226.
92. Hartshorn, K.L., *et al.*, *Blood* **79** (1992), 1049–1057.
93. Hartshorn, K.L., *et al.*, *J. Immunol.* **141** (1988), 1295–1301.
94. Coope,r Jr. J.A.D., Carcelen, R., Culbreth, R., *J. Infect. Dis.* **173** (1996), 279–284.
95. Abramson, J.S., *et al.*, *Blood* **64** (1984), 131–138.
96. Abramson, J.S., *et al.*, *J. Clin. Invest.* **9** (1982), 1393–1397.
97. Moore, D.L. and Mills, E.L., *Blood* **70** (1987), 351–355.
98. Abramson, J.S., *et al.*, *J. Infect. Dis.* **154** (1986), 456.
99. Abramson, J.S., *et al.*, *J. Leuk. Biol.* **50** (1991), 160–166.
100. Abramson, J.S. and Hudnor H.R., *Blood* **83** (1994), 1929–1934.
101. Thiele, J., *et al.*, *Analytical Cellular Pathology* **3** (1996), 141–157.
102. Rosenberg, Z.F. and Fauci ,A.S., *Adv. Immunol.* **47** (1989), 377–431.
103. Busch, M., Beckstead, J., Gantz, D., Vyas, G., *Blood* **68 (Suppl)** (1986), 122A.
104. Donahue, R.E., *et al.*, *Nature* **326** (1987), 200–203.
105. Folks, T.M., *et al.*, *Science* **242** (1988), 919–922.
106. Ganser, A., *Blut* **56** (1988), 49–53.
107. Spear, G.T., *et al.*, *J. Infect. Dis.* **162** (1990), 1239–1244.
108. Zon, L.I. and Groopman, J.E., Seminars in Hematology, **25** (1988), 208–218.
109. Scadden, D.T., Zon, L.I., Groopman, J.E., *Blood* **74** (1989), 1455–1463.
110. Hoxie, J.A., Rackowski, J.L., Haggarty, B.S., Gaulton, G.N., *J Immunol* **140** (1988), 786–795.
111. Maddon, P.J., *et al.*, *Cell* **54** (1988), 865–874.

112. Gabrilovich, D.I., et al., J. Acquired Immune Deficiency Syndromes 6 (1993), 587–591.

113. Gabrilovich, D.I., et al., Zhurnal Mikrobiologii, Epidemiologii Immunobiologii 5 (1995), 52–55.

114. Minchinton, R.M. and Frazer I., Lancet 1 (1985), 936–937.

115. Murphy, M.F., et al., Lancet 1 (1985), 217–218.

116. Celton, J.L., et al., Nouv. Rev. Fr. Hematol. 31 (1989), 187–188.

117. Klaassen, R.J.L., Vlekke, A.B.J., von dem Borne, A.E.G. Kr., British J. Haematology 77 (1991), 403–409.

118. Stroncek, D.F., et al., J. Lab. Clin. Med. 119 (1992), 724–731.

119. Valone, F.H., Payan, D.G., Abrams, D.J., Goetzl, E.J., J. Infect. Dis. 150 (1984), 267–271.

120. Nielsen, H., Kharazmi, A., Faber, V., Scand. J. Immunol. 24 (1986), 291–296.

121. Martin, L.S., Spira, T.J., Orloff, S.L., Holman, R.C., J. Leuk. Biol. 44 (1988), 361–366.

122. Lazzarin, A., et al., Clin. Exp. Immunol. 65 (1986), 105–111.

123. Roilides, E., et al., J. Pediatr. 117 (1990), 531–540.

124. Flo, R.W., et al., AIDS 8 (1994), 771–777.

125. Pos, O., et al., Clin. Exp. Immunol. 88 (1992), 23–28.

126. Sönnerborg, A. and Jarstrand, C., Scand. J. Infect. Dis. 18 (1986), 101–103.

127. Pitrak, D.L., et al., J. Infect. Di.s 167 (1993) 1406–1410.

128. Bandres, J.C., Musher, D.M., Rossen, R.D., J. Infect. Dis. 168 (1993), 75–83.

129. Elbim, C., et al., Blood 84 (1994), 2759–2766.

130. Laursen, A.L., Rungby, J., Andersen, P.L., J. Infect. Dis. 172 (1995), 497–505.

131. Pitrak, D.L., et al., J. Clin. Invest. 98 (1996), 2714–2719.

132. Murphy, P.M., Lane, H.C., Fauci, A.S., Gallin, J.I., J. Infect. Dis. 158 (1988), 627–630.

133. Roilides, E., et al., J. Infect. Dis. 167 (1993), 905–911.

134. Wenisch, C., et al., AIDS 10 (1996), 983–987.

135. Shah, T.P. and Sattler, F.R., J. Infect. Dis. 155 (1987), 594–595

136. Kinne, T.J. and Gupta, S., J. Clin. Lab. Immunol. 30 (1989), 153–156.

137. Szelc, C.M., Mitcheltree, C., Roberts, R.L., Stiehm, E.R., J. Infect. Dis. 166 (1992), 486–493.

CHAPTER 10

USE OF COLONY-STIMULATING FACTORS FOR TREATMENT OF NEUTROPENIA AND INFECTIOUS DISEASES

David C. Dale and Steve Nelson[1]

The "colony-stimulating factors" are growth-promoting substances for the hematopoietic cells. This term was introduced by Bradley & Metcalf in 1966, when they demonstrated that specific factors derived from living cells can stimulate hematopoietic precursors to form colonies and clusters of cells in an *in vitro* culture system [1]. In a series of critical experiments they demonstrated that these factors can be detected in serum, urine and other body fluids, using their colony-forming assay [2–4]. They also demonstrated that endotoxin injections and experimental infections, conditions known to increase blood neutrophil levels, are associated with enhanced production and secretion of these factors [4,5]. Currently three hematopoietic growth factors are called colony-stimulating factors (CSF). These are granulocyte-CSF (G-CSF), granulocyte macrophage colony-stimulating factor (GM-CSF) and macrophage-CSF (M-CSF). A fourth factor, originally called multi-CSF, is now usually referred to as Interleukin-3 (IL-3). A number of other interleukins (IL-1 through IL-18), as well as erythropoietin (EPO) and thrombopoietin (TPO), and several

---

[1]Correspondence to:Steve Nelson, MD, John H. Seabury Professor of Medicine, Pulmonary/ Critical Care Medicine, Louisiana State University Medical Center, 1901 Perdido Street, Suite 3205, New Orleans, LA 70112 1393, Telephone: 504-568-4634, Fax: 504-568-4295, Email: snelso1@lsumc.edu

other factors, are known regulators of the hematopoietic process. This chapter focuses on G-CSF and GM-CSF, the factors principally influencing neutrophil production and function.

1. Characteristics of G-CSF, GM-CSF and its Receptors

G-CSF was first described as a stimulatory factor present in serum of mice after endotoxin injections [6,7]. Murine and human G-CSF were subsequently identified and purified, and the G-CSF cDNA was subsequently isolated from a bladder carcinoma cell line [8–10]. Native human G-CSF is a glycosolated protein containing 174 amino acids, coded for by a gene on chromosome 17 [11]. Recombinant human G-CSF and the native molecule have similar functional and pharmacological effects *in vivo* and *in vitro*.

Murine and human GM-CSF were purified and characterized in 1977, several years before G-CSF [12]. Human GM-CSF is a glycoprotein containing 127 amino acids and is coded for by a gene on chromosome 5, contiguous to the genes for several hematopoietic growth factors [13]. In contrast to G-CSF, which shows close homologies across many species, GM-CSF shows greater sequence heterogeneity and is relatively species-specific in its activities. Both GM-CSF and G-CSF are composed of four anti-parallel, helical peptide segments connected by amino acid chains, which give the molecules their three-dimensional structure [14,15]. Specificity is determined by the CSF's amino acid sequence and the three dimensional structure of its binding domain, as well as the presence and integrity of the cellular receptor.

Humans have one class of high affinity receptors for G-CSF which are composed of two identical molecules, i.e., they are homodimers [16]. The binding of G-CSF to its receptor induces intracellular protein tyrosine phosphorylation and activates various signaling cascades leading to induction of gene transcription. The JAK tyrosine kinases, signal transducers and activators of transcription (STAT) proteins and the ras-MAP kinases are involved in this process [17]. Distinctive regions of the internal domain of the G-CSF receptor are required for the separable processes of proliferation and maturation of myeloid cells bearing the G-CSF receptor [18].

By contrast, the GM-CSF receptor is a heterodimer, i.e., composed of two dissimilar transmembrane proteins, an alpha and a beta chain [19,20]. The high affinity GM-CSF receptor is found on all types of granulocyte precursors, including eosinophils, as well as blood and marrow monocytes and their precursors. By contrast, G-CSF receptors are present only on cells of the neutrophilic lineage. GM-CSF also activates cells bearing its receptor through the JAK kinases, as well as the Jun kinase pathway to ras-MAP kinase activation [21,22]. Although low affinity G-CSF and GM-CSF receptors have been found on various non-hematopoietic and cancer cells, the functional significance of these receptors is largely unknown.

2. Neutrophil and Monocyte Development and Function

Neutrophils are derived from the common hematopoietic stem cells through processes of proliferation, differentiation and maturation. Overall this process normally takes ten to fourteen days, as estimated by *in vivo* radioisotopic labeling studies. Morphologically the earliest recognizable neutrophil precursors are the myeloblasts, large cells which have few cytoplasmic granules. Differentiation and maturation involves the condensation of the nuclear chromatin, development of primary and secondary granules, accumulation of cytoplasmic glycogen and actin filaments, acquisition of specific surface adherence proteins and receptors, and a number of other refinements in these cells. A unique feature for cells of the neutrophilic series is the production and storage in the marrow of a large population of relatively mature cells which are normally released from the marrow to the blood in response to infections. Their release can also be stimulated by glucocorticosteroid, endotoxin, G-CSF or GM-CSF administration [23–25].

Neutrophils are formed in the extravascular spaces of the marrow and enter the blood by movement through pores or fenestrae in the marrow vasculature. In the blood they are found in two pools in dynamic equilibrium. About half of the cells flow along with the circulating red blood and are regarded to be in the circulating pool. Other cells are in the marginal pool. The marginated cells are loosely adherent to vascular endothelial cells throughout the circulation, although the lung, spleen and tissues with capillaries with low blood flow rates may preferentially hold these cells. Adherence proteins, e.g., the selectins which are expressed on the surface of neutrophils, are thought to regulate the loose and reversible adherence of these cells, which creates the marginal pool. Firm adherence, mediated by leukocyte integrins, is a necessary and final step before neutrophils migrate from the blood to the tissues [26].

Neutrophils serve as the "first line" cells of the acute inflammatory response in all body tissues. The rapidity of this response is easily demonstrated by examining the cutaneous inflammatory response by the skin chamber or Rebuck skin window technique. Neutrophils can be measured to migrate to the site of injury and accumulate in large numbers over a few hours. Although bacteremia is a relatively common event in severely neutropenic patients, it is generally a consequence of an inadequate tissue response to contain infection. Ordinarily bacterial clearance from the blood is a function of the fixed phagocytes lining the vasculature in the spleen, liver, lung, marrow and other tissues.

At the inflammatory site, neutrophils engulf bacteria and other foreign debris in a phagocytic vacuole into which microbicidal and proteolytic enzymes are released, resulting in killing and digestion of the invading organism. Many details of this process have been dissected through the recognition of genetic diseases such as chronic granulomatous disease and disorders of neutrophil granule proteins such as myeloperoxidase. Most frequently, however, failure of neutrophils to adequately contain a tissue infection is attributable to a deficiency in their number, rather than their function. Because the colony-stimulating factors are potent agents to increase the rate of phagocyte production, as well as stimulators of phagocyte functions, there are many ways in which they may potentially be used to improve the outcome for infectious diseases

The hematopoietic growth factors play an important role in all stages of neutrophil development and deployment. The earliest precursors, the hematopoietic stem cells, appear to have multiple growth factor receptors [27]. As cells mature the number and function of these receptors evolves, but uniquely, G-CSF and GM-CSF receptors are present both early in the developmental process and on mature neutrophils [16,20]. In the *in vitro* colony-forming assay system, G-CSF predominantly stimulates the formation of neutrophilic cells from early precursors, whereas GM-CSF stimulates a more diverse pattern of cell formation, with colonies and clusters of cells of all lineages. Complete maturation of erythroid and megakaryocytic cells, however, requires the addition of other factors, i.e., erythropoietin and thrombopoietin.

In vitro incubation of G-CSF and GM-CSF with mature blood neutrophils primes these cells for an enhanced metabolic burst when exposed to a second agonist such as FMLP, opsonized zymosan particles, or other stimuli [28]. The respiratory burst which follows this response leads to production of microbicidal concentrations of superoxide anion and hydrogen peroxide, thus suggesting that these cytokines may play a direct role in enhancing the killing of bacteria and fungi [29–32]. In addition, neutrophils previously exposed to these CSFs have an enhanced antibody dependence, cell-mediated cytotoxicity against certain tumor cells (see Tables 1 and 2).

Our best information on the *in vivo* effects of G-CSF and GM-CSF comes from studies of the administration of these factors to normal human subjects or hematologically normal patients. In this setting it is known that the proliferation of hematopoietic precursor cells is enhanced by G-CSF and GM-CSF, as reflected *in vivo* by marrow cell numbers, the proportion of cells in mitosis, and a more rapid transit of cells through the marrow to the blood

Table 10.1   Effects of G-CSF on phagocytes

Precursor cells:
- Stimulation of proliferation and differentiation to neutrophils.

Effects on mature neutrophils:
- Enhanced respiratory burst
- Increased phagocytosis of bacteria and fungi
- Increased presence of C3bi receptor (CD-35)
- Upregulated affinity for the ligand of the LAM-1 receptor
- Stimulates chemotaxis at low concentrations, decreases at high concentrations
- Decreases migration in skin chamber assay
- Enhanced neutrophilic antibody-dependent cell-mediated cytotoxicity (ADCC) against certain tumor cells

Table 10.2   Effects of GM-CSF on phagocytes

Precursor cells:

• Stimulation of proliferation and differentiation of precursors to neutrophils, eosinophils and monocyte/macrophages.

Effects on mature neutrophil granulocytes:

• Enhanced respiratory burst
• Increased phagocytosis of bacteria and fungi
• Increased presence of C3bi receptor
• Loss of leukocyte adhesion molecule-1 (LAM-1)
• Upregulated affinity for the ligand of the LAM-1 receptor
• Stimulates chemotaxis at low concentrations, decreases at high concentrations
• Decreases migration on skin chamber assay
• Enhanced neutrophilic antibody-dependent cell-mediated cytotoxicity (ADCC) against certain tumor cells

Effects on mature macrophages/monocytes:

• Increased *in vitro* effect against M. avium and M. tuberculosis; Leishmania and Trypanosoma
• Increased cytokine expression/secretion
• Enhanced ADDC against tumor cells *in vitro*
• Enhanced antitumor response *in vitro* in combination with endotoxin, interferon gamma and lipopolysaccarides

---

[24,25]. Both G-CSF and GM-CSF can accelerate neutrophil maturation through the post mitotic/maturational compartment.

For example, administration of G-CSF at a dose of 300 μg/day will reduce the transit time for neutrophils through this compartment from approximately six to three days [24]. GM-CSF at a dose of 250 μg/kg/day, a dose frequently used clinically, has a somewhat lesser effect in accelerating this transit time [25]. Autologous studies using radioisotopically labeled neutrophils have shown that this dose of G-CSF will increase neutrophil production rates about six-fold [24]. GM-CSF at 250 μg/kg/day had a far lesser effect [25]. The production of monocytes, eosinophils and dendritic cells are also stimulated *in vivo* and *in vitro* by GM-CSF; G-CSF has relatively little effect on these cells. Some recent studies suggest that increased anti-tumor responses and treatment benefits in infectious diseases may accrue from the effects of GM-CSF on monocytes and dendritic cells [33,34], but human studies conclusively demonstrating such benefit are not yet available. Adverse effects are more frequently associated with GM-CSF treatment than with G-CSF therapy (i.e., local skin reactions, malaise and fever). This difference may be due to stimulation of cytokine production (e.g., gamma interferon, tumor necrosis factor) mediated through the monocyte receptors for GM-CSF.

3. Measurement of CSF Levels in Patients with Neutropenia and Infectious Diseases

Under basal conditions in normal subjects circulating concentrations of G-CSF and GM-CSF are usually undetectable, i.e., less than 50 to 100 nanograms per milliliter. Levels of these factors are also quite low in urine and other body fluids and generally only detectable if the fluids are concentrated. For this reason it has been difficult to identify genetic or clinical conditions attributable to low levels of the CSFs. Animal studies, including gene "knock-out" experiments, however, clearly show that deficiencies of G-CSF lead to severe neutropenia [35]. GM-CSF "knock-outs" are hematologically normal [36]. Deficiencies of G-CSF, the absence of its receptor, as well as deficiencies of the promoters for these genes, lead to neutropenia. Thus, it is clear that G-CSF is required for maintenance of a normal blood neutrophil count.

Endotoxin injection in normal human subjects and in other species has a profound effect on cytokine production and release, including the CSFs. In man and other species G-CSF levels are markedly elevated within the first few hours after endotoxin injection, the time course closely corresponding to that for increased IL-6 and IL-8 after endotoxin, and slightly follows the peaking of levels of tumor necrosis factor [37]. By contrast, GM-CSF levels are not significantly elevated in response to endotoxin administration [37]. Commercially available immunoassay systems, as well as bioassay systems, have been used to demonstrate these differences.

Patients with neutropenia may have elevation of G-CSF levels, but increases in GM-CSF are rarely observed [38,39]. Understanding the relationship of neutropenia and CSF levels is confounded by the frequency of fever and inflammation in neutropenic patients, thus making it unclear if changes in the CSFs are directly attributable to the circulating neutrophil level or have occurred secondarily in response to exogenous factors (e.g., microbial products or endotoxin) entering the tissues or blood. With current assay methods, most data suggests that neutropenia must be extreme, i.e., counts less than 0.2×10^9/L to have detectably increased G-CSF levels in patients without overt infections.

With naturally occurring infections in both normal and neutropenic subjects G-CSF levels are increased, although many details of the time course of this response in a clinical setting are yet unknown [40–42]. In general there is a correlation of levels with the severity of sepsis, the highest levels being detected in patients with bacteremia and septic shock [43,44]. Higher levels also appear to occur with gram-negative than with gram-positive infections [42]. By contrast, GM-CSF levels are rarely elevated even with severe infections. As patients improve, G-CSF levels gradually return to normal [43,44]. Many factors may be involved in determining the pattern of decline in G-CSF levels over the course of an infection. These include the binding of G-CSF by receptors on immature and mature cells produced in greater number in response to the infection [45], reduced production of G-CSF as the infection resolves, and reduced levels of other mediators such as tumor necrosis factor and interleukin-1, which may be modulators of the G-CSF response. It is puzzling that GM-CSF is not detected in the blood with inflammation because it is produced by the same types of cells which produce G-CSF, i.e., fibroblasts and endothelial cells, as well as by T-lymphocytes. Currently it is believed that it is produced locally, i.e., in the bone marrow or at sites of inflammation, and acts locally to modulate hematopoiesis and the inflammatory response at the tissue level.

4. G-CSF in Nonneutropenic Animal Models of Infection

Contrary to the widespread belief that infectious diseases are no longer a serious threat to life in any but developing countries, mortality from infections in the

United States has, in fact, increased in recent years [46]. Between 1980 and 1992, mortality attributable to infectious disease rose from 41 to 65 deaths per 100,000 population in the United States — a 58% increase. Deaths resulting from respiratory tract infections increased from 25 to 30 per 100,000, a 20% increase, while deaths from septicemia increased by 83%, from a mortality rate of 4.2 to 7.7 per 100,000. These statistics clearly underscore the need for adjuvant therapies in the treatment of severe infections, such as sepsis.

One promising strategy for upregulating the host defense system of the infected patient focuses on the use of G-CSF; this cytokine has been studied much more intensively than GM-CSF because of its clearer role in regulating the neutrophil response. The efficacy of G-CSF, either alone or in combination with antibiotic therapy, has been studied in a variety of nonneutropenic animal infectious disease models. (Table 3) These include neonatal sepsis, burn wound injury, surgical wound infection, bacteremia, intraabdominal sepsis and pneumonia.

Table 10.3   Effects of G-CSF in nonneutropenic animal infection models

Increased production of neutrophils during infection
Increased neutrophil delivery into the site of the infection
Additive to synergistic effects of G-CSF with antibiotic therapy
Reduction in the burden of the infection and mortality

4.1 *Neonatal sepsis*

Neonatal sepsis due to group B streptococci remains a significant cause of morbidity and mortality. Developmental immaturity in neonatal phagocytic defenses is a predisposing factor [47]. Depletion of the marrow neutrophil storage pool with profound neutropenia typically precedes death. Studies suggest that the observed deficit in neutrophil supply may be due to an inadequate endogenous G-CSF response [48]. *In vitro* stimulation of blood monocytes from preterm neonates produce less G-CSF than do monocytes recovered from term neonates or adults [49] As a result, during an infection, circulating levels of G-CSF may not rise appropriately in order to ensure a steady supply of neutrophils.

These observations suggest that exogenous G-CSF may be of benefit in the treatment of group B streptococcal infection in this patient population. In one study, neonatal rats were infected subcutaneously with group B streptococci and then treated with one of the following regimens: no antibiotics or G-CSF (control); G-CSF given once at the time of infection; ampicillin and gentamicin starting 24 hours after infection, or both G-CSF and antibiotics by these same dosing schedules [50]. At 72 hours, the survival rate for animals receiving both G-CSF and antibiotics was 91% versus 4% for the control group, 9% for animals treated with G-CSF alone, and 28% for animals treated with antibiotics only. When G-CSF was administered prophylactically prior to the bacterial challenge, a similar synergistic effect on survival was seen for G-CSF in addition to antibiotics compared to antibiotics alone. Randomized controlled clinical trials of both G-CSF and GM-CSF for neonates with sepsis are presently underway.

4.2 Burn wound injury

Infection continues to be a major problem following burn injury. Multiple immune defects have been demonstrated after thermal injury, including inhibition of both the production and function of neutrophils [51]. To study the effects of G-CSF after thermal injury, mice were burned and their wounds inoculated with *Pseudomonas aeruginosa* [52]. Animals were randomized to receive either G-CSF or placebo starting at the time of injury and bacterial seeding, then twice daily thereafter. Mice receiving G-CSF showed an enhanced myelopoietic response, as assessed by significant increases in the absolute neutrophil count, bone marrow cellularity, and numbers of myelopoietic progenitor cells. The addition of antibiotic therapy to G-CSF significantly improved survival compared to burn infected control mice or animals that received either G-CSF or antibiotic therapy alone.

4.3 *Surgical wound infection*

In an experimental model of surgical wound infection, *P. aeruginosa* was inoculated into the thigh muscle of mice [53]. G-CSF was administered immediately after infection and for 2 days thereafter. Greater than 90% of the control animals died, while only 50% of animals treated with G-CSF succumbed to their infection. G-CSF greatly enhanced the influx of neutrophils into the infected tissue site which resulted in a significant reduction in the number of viable bacteria compared to control animals.

In this study, the authors also examined the relationship between the number of circulating neutrophils and the efficacy of antibiotic therapy in this intramuscular infection model. Mice were treated with cyclophosphamide to make them granulocytopenic or with G-CSF to induce neutrophilia prior to the onset of infection. The therapeutic effect of the aminoglycoside netilmicin, was not significantly affected by the number of neutrophils in the blood. In contrast, the therapeutic effect of ceftazidime, a B-lactam antibiotic, was significantly affected by the number of circulating neutrophils at the time of the infection. Thus, selection of a particular antibiotic may also be an important consideration when utilizing G-CSF as an adjunct therapy.

Because some antibiotics are known to concentrate within neutrophils, McKenna et al recently hypothesized that G-CSF might increase the antibiotic uptake into these cells as a way of enhancing their function [54]. This effect would potentially result in "targeting" antibiotic delivery to an infected site and be particularly useful in parts of the body where antibiotic concentrations are typically lower compared to serum concentrations, such as the lung. Ciprofloxacin is a quinolone antibiotic which is known to concentrate within neutrophils three to four times greater than the extracellular concentration. McKenna et al isolated human neutrophils and incubated them with G-CSF for 1 hour. Ciprofloxacin was then added and the cells were incubated for an additional hour. G-CSF increased the intracellular-to-extracellular concentration of ciproflaxicin approximately 10-fold [54]. Further investigations of these important findings are now underway.

4.4 Bacteremia

In a recently published study by Haberstroh and colleagues, 15 intravenously catheterized pigs were given a constant infusion of live *P. aeruginosa*, reaching a final blood concentration of approximately 10^3 colony-forming units (CFU)/ml, not unlike the concentration observed in bacteremic patients [55]. Seven of the animals received G-CSF 30 minutes before the start of the bacterial infusion, and eight received placebo. Two animals in the placebo group died, whereas all of the animals treated with G-CSF survived. The blood endotoxin levels in control animals steadily increased during the first 24 to 36 hours, and then gradually declined. In the G-CSF treated animals, the peak endotoxin levels were approximately 50% lower compared to the peak values in control animals. A similar pattern was observed with levels of TNF in the circulation. Thus, the use of G-CSF in this model system resulted in lower systemic cytokine levels and improved survival.

As noted previously, it is important to appreciate that there are critical differences between hematopoietic growth factors. Whereas G-CSF is specific in stimulating the proliferation, differentiation, and functional activities of neutrophils, GM-CSF also exerts profound effects on cells of macrophage lineage. These differences can have dramatic effects in the infected host. Havill et al pretreated mice with either GM-CSF or G-CSF prior to an intravenous endotoxin challenge, and we monitored mortality over the following 72 hours [56]. Prior treatment with GM-CSF converted a nonlethal endotoxin challenge to one with 50% mortality. For these experiments, a dose of GM-CSF was selected which did not increase circulating neutrophil levels. G-CSF, which increased the absolute neutrophil count by approximately 80%, caused no enhancement of endotoxin induced lethality. Therefore, this effect on mortality was presumably due to the effect of GM-CSF on the mononuclear phagocyte cell population, priming them for enhanced release of pro-inflammatory cytokines. In this study, there was a 20 fold increase in the serum TNF levels in the animals receiving GM-CSF prior to the endotoxin challenge, whereas G-CSF had no effect on the TNF response. Similar to these observations, Tiegs et al. reported that GM-CSF enhanced endotoxin induced organ injury and mortality in mice [57]. Furthermore, administration of a neutralizing anti-GM-CSF monoclonal antibody prior to the endotoxin challenge significantly improved survival. These observations lend support to the hypothesis that the macrophage, as opposed to the neutrophil, may be the primary effector cell type mediating, in large part, the lethal consequences of sepsis.

4.5 Intraabdominal infection

Lundblad et al utilized a model of cecal ligation and puncture to simulate intraabdominal sepsis [58]. These investigators focused on the burden of bacterial infection and blood levels of cytokines and endotoxin, as well as evidence of neutrophil-mediated tissue injury. None of the organs examined in those animals that were treated with G-CSF showed histopathological evidence of neutrophil-mediated injury. Furthermore, as in the previous study, blood levels of bacteria , endotoxin, and TNF were consistently lower in the G-CSF-treated animals compared to placebo treated animals. In contrast to these observations, Toda et al. reported that in their model of cecal ligation and puncture, administration of GM-CSF failed to improve survival and appeared to cause the animals to succumb more rapidly to their infection [59] .

In a model of intraabdominal sepsis utilizing agar pellets implanted with live *Escherichia coli*, Zhang et al have recently shown that G-CSF increased the number of neutrophils responding to the infection within the peritoneum by approximately three-fold and increased survival from 38% to 78% [60]. Furthermore the bactericidal activity of these neutrophils recovered from the peritoneal cavity was significantly enhanced compared to vehicle treated animals. Studies in a model of cecal ligation and puncture have also shown that G-CSF increases the phagocytic function of both circulating and peritoneal neutrophils [61].

4.6 Pneumonia

Examination of the lung may be particularly useful in defining the role of the CSFs and other cytokines in the host response to infection. The cellular population of the uninfected lung is almost exclusively composed of alveolar macrophages and these cells can be readily obtained by bronchoscopy. Alveolar macrophages recovered by bronchoalveolar lavage from patients with pneumonia spontaneously release G-CSF, whereas alveolar macrophages from healthy controls produce G-CSF only after endotoxin stimulation [62]. This G-CSF response in patients with pneumonia most likely serves at least two purposes. It would act locally, along with other cytokines and inflammatory mediators, within the lung to increase the functional activity of neutrophils entering the infected lung. It would also function systemically to stimulate the bone marrow to ensure an ongoing supply of additional effector cells needed to eradicate the infection. In contrast to certain other cytokines, such as TNF , IL-1, and IL-8, G-CSF is not compartmentalized within the lung [63]. In studies of patients with unilateral pneumonia, these other cytokines have been shown to remain localized within the lung and remain undetectable in the serum of these pneumonia patients [64,65]. By contrast, serum levels of G-CSF rapidly rise following intrapulmonary administration of G-CSF and causes a similar increase in the blood neutrophils as does subcutaneous administration [66].

One important determinant of the specific patient populations that might benefit from CSF therapy is how host factors or underlying illness may affect the endogenous cytokine responses to infection. Alcohol is known to significantly increase patient susceptibility to a variety of infections, particularly bacterial pneumonia [67–69]. Although this relationship is widely appreciated, the basic mechanisms remain unclear. Numerous *in vitro* and *in vivo* studies have reported ethanol-induced defects in neutrophil function, including adherence, mobilization, and delivery [70–72]. Furthermore, alcohol-abusing patients frequently fail to initiate a leukocytosis in response to their infection, which markedly increases their likelihood of succumbing to the infection [73]. These observations suggest that the ability of the host to generate an appropriate neutrophil response is both essential for survival and may be impaired by alcohol abuse.

Nelson et al investigated the effects of G-CSF in ethanol-treated rats with experimentally induced pneumonia [74]. Rats were pretreated with G-CSF or placebo for 2 days, then administered intraperitoneal alcohol or saline, which was followed by an intratracheal challenge with *Klebsiella pneumoniae*. At 4 hours after the intratracheal challenge, G-CSF augmented the recruitment of neutrophils into the lungs of control animals and significantly attenuated the adverse effects of ethanol on neutrophil delivery into the infected lung. G-CSF also enhanced the bactericidal activity of the lung in both control and ethanol treated rats. Twelve of 12 intoxicated control rats with pneumonia died within 72 hours of infection, whereas only 1 of 12 rats treated with G-CSF died. Subsequently these investigatores showed that alcohol suppresses the normal serum G-CSF response to a bacterial infection *in vivo* and that G-CSF can attenuate the adverse effects of alcohol on several vital neutrophil functions *in vitro*, including the expression of adhesion molecules and phagocytosis [75–76].

Splenectomy is a known risk factor for increased morbidity and mortality resulting from pneumococcal pneumonia [77]. In a murine model, G-CSF administered from 24 hours before challenge to 3 days after challenge improved survival among splenectomized animals exposed to an aerosol challenge with *Streptococcus pneumoniae*. The survival rate among splenectomized G-CSF-treated mice was 70% compared to 20% in the splenectomized control animals [78].

Smith et al. studied the effect of G-CSF in a rabbit model of gram-negative pneumonia and sepsis [79]. Rabbits were inoculated transtracheally with *Pasteurella multocida* and treated 24 hours later with penicillin G and G-CSF or placebo once daily for up to 5 days. All rabbits underwent careful histologic examination at the time of death or when sacrificed on day 6. In these animals, sepsis-induced leukopenia was a predictor of significantly improved survival with G-CSF therapy (57% compared to 39% in controls). Interestingly, the majority of this survival benefit occurred within the first 24 hours of treatment with G-CSF which was prior to the onset of G-CSF-induced neutrophilia. Histologic examination of these animals did not demonstrate evidence of organ toxicity related to G-CSF therapy.

5. Clinical Studies of the CSFs in Infectious Diseases

5.1 *Neutropenia*

The CSFs have had a major impact upon the treatment of neutropenic patients. There are many types and causes for neutropenia, e.g., congenital and acquired neutropenias; acute and chronic neutropenias; and neutropenias occurring with and without other defects in host defenses. Mechanistically these disorders can also be described as abnormalities of production, maturation or distribution of these cells [80]. Severe neutropenia, i.e. blood neutrophil counts less than 0.5×10^9/liter, generally results in infections if it lasts more than a few days. Cancer chemotherapy and marrow ablation for bone marrow transplantation are common causes of this type of neutropenia. Randomized controlled trials have established that the CSFs are effective at ameliorating neutropenia in this setting by hastening marrow recovery and shortening the duration of severe neutropenia. Recently guidelines for the use of CSFs in these settings have been published [81,82].

Patients with congenital neutropenia, cyclic neutropenia and idiopathic neutropenia, sometimes referred to as "severe chronic neutropenia," have a defect in neutrophil production which leads to a life-long risk of recurrent infections [83], They frequently have mouth ulcers, gingivitis, sinusitis and cervical lymphadenopathy. Life-threatening infections, e.g., pneumonia, neutropenic colitis, deep tissue abscesses and bacteremia can also occur, especially in the most severely affected patients. The precise cellular or genetic causes for most disorders are not yet known. At present they are not attributable to recognized defects in the production of the CSFs or in the structure or function of the CSF receptors. Characteristically, bone marrow examination in these patients shows relatively normal numbers of other hematopoietic cells, but a deficiency in cells of the neutrophil lineage. Generally there are some early precursors, but a deficiency in the number of the more mature cells. In cyclic neutropenia the severity of this defect in the marrow varies in a regular oscillatory fashion [84].

Clinical trials of the CSFs for the treatment of severe chronic neutropenia were begun in 1987. A randomized controlled trial clearly established the effectiveness of G-CSF for these conditions, with more than 90% of patients responding to increase their blood neutrophil counts to normal levels with a concomitant decrease in the occurrence of fever and infections [85]. Detailed clinical studies have shown that patients with cyclic neutropenia and idiopathic neutropenia respond to relatively low doses of G-CSF, i.e., 1 to 3 μg/kg/day, administered subcutaneously on a daily or alternate day basis. Patients with congenital neutropenia generally have lower counts, a more severe marrow defect, and require higher doses of G-CSF [86]. There are now several hundred patients who have been treated generally with daily or alternate day G-CSF for more than five years, with few long-term adverse effects. One group of patients, patients with congenital neutropenia, were known to be at risk of conversion to acute myelogenous leukemia before the availability of the CSFs [87]. Since the availability of the CSFs this occurrence has been better documented, but it is unclear if treatment affects this evolution. GM-CSF is much less effective than G-CSF for these patients.

5.2 *G-CSF in nonneutropenic patients with pneumonia*

Three trials have recently been completed studying the effect of G-CSF in nonneutropenic patients with pneumonia. The first trial was a phase I study of 30 nonneutropenic patients hospitalized with community-acquired pneumonia (CAP) [89]. All patients received intravenous antibiotics in addition to G-CSF (75–300 ug) subcutaneously daily for a maximum of 10 days. Overall, the median change in the absolute neutrophil count from baseline was approximately 200% and the peak was achieved by day 4 of G-CSF administration. Aside from mild bone pain, no adverse pulmonary or systemic side effects occurred that were attributable to G-CSF.

A phase III, double-blind, placebo-controlled trial of recombinant human G-CSF for the treatment of hospitalized patients with CAP has recently been concluded [90]. This was a multicenter trial involving 756 patients enrolled in 71 centers in the United States, Canada, and Australia. Participants in this study were randomized to receive 300 ug/day G-CSF (376 patients) or placebo (380 patients) in addition to conventional antibiotic therapy. Treatment duration was up to 10 days and the length of the study observation period was 28 days or until death. The primary objectives of this study were to determine safety and the effect of G-CSF on TRM. TRM (time to resolution of morbidity) was defined as an index of several clinical variables which are useful in determining if a patient with pneumonia is benefiting from therapy [91]. In this study, in order to reach TRM a patient had to have either an improved or stable chest radiograph, resolve their tachypnea, become afebrile, and improve or normalize their oxygenation. Mortality was low (6%) in this study and length of stay was only 7 days. Both variables were unaffected by G-CSF treatment. Similarly, TRM was 4 days in each treatment group. In the intent-to-treat analysis, G-CSF did increase blood neutrophils 3-fold, significantly accelerated radiological resolution of pneumonia, and reduced serious complications (i.e. ARDS and disseminated intravascular coagulation (DIC). Post hoc analyses showed that these benefits were more pronounced in patients with multilobar (>2 lobes) pneumonia. In this study, there were 261 patients with multilobar pneumonia (G-CSF, n = 138; placebo, n = 123) and 28% of these patients were admitted to an ICU at study entry. G-CSF administration was safe and well-tolerated in this study.

G-CSF has also been studied in the treatment of patients with pneumonia and severe sepsis [92]. Eighteen patients were randomized in a 2:1 ratio to G-CSF (300 μg/day intravenously) or placebo for a maximum of 5 days in addition to standard therapy. Inclusion criteria included a chest radiograph compatible with pneumonia, a respiratory pathogen on gram stain or culture, fever, tachycardia, tachypnea or need for mechanical ventilation, and either hypotension despite volume resuscitation requiring vasopressors or, in the absence of shock, two end organ dysfunctions (metabolic acidosis, ARDS, acute renal failure, DIC). Three of 12 G-CSF treated patients and 4 of 6 placebo treated patients died. Septic shock resolved in 9 of 10 G-CSF treated patients and none of 4 placebo treated patients. ARDS resolved in 2 of 5 G-CSF treated patients and 1 of 4 placebo treated patients. G-CSF was well tolerated in these septic patients. Based on the favorable trends seen in these studies, additional trials in patients with multilobar pneumonia and in patients with severe pneumonia with sepsis are presently underway.

6. References

1. Bradley, T.R. and Metcalf, D. The growth of mouse bone marrow cells *in vitro*. *Aust. J. Exp. Biol. Med. Sci.* 1966; **44**:287–294.
2. Foster, R., Metcalf, D., Robinson, W.A. and Bradley, T.R. Bone marrow colony stimulating activity in human sera. *Br. J. Haematol.* 1968; **15**:147–159.

3. Metcalf, D. and Stanley, E.R. Quantitative studies on the stimulation of mouse bone marrow colony growth in vitro by normal human urine. *Aust. J. Exp. Biol. Med. Sci.* 1969; **47**:453–466.

4. Metcalf, D. The role of the colony-stimulating factors in resistance to acute infections. *Immunol. Cell. Biol.* 1987; **65**:35–43.

5. Cheers, C., Haigh, A.M. and Kelso, A., *et al.*, Production of colony-stimulating factors (CSFs) during infection: separate determinations of macrophage-, granulocyte-, and multi-CSFs. Infect. Immun. 1998; **56**:247–251.

6. Nicola, N.A., Metcalf, D., Johnson, G.R. and Burgess, A.W. Separation of functionally distinct human granulocyte-macrophage colony-stimulating factors. *Blood* 1979; **54**:614–627.

7. Burgess, A.W. and Metcalf, D. Characterization of a serum factor stimulating the differentiation of myelomonocytic leukemic cells. *Int. J. Cancer* 1980; **26**:547–554.

8. Nicola, N.A., Metcalf, D. and Matsumoto, M. Purification of a factor inducing differentiation in murine myelomonocytic leukemia cells. *J. Biol. Chem.* 1983; **258**:9017–9023.

9. Welte, K., Platzer, E. and Lu, L., *et al.*, Purification and biochemical haracterization of human pluripotent hematopoietic colony-stimulating factor. *Proc. Natl. Acad. Sci., USA* 1985; **82**.

10. Souza, L.M., Boone, T.C. and Gabrilove, J., *et al.*, Recombinant human granulocyte colony-stimulating factor: effects on normal and leukemic myeloid cells. *Science* 1986; **232** (4746):61–65.

11. Simmers, R.N., Webber, L.M. and Shannon, M.F., *et al.*, Localization of the G-CSF gene on chromosome 17 proximal to the breakpoint in the t(15;17) in acute promylocytic leukemia. *Blood* 1987; **70**:330–332.

12. Wong, G.G., Witek, J.S. and Temple, P.A., et al., Human GM-CSF: Molecular cloning of the complementary DNA and purification of the natural and recombinant proteins. *Science* 1985; **228**:910–915.

13. Huebner, K., Isobe, M., Croce, C.M., Golde, D.W., Kaufman, S,E. and Gasson, J.C. The human gene encoding GM-CSF is at 5q21-q32, the chromosome region deleted in the 5q anomaly. *Science* 1985; **230**:1282–1285.

14. Hill, C.P., Osslund, T.D. and Eisenberg, D.S. The structure of granulocyte colony-stimulating factor (r-hu-G-CSF) and its relationship to other growth factors. *Proc. Natl. Acad. Sci. USA* 1993; **90**:5167–5171.

15. Nicola, N.A., Smith, A., Robb, L., Metcalf, D. and Begley, C.G. The structural basis of the biological actions of the GM-CSF receptor. *Ciba Found Symp.* 1997; **204**:19–27.

16. Avalos, B.R., Gasson, J.C. and Hedvat, C., *et al.*, Human granulocyte colony-stimulating factor: biologic activities and receptor characterization on hematopoietic cells and small cell lung cancer cell lines. *Blood* 1990; **75**:851–857.

17. Tidow, N. and Welte, K. Advances in understanding postreceptor signaling in response to granulocyte colony-stimulating factor. *Cur. Opn. Hematol.* 1997; **4**:171–175.

18. Dong, F., Pouwels, K., Hoefsloot, L.H., Rozemuller, H., Lowenberg, B. and Touw, I.P. The C-terminal cytoplasmic region of the granulocyte colony-stimulating factor receptor mediates apoptosis in maturation-incompetent murine myeloid cells. *Exp. Hematol.* 1996; **24**:214–220.

19. DiPersio, J.F., Hedvat, C., Ford, C.F. and Golde, D.W. Characterization of the soluble human granulocyte-macrophage colony-stimulating factor receptor complex. *J. Biol. Chem.* 1991; **266**:279–286.

20. Nicola, N.A., Smith, A., Robb, L., Metcalf, D. and Begley, C.G. The structural basis of the biological actions of the GM-CSF receptor. *Ciba Found Symp.* 1997; **204**:19–27 and 27–32.

21. Watanabe, S., Itoh, T. and Arai, K. Roles of JAK kinases in human GM-CSF receptor signal transduction. *J. allergy Clin. Immunol.* 1996; **98**:S183–191.

22. Gomez-Cambonero, J. and Veatch, C. Emerging paradigms in granulocyte-macrophage colony-stimulating factor signaling. *Life Sci.* 1996; **59**:2099–2111.

23. Dale, D.C., Fauci, A.S., Guerry, D. and Wolff, S.M. Comparison of agents producing a neutrophilic leukocytosis in man: Hydrocortisone, prednisone, endotoxin and etiocholanolone. *J. Clin. Invest.* **56**; 808–813, 1975.

24. Price, T.H., Chatta, G.S. and Dale, D.C. The effect of recombinant granulocyte colony-stimulating factor on neutrophil kinetics in normal young and elderly humans. *Blood* **88**; 335–340, 1996.

25. Dale, D.C., Liles, W.C., Llewellyn, C. and Price, T.H. The effects of granulocyte macrophage colony-stimulating factor (GM-CSF) on neutrophil kinetics and function in normal human volunteers Am J Hematol (in press) 1997.

26. Babior, B.M. and Golde, D.W. "Production, distribution and fate of neutrophils." Hematology, 5th edition, Edited by W.J. Williams *et al.*, McGraw-Hill, New York 773–779, 1995.

27. Ogawa, M. Differentiation and proliferation of hematopoietic stem clls. *Blood* 1993; **81**:2844.

28. Sullivan, G.W., Carper, H.T. and Mandell, G.L. The effect of three human recombinant hematopoietic growth factors (granulocyte-macrophage colony-

stimulating factor, granulocyte colony-stimulating factor, and interleukin-3) on phagocyte oxidative activity. *Blood* 1993; **81**:1863–1870.

29. Dale, D.C., Liles, W.C., Summer, W. and Nelson, S. Granulocyte-colony-stimulating factor: Role and relationships in infectious diseases. *J. Inf. Dis.* 1995; **172**:1061–1075.

30. Harmenberg, J., H`glund, M., Hellstr`m, and Lindberg, E. G- and GM-CSF in oncology and oncological haematology. *Eur. J. Haematol.* 1994; **52**:1–28.

31. Turzanski, J., Crouch, S.P., Fletcher, J. and Hunter, A. Ex vivo neutrophil function in response to three different doses of glycosylated rHuG-CSF (lenograstim). *Br. J. Haematol.* 1997; **96**:46–54

32. Sullivan, G.W., Gelrud, A.K., Carper, H.T., Mandell, G.L. Interaction of tumor necrosis factor-α and granulocyte colony-stimulating factor on neutrophil apoptosis, receptor expression, and bactericidal function. *Proc. Assoc. Amer. Phys.* 1996; **108**:455–466.

33. Jones, T.C. The effect of granulocyte-macrophage colony-stimulating factor (rGM-CSF) on macrophage function in microbial disease. *Med. Oncol.* 1996; **13**:141–147.

34. Tarr, P.E. Granulocyte-macrophage colony-stimulating factor and the immune system. *Med. Oncol.* 1996; **13**:133–140.

35. Lieschke, G.J., Grail, D., Hodgson, G., Metcalf, D., Stanley, E., Cheers, C., Fowler, K.J., Basu, S., Zhan, Y.F. and Dunn, A.R. Mice lacking granulocyte colony-stimulating factor have chronic neutropenia, granulocyte and macrophage progenitor cell deficiency, and impaired neutrophil mobilization. *Blood* 1994; **84**:1737–1746.

36. Stanley, E., Lieschke, G.J., Grail, D., Metcalf, D., Hodgson, G., Gall, J.A., Maher, D.W., Cebon, J., Sinickas, V. and Dunn, A.R. Granulocyte/macrophage colony-stimulating factor-deficient mice show no major perturbation of hematopoiesis but develop a characteristic pulmonary pathology. *Proc. Natl. Acad. Sci. USA* 1994; **91**:5592–5596.

37. Kuhns, D.B., Alvord, W.G., Gallin, J.I. Increased circulating cytokines, cytokine antagonists, and E-selectin after intravenous administration of endotoxin in humans. *J. Infect. Dis.* 1995; **171**:145–152.

38. Mempel, K., Pietsch, T., Menzel, T., Zeidler, C. and Welte, K. Increased serum levels of granulocyte colony-stimulating factor in patients with severe congenital neutropenia. *Blood* 1991; **77**:1919–1922.

39. Kojima, S., Matsuyama, T., Kodera, Y., Nishihira, H., Ueda, K., Shimbo, T. and Nakahata, T. Measurement of endogenous plasma granulocyte colony-stimulating

factor in patients with acquired aplastic anemia by a sensitive chemiluminescent immunoassay. *Blood* 1996; **87**:1303–1308.

40. Kragsbjerg, P., Vikerfors, T. and Holmberg, H. Diagnostic value of blood cytokine concentrations in acute pneumonia. *Thorax* 1995; **50**:1253–1257.

41. Pauksen, K., Elfman, L., Ulfgren, A.K. and Venge, P. Serum levels of granulocyte-colony-stimulating factor (G-CSF) in bacterial and viral infections, and in atypical peumonia. *Br. J. Haematol.* 1994; **88**:256–260.

42. Cebon, J., Layton, J.E., Maher, D. and Morstyn, G. Endogenous haemopoietic growth factors in neutropenia and infection. *Br. J. Haematol.* 1994; **86**:265–274.

43. Kawakami, M., Tsutsumi, H., Kumakawa, T., Abe, H., Hirai, M., Kurosawa, S., Mori, M. and Fukushima, M. Levels of serum granulocyte colony-stimulating factor in patients with infections. *Blood* 1990; **76**:1962–1964.

44. Waring, P.M., Presneill, J., Maher, D.W., Layton, J.E., Cebon, J., Waring, L.J. and Metcalf, D. Differential alterations in plasma colony-stimulating factor concentrations in meningococcaemia. *Clin. Exp. Immunol.* 1995; **102**:501–506.

45. Layton, J.E., Hockman, H., Sheridan, W.P. and Morstyn, G. Evidence for a novel *in vivo* control mechanism of granulopoiesis: mature cell-related control of a regulatory growth factor. *Blood* 1989; **7**:1303–1307.

46. Pinner, R.W., Teutsch, S.M. and Simonsen, L., *et al.*, Trends in infectious diseases mortality in the United States. *JAMA* 1996; **275**:189–193.

47. Cairo, M.S. Neonatal neutrophil host defense. *Am. J. Dis. Child* 1989; **143**:40–46.

48. Liechty, K.W., Schibler, K.R. and Ohls, R.K., *et al.*, The failure of newborn mice infected with *Escherichia coli* to accelerate neutrophil production correlates with their failure to increase transcripts for granulocyte colony-stimulating factor and interleukin-6. *Biol. Neonate* 1993; **64**:331–340.

49. Schibler, K.R., Liechty, K.W., White, W.L. and Christensen, R.D. Production of granulocyte colony-stimulating factor *in vitro* by monocytes from pre-term and term neonates. *Blood* 1993; **82**:2478–2484.

50. Cairo, M.S., Mauss, D. and Kommareedy, S., *et al.*, Prophylactic or simultaneous administration of recombinant human granulocyte colony-stimulating factor in the treatment of group B streptococcal sepsis in neonatal rats. *Pediatr. Res.* 1990; **27**:612–616.

51. Nelson, S. The effects of thermal injury on systemic and pulmonary host defenses. *Crit. Care Rep.* 1991; **2**:241–243.

52. Mooney, D.P., Gamelli, R.L., O'Reilly, M. and Hebert, J.C. Recombinant human granulocyte colony-stimulating factor and *Pseudomonas* burn wound sepsis. *Arch. Surg.* 1988; **123**:1353–1357.

53. Yasuda, H., Ajiki, L. and Shomozato, T., *et al.*, Therapeutic efficacy of granulocyte colony-stimulating factor alone and in combination with antibiotics against *Pseudomonas aeruginosa* infections in mice. *Infect. Immun.* 1990; **58**:2502–2509.

54. McKenna, P.H., Nelson, S. and Andresen, J. Filgrastim (rhuG-CSF) enhances ciprofloxacin uptake and bactericidal activity of human neutrophils *in vitro. Am. J. Respir. Crit. Care Med.* 1996; 153S:A535.

55. Haberstroh, J., Breuer, H. and Lücke, I., *et al.*, Effect of recombinant human granulocyte colony-stimulating factor on hemodynamic and cytokine response in a porcine model of *Pseudomonas* sepsis. *Shock* 1995; **4**:216–224.

56. Havill, A.M., Anderson, J.W., Karoch, J.W. and Nelson, S. Enhancement of endotoxin-induced lethality in the mouse by GM-CSF [abstract]. *Am. Rev. Respir. Dis.* 1991; **143**(suppl):236.

57. Tiegs, G., Barsig, J. and Matiba, B., *et al.*, Potentiation by granulocyte macrophage colony-stimulating factor of lipopolysaccharide toxicity in mice. *J. Clin. Invest.* 1994; **93**:2616–2622.

58. Lundblad, R., Nesland, J.M. and Giercksky, K.-E. Granulocyte colony-stimulating factor improves survival rate and reduces concentrations of bacteria, endotoxin, tumor necrosis factor, and endothelin-1 in fulminant intraabdominal sepsis in rats. *Crit. Care Med.* 1996; **24**:820–826.

59. Toda, H., Murata, S. and Oka, Y., *et al.*, Effect of granulocyte-macrophage colony- stimulating factor on sepsis-induced organ injury in rats. *Blood* 1994; **83**:2893–2898.

60. Dunne, J.R., Dunkin, B.J., Nelson, S. and White, J.C. Effects of granulocyte colony-stimulating factor in a nonneutropenic rodent model of *Escherichia coli* peritonitis. *J. Surg. Res.* 1996; **61**:348–354.

61. Zhang, P., Bagby, G.J. and Stoltz, D.A., et al., Enhancement of peritoneal leukocyte function by granulocyte colony-stimulating factor in rats with abdominal sepsis. *Crit. Care Med.* (in press).

62. Tazi, A., Nioche, S. and Chastre, J., *et al.*, Spontaneous release of granulocyte colony- stimulating factor (G-CSF) by alveolar macrophages in the course of bacterial pneumonia and sarcoidosis: endotoxin-dependent and endotoxin-independent G-CSF release by cells recovered by bronchoalveolar lavage. *Am. J. Respir. Cell Mol. Biol.* 1991; **4**:140–147.

63. Nelson, S., Bagby, G.J. and Bainton, B.G., *et al.*, Compartmentalization of intra-alveolar and systemic lipopolysaccharide-induced tumor necrosis factor and the pulmonary inflammatory response. *J. Infect. Dis.* 1989; **159**:189–194.

64. Dehoux, M.S., Boutten, A. and Ostinelli, J., *et al.*, Compartmentalized cytokine production within the human lung in unilateral pneumonia. *Am. J. Repir. Crit. Care Med.* 1994; **150**:710–716.

65. Boutten, A., Dehoux, M.S. and Seta, N., *et al.*, Compartmentalized IL-8 and elastase release within the human lung in unilateral pneumonia. *Am. J. Respir. Crit. Care Med.* 1996; **153**:336–342.

66. Nelson, S., Bagby, G. and Andresen, J., *et al.*, Intratracheal granulocyte colony-stimulating factor enhances systemic and pulmonary host defenses. *Am. Rev. Respir. Dis.* 1991; **143S**:398.

67. Capps, J.A. and Coleman, G.H. Influence of alcohol on prognosis of pneumonia in Cook County Hospital. *JAMA* 1923; **80**:750.

68. Kolb, D. and Gunderson, E.K.E. Alcohol-related morbidity among older career navy men. *Drug Alcohol Depend* 1982; **9**:181–189.

69. Olser, W. The Principles and Practices of Medicine. New York: D. Appleton, 1905.

70. Brayton, R.G., Stokes, P.E., Schwartz, M.S. and Louria, D.B. Effect of alcohol and various diseases on leukocyte mobilization, phagocytosis, and intracellular bacterial killing. *N. Eng. J. Med.* 1970; **282**:123–128.

71. Hallengren, B. and Forsgren, A. Effect of alcohol on chemotaxis, adherence, and phagocytosis of human polymorphonuclear leukocytes. *Acta Med. Scand.* 1978; **204**:43–48.

72. MacGregor, R.R. and Gluckman, S.G. Effect of acute alcohol intoxication on granulocyte mobilization and kinetics. *Blood* 1979; **52**:551–559.

73. Limson, B.M., Romansky, M.J., Shea, J.G. Acute and chronic pulmonary infection with the Friedlander bacillus: a persistent problem in early diagnosis and therapy. In: Antibiotics Annual 1955–56, New York: Medical Encyclopedia, 1956; 86–93.

74. Nelson, S., Summer, W. and Bagby, G., *et al.*, Granulocyte colony-stimulating factor enhances pulmonary host defenses in normal and ethanol-treated rats. *J. Infect. Dis.* 1991; **164**:901–906.

75. Nelson, S., Bagby, G., Mason, C. and Summer, W. *Escherichia coli*-induced plasma granulocyte colony-stimulating factor. *Am. J. Respir. Crit. Care Med.* 1995; **151S**:A14.

76. Zhang, P., Summer, W.R. and Bagby, G.J., *et al.*, Ethanol inhibits neutrophil $_2$-integrin expression and phagocytosis during endotoxemia. *Am. J. Respir. Crit. Care Med.* 1997; **155S**:A292.

77. Gopal, V. and Bisno, A.L. Fulminant pneumococcal infection in "normal" asplenic hosts. *Arch. Intern. Med.* 1977; **137**:526–530.

78. Herbert, J.C., O'Reilly, M. and Gamelli, R.L. Protective effect of recombinant human granulocyte colony-stimulating factor against pneumococcal infections in splenectomized mice. *Arch. Surg.* 1990; **125**:1075–1078.

79. Smith, W.S., Sumnicht, G.E. and Sharpe, R.W., *et al.*, Granulocyte colony-stimulating factor versus placebo in addition to penicillin G in a randomized blinded study of gram-negative pneumonia sepsis: analysis of survival and multisystem organ failure. *Blood* 1995; **86**:1301–1309.

80. Dale, D.C. "Neutropenia" in Hematology, 5th edition, Edited by W.J. Williams *et al.*, McGraw-Hill, New York 815–824, 1995.

81. American Society of Clinical Oncology recommendations for the use of hematopoietic colony-stimulating factors: evidence-based, clinical practice guidelines. *J. Clin. Oncol.* 1994; **12**:2471–2508.

82. Boogaerts, M., Cavalli, F., Cortès-Funes, H., Gatell, J.M., Gianni, A.M., Khayat, D., Levy, Y. and Link, H. Granulocyte growth factors: achieving a consensus. *Ann. Oncol.* 1995; **6**:237–244.

83. Welte, K. and Dale, D.C. Pathophysiology and treatment of severe chronic neutropenia. Ann. Hematol. 1996; **72**:158–165.

84. Dale, D.C., Hammond, W.P.: Cyclic Neutropenia: A Clinical Review. *Blood Reviews* 1988; **2**:178–185.

85. Dale, D.C., Bonilla, M.A., Davis, M.W., Nakanishi, A., Hammond, W.P., Kurtzberg, J., Wang, W., Jakubowski, A., Winton, E., Lalezari, P., Robinson, W., Glaspy, J.A., Emerson, S., Gabrilove, J., Vincent, M. and Boxer, L.A. A randomized controlled phase III trial of recombinant human G-CSF for treatment of severe chronic neutropenia. *Blood* 1993; **81**:2496–2502.

86. Dale, D.C. Hematopoietic growth factors for the treatment of severe chronic neutropenia. *Concise Review. Stem Cells* 1995; **13**:94–100.

87. Bonilla, M.A., Dale, D.C., Zeidler, C., Ruggeiro, M., Reiter, A., Last, L., Davis, M., Koci, B., Hammond, W., Riehm, H., O'Reilly, R. and Welte, K. Long-term treatment with recombinant human colony-stimulating factor in patients with severe chronic neutropenia. *British J. Hematol.* 1994; **88**:723–730.

88. Freedman, M.H. Safety of Long-term administration of granulocyte colony-stimulating factor for severe chronic neutropenia. *Cur. Opn. Hematol.* 1997; **4**:217–224.

89. DeBoisblanc, B.P., Mason, C.M. and Andresen, J., *et al.*, Phase I safety trial of filgrastim (r- metHuG-CSF) in non-neutropenic patients with severe community-acquired pneumonia. *Respir. Med.* 1997; **91**:387–394.

90. Nelson, S., Farkasm S. and Fotheringham, N., *et al.*, Filgrastim in the treatment of hospitalized patients with community acquired pneumonia (CAP). *Am. J. Respir. Crit. Care Med.* 1996; 153S:A535.

91. Daifuku, R., Movahhed, H. and Fotheringham, N., *et al.*, Time to resolution of morbidity: an endpoint for assessing the clinical cure of community-acquired pneumonia. *Respir. Med.* 1996; **90**:587–592.

92. Wunderink, R.G., Leeper, K.V. and Schein, R.M.H., *et al.*, Clinical response to filgrastim (r- metHuG-CSF) in pneumonia with severe sepsis. *Am. J. Respir. Crit. Care Med.* 1996; 153S:A123.

CHAPTER 11

NEUTROPHIL TRANSFUSION THERAPY

Ronald G. Strauss[1]

1. Introduction

Current cytapheresis technology permits collection of highly enriched fractions of several types of blood leukocytes from healthy donors and patients either for transfusion and transplantation or for further processing (e.g., positive or negative cell selection, *ex vivo* expansion, genetic manipulation, etc.) and storage. Neutrophils (PMNs) are leukocytes that are collected routinely and issued as a standard blood component (Granulocytes, pheresis) to support patients with infections. This chapter analyzes use of PMN transfusions — called granulocyte transfusions (GTX) by convention — as an adjunct to antimicrobial drugs in the treatment and possible prevention of certain types of infections.

Serious and repeated infections with bacteria, yeast and fungus continue to be a consequence of severe neutropenia ($<0.5 \times 10^9$/L blood PMNs) or PMN dysfunction. In the recent multicenter TRAP study (Autoimmunization and refractiveness to platelet transfusion. New England J. Medicine, 1997, 337: 1861–1869), 7% of adult patients with acute nonlymphocytic leukemia died of infection during first remission induction therapy — despite use of modern antibiotic therapy. Previous attempts to prevent infections in severely

---

[1]Correspondence: Ronald. G. Strauss, Department of Pathology, 153A MRC, University of Iowa College of Medicine, Iowa City, IA 52242-1182, Fax: (319)335-6555, Telephone: (319)335-8150, e-mail: ronald-strauss@uiowa.edu

neutropenic patients using prophylactic GTX achieved only modest success (i.e., rates of certain infections were reduced, but GTX failed to prevent all infections), and GTX were toxic and expensive. Similarly, use of therapeutic GTX has diminished strikingly over the past several years — despite many reports that have shown them to offer benefit in certain experimental and clinical settings (1). This lack of enthusiasm for GTX can be explained, at least in part, by diminished need due to the development of effective antimicrobial drugs to prevent and treat infections and by the availability of recombinant hematopoietic growth factors and peripheral blood hematopoietic progenitor cell transfusions to hasten marrow recovery.

Recombinant myeloid growth factors such as granulocyte colony stimulating factor (G-CSF) and granulocyte/macrophage colony stimulating factor (GM-CSF) are glycoprotein cytokines that enhance the production, differentiation and function of myeloid cells (2). Both G-CSF and GM-CSF have been used to accelerate marrow recovery following chemotherapy and to successfully diminish the rate of acquiring infections and need for prolonged hospitalization (2). In contrast to this success in preventing neutropenic infections, the role of G-CSF and GM-CSF as treatment for already established infections is not as firmly documented. These growth factors frequently are given to patients with neutropenia and severe infections, and it seems reasonable to consider adding therapeutic GTX when severe bacterial, yeast or fungal infections are progressing in neutropenic patients despite use of appropriate antibiotics plus recombinant myeloid growth factors.

The preference of combination antibiotic therapy and use of myeloid growth factors plus the strong negative opinions about the value of GTX — held by many physicians — have been reinforced by knowledge that PMN concentrates collected for transfusion, historically, contained woefully inadequate numbers of PMNs. It is now possible to collect relatively large numbers of PMNs from normal donors stimulated with G-CSF using large volume leukapheresis. This fact, along with the historical success of GTX in treating bacterial infections, even when given in relatively low doses, suggests that a critical reassessment of therapeutic GTX is warranted. Further, because of relatively rapid engraftment following use of peripheral blood progenitor cell transfusions, as replacement for either autologous or allogeneic bone marrow transplantation, it is reasonable to hypothesize that severe neutropenia following intense myeloablative therapy might even be eliminated by prophylactic GTX used in this setting.

2. Therapeutic Granulocyte Transfusions in Neutropenic Patients

Recently, 34 papers that reported use of therapeutic GTX in severely neutropenic patients ($<5 \times 10^9$/L blood PMNs) were reviewed (3). Patients were tabulated (Table 11.1) according to the index infection that prompted GTX therapy and were counted only once (e.g., patients with septicemia were listed only in the septicemia section, even if they had another infection such as pneumonia). As an exception, all patients with invasive fungal infections were counted together because it was impossible to accurately separate sepsis, pneumonia, sinusitis, etc., into distinct categories. All patients given GTX for a designated type of infection were listed under the "Treated" heading. Of the treated patients, those for whom the actual course and mortality of the index infection could be clearly documented were listed again under the "Evaluable" heading. GTX therapy was considered successful if so stated by the author. Several of the 34 reports described uncontrolled studies of small numbers of patients with a diversity of underlying diseases, types of infections, antimicrobial therapies, GTX

Table 11.1   Infections treated in Neutropenic Patients with GTX in 34 Studies*

Type of Infection	Treated	Evaluable	Succes Rate
Bacterial septicemia	298	206	127/206 = 62%
Sepsis organism unspecified	132	39	18/39 = 46%
Invasive fungus and yeast	83	77	28/77 = 36%
Pneumonia	120	11	7/11 = 64%
Localized infections	143	47	39/47 = 83%
Fever etiology unknown	184	85	64/85 = 75%

*Individual references cited in reference 3.

management strategies (i.e., variable dose and quality of PMNs), as well as varying definitions of success. Because of these confounding factors, combining data from multiple reports is of limited value in drawing conclusions, and it was done simply to document the breadth of experience reported.

To obtain more definitive information regarding efficacy, the seven controlled studies (4–10) are analyzed in more detail in Table 11.2. In these seven studies, the response of infected neutropenic patients to treatment with GTX plus antibiotics (study group) was compared to that of comparable patients given antibiotics alone and evaluated concurrently (control group).

Table 11.2   Seven Controlled Studies of Therapeutic GTX in Neutropenic Patients

	Study (GTX) Group				**Control (No GTX) Group**		
Ref	**Patients**	**Survival**	**Dose × 10^{10}**	**HLA-WBC***	**Patients**	**Survival**	**Success**
4	17	76%	2.2 (F)[†]	No-Yes	19	26%	Yes
5	17	59%	2.7 (C)	Yes-Yes	13	15%	Yes
6	13	75%	1.7 (F)	No-Yes	14	36%	Yes
		0.4 (C)					
7	12	82%	5.9 (F)	No-No	19	62%	Partial
8	39	46%	2.0 (F)	No-Yes	37	30%	Partial
		0.6 (C)					
9	48	63%	0.5 (C)	No-No	47	72%	No
10	17	78%	0.4 (C)	No-Yes	2	80%	No

*Donor-recipient compatibility was enhanced by HLA matching or white blood cell crossmatching.
[†]F = filtration leukapheresis; C = centrifugation leukapheresis

Three of the seven controlled studies reported a significant overall benefit for GTX (4–6). In two additional studies (7,8), overall success was not demonstrated for GTX, but certain subgroups of patients were found to benefit significantly. For example, in the first controlled study (8), many patients received an inadequate dose of GTX by current standards, and overall success was not demonstrated. However, 100% of patients who received GTX on at least four occasions and 80% of those receiving at least three, survived, as compared to only 30% survival among controls. In the other study that found partial benefit (7), no advantage for GTX could be demonstrated when all patients were analyzed. However, when the subgroup of patients with persistent bone marrow failure were analyzed separately, 75% of those receiving GTX responded favorably, compared with only 20% of controls. Thus, some measure of success for GTX was evident in five of the seven controlled studies. However, this was counterbalanced by four studies that were negative in some respect — two totally (9,10) and two partially negative (7,8).

An explanation of these inconsistent results is evident on critical analysis of the adequacy of GTX support (Table 11.2). Patients in the three successful trials received relatively high doses of PMNs (generally $\geq 1.7 \times 10^{10}$/day) (4–6). Moreover, donors were selected to be both erythrocyte and leukocyte compatible. In contrast, the four negative controlled studies can be legitimately criticized in light of current technology. Data for three (7,8,10) of the four negative studies were collected before 1977, when both the quality and quantity of PMNs transfused were clearly inferior to those available today. Two of the four negative studies used PMNs collected by filtration leukapheresis for at least some patients (7,8). These PMNs are now known to be defective and are no longer transfused. Although three of the four negative studies used PMNs collected by centrifugation leukapheresis for some patients (8–10), the dose was extremely low ($0.41–0.56 \times 10^{10}$ per concentrate). This daily dose is approximately one-tenth the number that could be transfused currently, and it is not surprising that GTX were unsuccessful, when given in such a grossly inadequate fashion. As another factor, investigators in two of the four negative studies (7,9) made no provisions for the possibility of leukocyte alloimmunization and selected donors solely on the basis of erythrocyte compatibility. Finally, control subjects responded reasonably well to antibiotics alone in three of the four negative studies (7,9,10), suggesting that some patients have no apparent need for additional therapeutic modalities.

The preceding analysis is qualitative and suffers from the imprecision of combining data from studies that, although controlled, are not truly comparable (i.e., nonuniformity among factors such as the selection of control subjects, patient clinical status, GTX dose, compatibility, etc.). Recently, data from the seven controlled GTX trials were analyzed quantitatively by formal meta-analysis (11), and many of impressions of the preceding qualitative analysis were confirmed — specifically, that the dose of PMNs transfused and the survival rate of the nontransfused control subjects were primarily responsible for the differing success rates of the studies. In clinical settings in which the survival rate of nontransfused control subjects was low, study subjects were benefited by adequate doses of GTX. The authors concluded that severely neutropenic patients, with infections known to carry a high mortality rate, be considered for GTX given in an adequate dose (11).

The most frequent infection for which GTX were prescribed previously is bacterial sepsis (Table 1.11). Most neutropenic patients with bacterial sepsis, who experience bone marrow recovery during the early days of infection, will respond to antibiotics alone (1,3). Most patients with newly diagnosed acute leukemia, who experience successful induction chemotherapy, fit into this category of relatively brief severe neutropenia and will not require GTX. In contrast, septic patients with persistent neutropenia due to continuing marrow failure may benefit from GTX added to antibiotic therapy (1). Examples are patients in the later stages of leukemia undergoing investigational chemotherapy or recipients of marrow grafts in whom hematopoietic recovery may be delayed for >2–3 weeks.

Regarding the other infections listed in Table 11.1, information published to date is insufficient to determine definitively whether therapeutic GTX offer benefits over those of antibiotics alone. Currently, yeast and fungal infections pose difficult problems that deserve additional discussion. Occasional case reports, experimental studies in animals, and experience in treating patients with chronic granulomatous disease (12,13) support the success of GTX in some patients with yeast and fungal infections. In addition, an uncontrolled study of 15 patients (14) documented a 60% favorable response to GTX collected from G-CSF stimulated donors when given to neutropenic patients with fungal infections — a rate of success higher than expected per usual clinical experience. In contrast, a large clinical study (15) comparing infected bone marrow transplant patients given GTX (N = 50) to those treated without GTX (N = 37) found no benefit for GTX in treating fungal and yeast infections. This study was not designed to provide definitive answers. It was a retrospective review. Patients were not randomly selected for therapy — instead, the decision to use GTX or not was determined per individual physician preferences, making it impossible to exclude selection bias. Neither patient characteristics nor the types of infection being treated were evenly distributed between the GTX group and patients not given GTX. The dose of PMNs transfused was known for only 15% of the GTX administered and, likely, was quite low because of the collection techniques used (15).

To determine the optimal role for therapeutic GTX, individual physicians must survey the outcome of life-threatening infections with bacteria, yeast and fungi in their own neutropenic patients. If infections in their patients respond promptly to antibiotics alone and survival approaches 100%, GTX are unnecessary and should not be used, as the benefits would not outweigh potential risks. However, if significant numbers of infected neutropenic patients fail to respond to antibiotics alone, the addition of GTX should be considered, along with other modifications of therapy (e.g., selection of different antibiotics, closer monitoring of antibiotic blood levels, intravenous immunoglobulin therapy, G-CSF or other recombinant growth factors and immune modulating agents). Once the decision to use therapeutic GTX has been made, they must be given effectively, and recommendations for PMN collection are discussed later in this chapter. A daily infusion of approximately $5-8 \times 10^{10}$ PMNs should be given to patients with persistent neutropenia ($<0.5 \times 10^9$/L blood PMNs) and infections that have failed to respond to a reasonable course (approximately 48 hours) of combination antimicrobial agents. GTX are continued until the infection has resolved or until the blood PMN count is maintained at $>0.5 \times 10^9$/L. This endpoint may be difficult to detect because transfused PMNs — when collected from G-CSF stimulated donors and transfused at doses of $5-8 \times 10^{10}$ PMNs — may elevate the recipient's blood PMN count to $1-2 \times 10^9$/L for several hours postinfusion. Thus, accurately distinguishing transfused PMNs from those produced endogenously during marrow recovery is challenging and must be based on a sustained increase in blood PMN counts.

3. Therapeutic Granulocyte Transfusions for Neonates

Neonates (infants within the first month of life) may suffer life-threatening bacterial infections caused, at least in part, by neutropenia and PMN dysfunction (16,17). Neutropenia must be viewed differently in neonates than in older patients, in whom GTX are considered usually when the blood PMN count falls to $<0.5 \times 10^9$/L. In contrast, absolute blood PMN counts as high as 3.0×10^9/L might prompt consideration for GTX in neonates (16). The blood neutrophil count varies greatly during the first days of life, and a transient neutrophilia with absolute PMN counts of $10\text{--}25 \times 10^9$/L is commonly seen in healthy neonates. Although not completely specific, sepsis should be suspected in any sick neonate with an absolute PMN count of $<3.0 \times 10^9$/L during the first week of life. The mechanism of neutropenia cannot always be identified, but in some infants a marked decrease in the marrow PMN storage pool can be demonstrated. For example, these forms (metamyelocytes and segmented PMNs) account for 26–65% of all nucleated cells in normal marrow, but in some neonates with sepsis this value will be <10% of nucleated marrow cells.

Several investigators have reported use of GTX to treat neonatal sepsis. Four (18–21) of the six controlled studies (18–23) demonstrated a significant benefit of GTX (Table 11.3). However, these studies can be criticized for small size, faulty design, and heterogeneity of both patients and quality of GTX. Thus, the use of GTX for neonatal sepsis remains controversial, and alternative therapies must be considered.

Table 11.3   Five Controlled Trials (Six Reports) of Neonatal Granulocyte Transfusions

Reference	Randomized	Infants Transfused	Survival (%)	Infants Not Transfused	Survival (%)
18	No	20	90[a]	18	28
19	Yes	7	100[a]	9	11
	No[b]	–	–	10	100
20	Yes	13	100[a]	10	60
21	Yes[c]	21	95[a]	14	64
22	Yes	12	58	13	69
23	Yes	4	50	5	40
	No[b]	–	–	11	91

[a]Transfused infants survival significantly better than nontransfused.
[b]Additional nontransfused infants who were not randomized because all had adequate marrow storage pools.
[c]Expanded version of study reported earlier by Cairo et al.[20]

Intravenous immunoglobulin (IVIG) has been studied extensively as an alternative therapy to GTX and, although success has been reported by some investigators, data are inconsistent and insufficient to recommend IVIG — particularly at pharmacologic doses — as routine therapy for all neonates. Although controversial, some rationale exists for prescribing physiologic doses of IVIG to neonates with birth weight <1.5 kg because they are born before the bulk of maternal IgG is transported across the placenta and frequently are hypogammaglobulinemic. In studies of experimental infections, IVIG proved beneficial by increasing opsonic activity and by improving PMN kinetics in animals (24–26). Although the precise role for IVIG in the management of human infants is incompletely defined, this therapy has been given with mixed results both to prevent and to treat infections. Most prophylactic studies evaluating IVIG to prevent infections have found little or only modest benefit (27) — with a few studies suggesting true benefit (28–30). In contrast, several therapeutic studies reported benefit for adding IVIG to antibiotics during treatment of neonatal infections (27). However, data remain insufficient to justify the routine use of IVIG as standard therapy to prevent and/or to treat infections in preterm infants. Moreover, caution is warranted before IVIG is broadly applied as treatment for neonatal sepsis. At high doses, IVIG has been demonstrated to impair body defense mechanisms and to increase susceptibility to fatal infections (48–50). IVIG has great appeal because of the ease with which it can be prescribed, its apparent benefits to multiple body defense systems and, finally, its safety in terms of only rarely transmitting donor infectious diseases. However, the genuine benefits and risks of IVIG must be carefully examined before it is prescribed with impunity.

Recombinant myeloid growth factors offer another alternative to GTX. Preliminary studies of G-CSF and GM-CSF in newborn animals and in human neonates have shown beneficial effects on PMN production and functions. In neonates, studies of cytokine production have yielded conflicting results, with investigators finding values reported that are higher than, equal to, or lower than adult values (34–41). Generally, G-CSF and GM-CSF levels are lower in preterm versus term neonates, and the ability of preterm leukocytes to further increase production when stimulated is diminished. Plasma G-CSF levels were reported to be markedly elevated in neonates with infection (35,36), but other investigators found G-CSF mRNA expression and protein production to be decreased in neonatal leukocytes — particularly, in activated cells (37,38). In a controlled study (42), 42 neonates with presumed bacterial sepsis were randomized to receive three doses of either G-CSF or placebo. Therapy with G-CSF significantly increased the marrow PMN storage pool, blood PMNs and expression of PMN membrane C3bi (42). In a similar study of GM-CSF (43), 20 preterm neonates were randomized within 72 hours of birth to receive either GM-CSF or placebo for 7 days; GM-CSF increased marrow PMNs, blood PMNs and C3bi receptor expression. However, the efficacy of these agents to diminish infections and the potential for adverse effects have not been defined.

Thus, the role of GTX, IVIG and recombinant myeloid growth factors in the treatment of neonatal infections is unclear, none can be recommended as a standard of routine neonatal practice. Moreover, in many studies, standard supportive care with antibiotics seems to provide adequate therapy. Each institution must assess its own experience with neonatal sepsis and local management. If nearly all infants survive without apparent long-term morbidity, GTX and/or alternative therapies are unnecessary, and attention should be focused on prompt diagnosis and optimal antibiotic therapy. If the outcome of standard supportive therapy is less than optimal, additional therapies such as GTX must be explored.

4. Prophylactic Granulocyte Transfusions in Neutropenic Patients

Based on existing reports, prophylactic GTX are of marginal value. In 12 reports (44–55), benefits were few, while risks and expenses were substantial. However, partial success was demonstrated when certain subgroups of patients were examined separately. Some measure of success was found in 7 of 12 studies; the remaining 5 studies failed to show a benefit for prophylactic GTX (51–55). In none of these five negative studies were large numbers of PMNs obtained from matched donors and transfused daily. Thus, in a situation analogous to that for the negative therapeutic GTX trials, the failure of prophylactic GTX might be explained, at least in part, by inadequate transfusions.

A major concern raised by prophylactic GTX has been that of transfusion-related risks, a concern heightened because of the marginal benefits of prophylactic GTX (i.e., an unfavorable benefit to risk ratio). In the therapeutic setting, where GTX efficacy is more apparent, risks are more acceptable. Leukocyte alloimmunization poses a risk of special importance for GTX therapy. Although reports are controversial, it seems likely that most patients receiving multiple GTX from random donors will develop antileukocyte antibodies. Antileukocyte antibodies mediate transfusion reactions and alter the circulating kinetics of transfused PMNs to decrease post-transfusion increments and to decrease the antimicrobial effects of GTX (56–59). Many of the other risks of GTX have been greatly diminished by current practices, such as gamma-irradiation to prevent graft-versus-host disease and the use of cytomegalovirus-seronegative units to eliminate cytomegalovirus transmission.

Clearly, prophylactic GTX cannot be recommended at this time to treat patients with acute leukemia undergoing first remission induction or consolidation therapy. However, consideration should be given to use of prophylactic GTX in bone marrow transplant patients. Progressive infections, particularly with yeast and fungus, occur frequently in bone marrow transplant recipients who are neutropenic, exhibit PMN dysfunction, and manifest defective cellular and humoral immunity for months following transplantation. Altered immunity is particularly profound when marrow is T-lymphocyte depleted to diminish graft-vs-host disease. Although all types of infection pose a threat, 10% of 1186 marrow transplant patients developed a noncandidal fungal infection, with only 17% of infected patients surviving (60). Thus, the possible role of GTX, collected by modern techniques from G-CSF stimulated donors, needs to be reexamined as a means to approach this important clinical problem.

Autologous bone marrow transplantation has been supplanted by transfusion of peripheral blood hematopoietic/immunologic progenitor cells collected following cytokine (usually G-CSF) stimulation. This technique is being used increasingly in the allogeneic setting because it is convenient, economical and, very importantly, leads to relatively rapid engraftment (61,62). Recovery to a blood PMN count $\geq 0.5 \times 10^9$/L occurs within 6 to 14 days post-transfusion of progenitor cells. In some patients, the period of severe neutropenia

($<0.2 \times 10^9$/L) persists only a few days — particularly, when G-CSF is given to the patients following myeloablation. Thus, the complete elimination of severe neutropenia using this "transplantation" approach plus prophylactic GTX is a distinct possibility that deserves careful study.

Allogeneic peripheral blood progenitor cell donors receive G-CSF daily for 4 to 7 days with leukapheresis usually being performed on days 5 to 7 to collect sufficient progenitor cells for transfusion. Donor blood PMN counts increase, often to $>50 \times 10^9$/L, with G-CSF, and extraordinarily large doses of PMNs could be collected on the days following progenitor cell leukapheresis. Obviously, systematic studies are needed to define optimal G-CSF dose and schedule; the proper timing of leukapheresis procedures, first to collect progenitor cells for transplantation and then PMNs for GTX; the coordination of myeloablation, progenitor cell collection, storage and transfusion and subsequent PMN collection and transfusion; and the potential risks and inconvenience to the donor of prolonged G-CSF stimulation and multiple leukapheresis procedures. Preliminary studies have been reported to establish the feasibility and to develop methods (62). However, the efficacy of prophylactic GTX used as part of this progenitor cell then PMN transfusion approach versus peripheral blood progenitor cell transfusion followed by cytokine therapy of the patient without GTX must be investigated by properly designed randomized trials.

5. Preparation and Storage of Neutrophil Concentrates

To ensure adequate numbers and quality of PMNs, granulocyte concentrates must be collected from stimulated donors per automated leukapheresis using an erythrocyte sedimenting agent such as hydroxyethyl starch (HES) (63). A major limitation of GTX efficacy has been the inability to transfuse adequate numbers of perfectly functioning PMNs. Under the stress of a severe bacterial infection, the marrow of an otherwise healthy adult will produce between 10^{11} and 10^{12} PMNs in 24 hours. Granulocyte concentrates collected from healthy donors, who are not stimulated with corticosteroids or G-CSF, will contain between 0.2 to 0.8×10^{10} PMNs — about 1% of a healthy marrow's output.

Hence, donor stimulation is mandatory to achieve even a hope of a reasonable PMN dose per GTX. Donor stimulation with properly timed corticosteroids (≥ 4 hours before leukapheresis) will increase the yield to about 2×10^{10} PMNs (64). Stimulation with G-CSF alone or in combination with corticosteroids will produce higher, but variable PMN yields, depending on G-CSF dose and schedule of administration. Yields of $5-8 \times 10^{10}$ PMNs are achieved regularly, and post-transfusion blood PMN counts frequently increase to $1-2 \times 10^9$/L — with PMNs detected in the recipient's bloodstream for several hours following GTX (65–67,73). Thus, PMN donors are optimally 300 to 600 micrograms of G-CSF given 12 hours before leukapheresis plus corticosteroid, with dose and schedule determined best by local needs (66).

The optimal type of HES for granulocyte collection is controversial. In an uncontrolled multicenter trial, pentastarch appeared to be an efficacious and safe erythrocyte-sedimenting agent for use during centrifugation leukapheresis (64). The efficacy of pentastarch seemed established within granulocyte concentrates, prepared by a variety of centrifugation leukapheresis techniques in four cytapheresis centers, were found to contain quantities of total leukocytes and PMNs comparable to quantities found in concentrates prepared previously (historical controls) at participating centers using hetastarch. Most concentrates contained at least 2×10^{10} PMNs, if collected by a continuous-flow device (8 L of blood processed) from donors stimulated with steroids several hours before beginning leukapheresis.

Recently, however, the efficacy of pentastarch for PMN collection has been challenged. In two studies (68,69), the effects of pentastarch and hetastarch on the erythrocyte sedimentation rate were measured separately and later compared. In another study (70), the effects of pentastarch and hetastarch on PMN yields were compared directly during paired leukapheresis procedures of normal donors. In the first two studies (68,69), pentastarch was thought to exert lesser effects on donor erythrocyte sedimentation rates than hetastarch and, consequently, pentastarch was predicted by a granulocyte collection efficiency equation to be less effective in enhancing PMN yields. This prediction was supported later by a controlled clinical trial (70) in which steroid-stimulated donors underwent paired granulocyte collections — separated by 2 weeks to 7 months — in which they received 500 mL of either 10% pentastarch or 5%

hetastarch. Approximately 7 L of donor blood were processed at a 1:13 starch:donor blood ratio. In 92% of donors, hetastarch procedures were more efficient. The PMN yield (mean ± SD) was $2.3 ± 0.7 × 10^{10}$ with hetastarch vs $1.4 ± 0.076 × 10^{10}$ with pentastarch.

It is unclear why pentastarch performed so poorly in these recent studies (68–70), when compared with performance results in the initial multicenter trial (64) and with data from the DeGowin Blood Center (Table 11.4).

Table 11.4   Granulocyte Units at the DeGowin Blood Center, University of Iowa Hospitals and Clinics.*

Yield × 10^{10}	Prednisone (N = 353)	Prednisone + G-CSF (N = 113)
Total Leukocytes		
Mean ± SD	2.15 ± 1.15	7.04 ± 3.04
Median	1.97	7.05
Neutrophils		
Mean ± SD	1.53 ± 1.10	5.79 ± 2.70
Median	1.40	5.57

*Donors were stimulated either with prednisone alone (60 mg total dose given orally as 20 mg approximately 18, 12 and 4 hours before beginning leukapheresis) or prednisone (as described) plus G-CSF given subcutaneously as 300 mg approximately 12 hours before beginning leukapheresis. Each leukapheresis procedure is performed by continuous-flow centrifugation, using pentastarch at a 1:13 starch:donor blood ratio, until 10 L of donor blood is processed

The pentastarch solutions studied by both centers appear to have similar biochemical properties, but true identity cannot be established. In particular, information about the C2/C6 hydroxyethylation ratio — a property that can influence erythrocyte sedimentation (71) — is not given in any report, and the possibility that different pentastarch solutions were studied by the different groups cannot be excluded. Until the issue is resolved, it is prudent for each center preparing granulocyte concentrates to perform continuing quality assessment of its leukapheresis program. The average PMN yield obtained by processing 10 L of donor blood following corticosteroid stimulation and using pentastarch at a 1:13 starch:donor blood ratio should be between 1.5 and 2.5×10^{10}; after G-CSF stimulation, the PMN yield should be between 5.0 and 8.0×10^{10}. If this is achieved, it seems reasonable to use pentastarch because of its more rapid elimination from the bloodstream and its lesser effects on coagulation (72).

6. Conclusion. Future of Neutrophil Transfusions

Because a major criticism of granulocyte transfusions has been the relatively small doses of PMNs available in granulocyte concentrates, the feasibility of stimulating normal donors with G-CSF to obtain markedly increased numbers of PMNs for transfusion has renewed interest in this therapy as a treatment for infections in neutropenic patients. However, other medical advances — including treatment of patients with G-CSF and other recombinant growth factors, the availability of more effective antimicrobial agents, and the use of hematopoietic progenitor cell transfusions — have lessened the likelihood of progressive and unresponsive infections in severely neutropenic patients. Thus, it is ironic that now, when more effective doses of PMNs could be transfused therapeutically, they seem to be needed only occasionally. However, the potential to use prophylactic GTX — in the setting of bone marrow reconstitution using allogeneic peripheral blood progenitor cells — offers an exciting new area for investigation and possible clinical application.

7. References

1. Strauss, R.G., *Blood* **81** (1993), 1675–1678.
2. Gabrilove, J., *Blood* **80** (1992), 1382–1387.
3. Strauss, R.G., in *Apheresis: Principles and Practice*, ed. McLoed, B.C., Price, T.H. and Drew, M.J. (AABB Press, Bethesda, MD, 1997.), in press.
4. Higby, D.J., Yates, J.W., Henderson, E.S. and Holland J.F., *N. Engl. J. Med.* **292** (1975), 761–766.
5. Vogler, W.R. and Winton, E.F. *Am. J. Med.* **63** (1977), 548–555.

6. Herzig, R.H., *et al.*, *N. Engl. J. Med.* **396** (1977), 701–705.
7. Alavi, J.B., *et al.*, *N. Engl. J. Med.* **296** (1977), 706–711.
8. Graw, R.G. Jr., Herzig, G., Perry, S. and Henderson, I.S., *N. Engl. J. Med.* **287** (1972), 367–376.
9. Winston, D.J., Ho, W.G. and Gale, R.P., *Ann Intern Med* **97** (1983) 509–515.
10. Fortuny, I.E., *et al.*, *Transfusion* **15** (1975), 548–558.
11. Vamvakas, E.C. and Pineda, A.A., *J. Clin. Apheresis* **11** (1996), 1–9.
12. Yomtovian, R., Abramson, J., Quie, P. and McCullough, J., *Transfusion* **21** (1981), 739–744.
13. Buescher, E.S. and Gallin, J.I., *N. Engl. J. Med.* **307** (1982), 800–804.
14. Hester, J.P., *et al.*, *J. Clin. Apheresis* **10** (1995), 188–192.
15. Bhatia, S. *et al.*, *Transfusion* **34** (1994), 226–231.
16. Strauss, R.G., in *Developmental and Neonatal Hematology*, ed. Stockman, J.A. and Pochedly, C. (Raven Press, New York, 1988), 88–98.
17. Strauss, R.G., *J. Clin. Apheresis* **5** (1989), 25–30.
18. Laurenti, F. *et al.*, *J. Pediatr.* **98** (1981), 118–123.
19. Christensen, R.D., Rothstein, G., Anstall, H.B. and Bybee, B., *Pediatrics* **70** (1982), 1–6.
20. Cairo, M.S. *et al.*, *Pediatrics* **74** (1984), 887–892.
21. Cairo, M.S. *et al.*, *J, Pediatr,* **110** (1987), 935–941.
22. Baley, J.E., Stork, E.K., Warkentin, P.I. and Shurin, S.B., *Pediatrics* **80** (1987), 712–720.
23. Wheeler, J.C. *et al.*, *Pediatrics* **79** (1987), 422–425.
24. Kim, K.S., *Pediatr. Res.* **21** (1987), 289–291.
25. Harper, T.E., Christensen, R.D. and Rothstein ,G., *Pediatr. Res.* **22** (1987), 255–258.
26. Redd, H., Christensen, R.D. and Fischer, G.W., *J. Infect. Dis.* **157** (1988), 705–709.
27. Strauss, R.G., in *New Directions in Pediatric Hematology*, ed. Capon, S.M., Chambers, L.A. and Manno, C.S. (American Association of Blood Banks, Bethesda, MD, 1996), 121–129.
28. Haque, K.N. *et al.*, *Pediatr. Infect. Dis.* **5** (1986), 622–627.
29. Chirico, G., *et al.*, *J. Pediatr.* **110** (1987), 437–440.
30. Conway, S. *et al.*, *Vox Sang* **59** (1990), 6–11.
31. Cross, A.S., *et al.*, *Clin. Exp. Immunol.* **76** (1989), 159–163.
32. Weisman, L.E., Weisman, E. and Lorenzetti, P.M., *J. Pediatr.* **115** (1989), 445–449.

33. Cross, A.S., *et al.*, *Lancet* **1** (1984), 912–913.
34. Bailie, K.E.M., Irvine, A.E., Bridges, J.M. and McClure, B.G., *Pediatr. Res.* **35** (1994), 164–167.
35. Bedford-Russell, A.R., et al., *Br. J. Haematol.* **86** (1994), 642–646.
36. Gessler, P., *et al.*, *Blood* **82** (1993), 3177–3179.
37. Ohls, R.K., *et al.*, *Pediatr. Res.* **37** (1995), 806–809.
38. Schibler, K.R., Liechty, K.W., White, W.L. and Christensen, R.D., *Blood* **82** (1993), 2478–2482.
39. Min Lee, S., Knoppel, E., van de Ven, C. and Cairo, M.S., *Pediatr Res* **34** (1993), 560–564.
40. English, B.K., *et al.*, *Pediatr. Res.* **31** (1992), 211–215.
41. Cairo, M.S., *et al.*, *Pediatr. Res.* **30** (1991), 362–365.
42. Gillan, E.R., *et al.*, *Blood* **94** (1994), 1427–1430.
43. Cairo, M.S., *et al.*, *Blood* **86** (1995), 259–263.
44. Mannoni, P., *et al.*, *Blood Transfus Immunohaematol* **22** (1979), 503–508.
45. Gomez-Villagran, J.L., *et al.*, *Cancer* **54** (1984), 734–738.
46. Clift, R.A., *et al.*, *N. Engl. J. Med.* **298** (1978), 1052–1056.
47. Strauss, R.G., *et al.*, *N. Engl. J. Med.* **305** (1981), 597–603.
48. Hester, J.P., McCredie, K.B. and Freireich, E.J., *Care of the Child with Cancer* (American Cancer Society, Atlanta, 1979), 93–97.
49. Buckner, C.D., *et al.*, *Infection* **11** (1983), 243–247.
50. Curtis, J.E., Hasselback, R. and Bergsagel, D.E., *Can. Med. Assoc. J.* **117** (1977), 341–346.
51. Schiffer, C.A., *et al.*, *Blood* **54** (1979), 766–770.
52. Sutton, D.M.C., Shumak, K.H. and Baker, M.A., *Plasma. Ther. Transfus. Technol.* **3** (1982), 45–52.
53. Ford, J.M., *et al.*, *Transfusion* **22** (1982), 311–315.
54. Cooper, M.R., Personal communication update of earlier study, Cooper, M.R. *et al.*, in *Leukocytes: Separation, Collection and Transfusion*, ed. Goldman, J.M. and Lowenthal, R.M. (Academic Press, San Diego, 1981), 436–439.
55. Winston, D.J., Ho, W.G., Young, L.S. and Gale, R.P., *Am. J. Med.* **68** (1982), 893–900.
56. Goldstein, I.M., *et al.*, *Transfusion* **11** (1971), 19–24.
57. McCullough, J.J., Weiblen, B.J., Clay, M.E. and Forstrom, L., *Blood* **58** (1981), 164–169.
58. Dutcher, J.P., *et al.*, *Blood* **62** (1983), 354–360.
59. Dahlke, M.B., *et al.*, *Transfusion* **22** (1982), 347–353.

60. Pirsch, J.D. and Maki, D.G., *Ann. Intern. Med.* **104** (1986), 619–624.
61. Urbano-Ispizua ,A. *et al.*, *Bone Marrow Transplant* **18** (1996), 35–39.
62. Adkins, D., *et al.*, *Transfusion* **37** (1997), 737–748.
63. Strauss, R.G., Rohert, P.A., Randels, M.J. and Winegarden, D., *J. Clin. Apheresis* **6** (1991), 241–245.
64. Strauss, R.G., *et al.*, *Transfusion* **26** (1986), 258–262.
65. Bensinger, W.I., *et al.*, *Blood* **81** (1993), 1883–1888.
66. Liles, W.C., *et al.*, *Transfusion* **37** (1997), 182–188.
67. Caspar, C.B., Seger, R.A., Burger, J., and Gmur, J., *Blood* **81** (1993), 2866–2871.
68. Lee, J.H., Cullis, H., Leitman, S.F. and Klein, H.G., *J. Clin. Apheresis* **10** (1995), 198–202.
69. Lee, J.H. and Klein, H.G., *Transfusion* **35** (1995), 384–388.
70. Lee, J.H., Leitman, S.E. and Klein, H.G., *Blood* **86** (1995), 4662–4666.
71. Treib, J., *et al.*, *Thromb Haemost.* **74** (1995), 1452–1456.
72. Strauss, R.G., *J. Cardiothorac. Anesth.* **2** (1988), 24–32, S1.
73. Dale, D.C. *et al.*, *Transfusion* **38** (1998), 713–721.

WITHDRAWN